MW00565578

HYPNOSIS
AND
IMAGINATION

Editors

Robert G. Kunzendorf
University of Massachusetts Lowell

Nicholas P. Spanos
Carleton University

Benjamin Wallace
Cleveland State University

Imagery and Human Development Series
Series Editor: Anees A. Sheikh

Baywood Publishing Company, Inc.
AMITYVILLE, NEW YORK

Library of Congress Catalog Card Number 95-35997

ISBN: 0-89503-139-6 (Cloth)

Library of Congress Cataloging-in-Publication Data

Hypnosis and imagination / editors, Robert G. Kunzendorf, Nicholas P.
    Spanos, Benjamin Wallace.
        p.   cm. - - (Imagery and human development series)
    Includes bibliographical references and index.
    ISBN 0-89503-139-6 (cloth)
    1. Hypnotism. 2. Imagination. I. Kunzendorf, Robert G.
II. Spanos, Nicholas P.   III. Wallace, Benjamin.   IV. Series :
Imagery and human development series (Unnumbered)
BF1156.I53H86   1996
154.7- -dc20   95-35997
                                                                    CIP

In Memory of
Nick

In Memoriam to Nicholas P. Spanos

We dedicate this book to our late co-editor, Nick Spanos, who tragically died in a plane crash on June 7, 1994. Nick's unique blend of generosity, irreverence for authority, and commitment to scientific truth will long be missed by all of us who came to know Nick personally. Nick's research will continue to influence our field for years and years to come, and his dedication to teaching will live on forever through his students, and through their students. In ultimate tribute, the two students with whom Nick co-authored chapters in this book offer these reflections on their teacher.

Nick Spanos was one of the most enigmatic, unconventional individuals that one was likely to meet; however, he was very successful in the conventional confines of academia and scientific investigation. He was a man of many interests; a passionate reader who loved a good informal debate. I learned soon after meeting Nick that you had better be well armed if you would venture to engage him in a debate on practically any issue. He had in-depth knowledge of a multitude of topics: from experimental hypnosis to law and psychology; from claims of UFO abductions to JFK assassination conspiracies; from the Bible to the *National Enquirer.*

Nick was never content to let sleeping dogs lie, or to follow along with the status quo either socially or academically. He reveled in shaking foundations not only to see how others would react to his heresy, but because he firmly believed that there were flaws in the structures of these foundations, and he wanted to point them out for the world to see.

Nick served as an academic advisor to more than 100 graduate and undergraduate students over the years; I count myself lucky to be included among them. He always encouraged his advisees to rise up to and triumph over the challenges that we were (seemingly constantly) up against, not only the familiar challenges involving the hoops and hurdles of academia, but also the more general challenges of mastering the art of critical scientific thinking. His helpful advice concerning those academic challenges was at the time invaluable to me; his vital advice on scientific thinking and inquiry will remain with me always.

Nick was a prolific writer who was able to produce a manuscript of outstanding quality and insight in nary the blink of an eye. I remember more than once, Nick and I would spend a number of days (not to mention late nights) reviewing the analyses of a certain study we had just completed. I would head off, content with the day's work, and "waste away" the next eight hours in such mundane tasks as traveling home, sleeping, and eating. But not so for Nick. I'd arrive back at the lab the next morning, and there he would be, affixed to his desk, greeting me with, "I've got a draft of that paper for JPSP; let's go over it," and he'd hand me an almost letter-perfect handwritten manuscript. Did this man ever sleep? After working with Nick for ten years, I was almost able to read all of his (for lack of a better term) handwriting. His students eventually pushed Nick kicking and screaming into the computer age, and he bought his first computer for word processing, which, of course, accelerated his fantastic rate of output even more.

Nick was a generous man who gave freely, not only of his material possessions, but of his time, his knowledge, and his insight. To be a complete academic advisor to a single student is challenge enough for most of us. His ability to give his seemingly undivided attention to as many as thirty students at a time astounds me. We all owe an enormous debt of gratitude to Nick for fostering our fledgling interests, and instilling in us the desire to disengage fiction from fact, myth from reality. He has produced a new generation of psychological researchers; at least a dozen of his apprentices now hold faculty or professional research positions of their own. Mary Shelley's famous fictional doctor was a scientist who devoted his life to creating a man; Dr. Nicholas Spanos was a man who devoted his life to creating scientists.

I will always remember the loyalty, kindness, and benevolence Nick showed toward me, feelings that I'm confident are shared by all those whose lives Nick touched. The man may be gone, but his friendship, teachings, and spirit will guide me unendingly. For these and so many other reasons, I yearn to express once more, "Nick, thanks for everything."

Max Gwynn

To be the recipient of good mentoring seems to be a privilege rather than a right, as many graduate students can attest. The students of Nick Spanos were a privileged lot. Graduate school, for us, was a form of childhood, in which Nick served as both parent and teacher, guide and sage. He socialized us into the world of academia, helping form that invisible tribunal that guides our professional conduct. In this role, he created the mental benchmarks and standards of success that define academic integrity and excellence. Like our parents, he has left indelible marks on our character and will forever reside as the chief justice in this most supreme of courts: our professional conscience.

He imparted on us the skills, knowledge, and values of the discipline, and what is more, he empowered us to transfer this knowledge onto other students. Herein was his most valuable gift to us, for it was a gift whose value rested in it being imparted on another. Like myself, several of his graduate students went on to academic careers, and today our students are the recipients of Nick's gift to us. And what is precious here is that these recipients will never know the benefactor of these gifts.

He was reticent when his well-being and prosperity were at stake but was ardently outspoken when the truth was at stake. While iconoclastic and denying adherence to any ideology, to know Nick was to truly understand Henry David Thoreau when he said:

> I wanted to live deep and suck out all the marrow of life . . . to drive life into a corner, and reduce it to its lowest terms, and, if it proved to be mean, why then to get the whole and genuine meanness of it, and publish its meanness to the world; or if it were sublime, to know it by experience, and be able to give a true account of it in my next excursion . . . that is where I lived and what I lived for [1, p . 91].

He was intellectually courageous, confronting those issues which were previously cloaked in mystery and misunderstanding: witchcraft, glossolalia, dream healings, multiple personality, hypnosis, false memories, abduction experiences. In doing so, he introduced a "new" language replete with fascinating inferences and conclusions. He saw connections and relations among seemingly disparate constructs, a hallmark of the true visionary. He was not naive about the practice of science, fully aware of its adversarial and competitive nature; accordingly, he neither expected immediate approval nor received it. He was known to personalize his disagreements and was tenacious in his efforts to systematically challenge his adversaries. Despite this approach, or perhaps because of it, there are few of his contemporaries that have not been influenced by his ideas and writings.

Notwithstanding his enormous impact on the discipline, he was harshly humble about his accomplishments and loathed both titles and the reverence that others had of him. Toward his students, he was relentless in his demands for excellence, yet still patient about our personal and professional development. While many of his students emulated and envied him, none succeeded in imitating him. Those that tried, he derided for he was never driven to produce clones of himself, a temptation that many academics find difficult to resist. Perhaps he would be amused at the course his proteges have followed after their departure from his tutelage.

Like him, they speak better about absent than about present people. Like him, they do so from the basement offices of the ivory towers, marginal in status and thought. Like him, they are uninterested and unlikely to attain public office. And like him, frankly outspoken when the truth is at stake. The truth *is* that Nicholas Spanos was a visionary, a sage who forged a road "less traveled." And as one who pursued him on such a road, I can confidently say that he has made "all the difference."

As his student, he is among the most important figure in my life. His physical absence has strengthened his presence in the hallowed halls of my professional conscience, still forging the standards of intellectual excellence. He was, and will continue to be, my parent and teacher, guide and sage. He was my friend, one whom I loved very much. I will miss him dearly.

REFERENCE

1. H. D. Thoreau, *Walden,* L. Shanley (ed.), Princeton University Press, Princeton, New Jersey, 1971. (Original work published 1854.)

Arthur Perlini

Table of Contents

Preface

Students of both clinical and experimental hypnosis have long been concerned with the extent to which, and the manner in which, hypnotic responding and imaginal activity are related. For example, for over a decade, clinicians have debated whether progressive relaxation and guided imagery constitute hypnosis or whether, instead, the effects of induction procedures and hypnotic suggestions can be usefully understood in terms of relaxation and guided fantasy. Other debates have revolved around individual differences in hypnotizability, the utility of conceptualizing hypnotizability as a trait, and the degree to which stability in hypnotizability reflects stable individual differences in fantasy proneness, absorption, or other indices of imaginative functioning. The chapters in this book indicate that investigators with widely different theoretical interpretations of hypnosis are coming to the conclusion that hypnotic responding is multifaceted and that relationships between hypnotic responding and imaginal activity are complex and often moderated by numerous contextual and other variables.

The first three chapters examine relationships among hypnotic responding, imagination, and belief. Sheehan and Robertson emphasize the importance of belief in imaginings, as a characteristic of hypnotic responding. Wagstaff, on the other hand, emphasizes compliance—purposefully misdescribing images and other experiences in order to meet contextual demands—as a central component in hypnotic responding. Council, Kirsch, and Grant take a middle ground and focus on expectancies as moderators of the relationships between imaginative activity and hypnotic responding.

The next three chapters explore the hypnotic and clinical significance of belief in imaginings. Lynn, Neufeld, Green, Rhue, and Sandberg review evidence which suggests that hypnotizability, fantasy-proneness, the reporting of dissociative experiences, and some personality disorders involving distorted beliefs are related, albeit in some circumstances only weakly related. Rader, Kunzendorf, and Carrabino present data in support of the hypothesis that high hypnotizability entails dissociated reality-testing, whereas absorption in fantasy entails adaptive regression to "primary process" thinking. Relatedly, Barrett distinguishes the high hypnotizability of "dissociaters" and the high hypnotizability of "fantasizers."

Three subsequent chapters more closely examine the role of compliance, imagination, and suggestibility in various hypnotic phenomena. Coe examines the roles of contextual and skill variables in inducing both deception and self-deception during hypnotic amnesia. Gwynn and Spanos review the concept of suggestibility, the varied meanings applied to this concept, and the role of contextual factors in moderating relationships between various measures of suggestibility and hypnotizability. Gorassini also deals with the issues of deception and self-deception, and with the conditions that both facilitate and impede the ease with which people can lie to themselves about their imaginings.

The following two chapters examine evidence concerning negative hallucinations: suggested experiences which purportedly "block out" the perception of external events. Perlini, Spanos, and Jones examine both electrophysiological and behavioral correlates of hypnotic negative hallucination responding and conclude that such responding can be accounted for adequately in terms of attentional shifts and demand-induced reporting biases. Kunzendorf and Boisvert examine the effects of suggested imagery for deafness on brainstem components of the auditory evoked potential and conclude that brainstem blocking occurs only in vivid auditory imagers, whose blocked percepts are totally unavailable rather than hypnotically accessible to a "hidden observer."

The remaining three chapters pursue other physiological concomitants and relationships between hypnotic responding and imagination. Wallace and Turosky review psychophysiological evidence for bilateral activation, rather than right-hemisphere activation, during hypnotic and nonhypnotic imaging. Crawford presents cerebral blood flow evidence for frontal-lobe activation during hypnotic imaging. Finally, Persinger examines relationships among frontal and temporal lobe lability, partial epileptic-like signs, and hypnotic imagination.

As coeditors, we are grateful to all of the above contributors, to Baywood's series editor, Anees Sheikh, and to Baywood's president, Stuart Cohen. We hope that this book promotes further understanding and inspires further study of the relationships between hypnosis and imagination.

Robert G. Kunzendorf
Nicholas P. Spanos
Benjamin Wallace

CHAPTER 1

Imagery and Hypnosis: Trends and Patternings in Effects

PETER W. SHEEHAN
AND ROSEMARY ROBERTSON

Imagining is a rich and creative process that has occupied the attention of poets, philosophers, and psychologists throughout the ages. It is theoretically intriguing to hypothesize about the meaning of mental events that have such obvious "thing-quality." Controversy still abounds about whether the thing-quality of so-called images is an illusion, and about the essential relationship between "what we see" and "what we think we see." In fact, the nature of the relationship between what we say we see and what exists "out there," and the fact that there is such a discrepancy at times between the two defines, I think, one of the most intriguing aspects of hypnosis. It is not surprising in this sense, also, that the dominant theoretical issue throughout the history of nonhypnotic research into imagery is "how closely do imagery and perception really correspond—structurally, functionally, and interactively?" [1].

INTRODUCTION

It seems important at the outset to look by way of introduction at this link between imagery and perception. Outside the field of hypnosis, Finke's tripartite classification of theories addresses the issue in a useful, comprehensive fashion.

Structural theories dealing with the correspondence of imagery and perception usually focus on the explanation of the apparent spatial and pictorial qualities of mental imagery [2]. Typically, in experiments aiming to support this theory, subjects are asked to form mental images of objects and are then instructed to cognitively inspect the objects being imaged so as to make a perceptual judgment or to find specific items [3].

Functional theories are much more concerned with the dynamic properties of the image. A relevant question would be: Are the image and the percept

2 / HYPNOSIS AND IMAGINATION

functionally equivalent in terms of their formation and transformations? They attempt to explain, for example, the dynamics involved in the recognition of physical objects and the facilitation thereof by the formation and transformation of mental images. Representative of this approach is the work of Shepard and Cooper where the subject is asked to imagine a rotating object, the assumption being that the imagined object will rotate much like a real object would rotate [4].

Interactive theories attempt to explain how ongoing perceptual processes are influenced by mental imagery [5]. People sometimes imagine seeing an object when they expect to see it and this can lead to confusion between real and imagined objects [6, 7]. Support for the interactive viewpoint comes from the work of Finke and Schmidt [8] and Reeves [9]. This laboratory work has looked at how perception and imagery interfere with each other, and at the concept of perceptual aftereffects subsequent to imagination.

Finke concluded his review of mental imagery theories by stating that none of these three major approaches to theorizing about the relationship between imagery and perception is immune to challenge [5]. Each theory is vulnerable to the operation of particular artifacts. Structural theories, for example, are susceptible especially to the possible influence of experimenter bias [10]; functional theories seem most open to tacit knowledge [11], while interactive theories are thought to be susceptible to experimenter bias and/or eye movement artifact [12].

It is interesting in a way that theorizing which states a structural link between imagery and perception has actually had more support in the nonhypnosis than in the hypnosis literature. The strongest statement in the hypnotic literature of a structural link would probably be Sutcliffe's original formulation of the "credulous" view of hypnosis [13]. This posited (for later refutation) that hypnotic suggestion reinstitutes the physiological processes of perception: the consequences of suggestion parallel exactly the effects of real stimulation. Following this view, hallucinated colors can be expected to produce actual negative afterimages, regression should result in the actual revivification of past experience, and amnesia suggestion in hypnosis ought to result in the obliteration of memory traces. The extremity of this view is no longer held in the field, even though the "link" between imagery and perception is constantly stressed in what a hypnotist both says and does.

Finke's view that imagery equates structurally with perception is the most intriguing of the three approaches, and there is some consistency between this view and the data on hypnosis and the creation of subjective contours. Wallace, Persanyi, and Gerboc, working with subjective contours of geometric stimuli, found that mechanisms which are active in the information processing of perceptual events seem also to be active in the "imagery version" of the same event, at least for some subjects [14]. A number of studies [15-17] point to demand characteristics [18] and experimenter bias [10] as simpler explanations of the results. However, Wallace et al. claim that the quantity of evidence collected militates against all of the data being discounted by hypotheses that appeal only to the influence of social artifacts.

It is quite possible that the resolution of the ties between imagery and perception still awaits study of the physiological events which underlie the process of imaging. Farah [19] has attempted to unravel the view held by Finke [20] and Shepard [21] that representations used in imagery are the same as those used in perception, and has looked at this theory with respect to the opposite view held by theorists such as Pylyshyn [22]. The physiological complexity of the processes of imaging and perceiving are not to be underestimated according to studies of Kosslyn et al. [23, 24]. They showed that the two hemispheres of the brain process different aspects of the image; spatial arrangement of parts of the image being dealt with by the left hemisphere and the inspection, or evaluation of distances between points occurring in the right hemisphere. In 1985, the researchers demonstrated a functional dissociation between the kinds of imagery tasks which could be performed in the two cerebral hemispheres of so-called "split-brain" patients (ones with surgical transection of their corpus callosa). In 1989, the previous evidence was supported by visual processing experiments on university students.

This chapter essentially explores the relationship between hypnosis and imagery through analysis of the factors that affect the strength of the link between the two. Overall, it is argued that the relationship between imagery and hypnosis is a very complex one and that a range of factors actually defines the kind of influence imagery has on hypnotic performance. The common view that imagery is the dominant trait variable in understanding hypnosis has tended to obscure essential variability in the data. It is this variability, however, which offers us the greatest theoretical challenge for future research.

Let us set the stage, as it were, by first discussing imagery as a correlate of hypnosis. For the most part, this view emphasizes the trait-character of imagery response.

IMAGERY AS A MAJOR CORRELATE
OF HYPNOSIS

In a previous paper, it was argued that the most dominant view of imagery in the field of hypnosis is the notion that imagery is a reliable and stable correlate of hypnotizability [25]. Since that time, research has continued to focus on the nature of imagery and how different measures of imagery are related to hypnotizability [26, 27]. There are many measures of imagery (see Table 1) that help explain the prevalence of the view that imagery is a major, reliable correlate of hypnotizability.

The first thing that impresses one about the tests listed in Table 1 is the variety of the content and differences in format of the measures. For the most part, they all stress the importance of assessing individual differences in imagery, but they range widely across different dimensions of experience such as controllability,

Table 1. Sample of Measures of Imagery

Betts Questionnaire upon Mental Imagery (QMI) [71]
Creative Imagination Scale (CIS) [72]
Gordon Test of Imagery Control [73]
Imaginal Processes Inventory [74]
Individual Differences Questionnaire (IDQ) [75]
Inventory of Childhood Memories and Imaginings (ICMI) [76]
Phenomenology of Consciousness Inventory (PCI) [77]
Preference for Imagic Cognitive Style (PICS) [78]
Questionnaire on Subjective Experiences in Hypnosis (QSEH) [79]
Shortened version of QMI [80]
Tellegen Absorption Scale (TAS) [69]
Verbalizer-Visualizer Questionnaire (VVQ) [81]
Visual Elaboration Scale (VES) [82]
Vividness of Visual Imagery Questionnaire (VVIQ) [66]

vividness and cognitive style, and involve different sensory modes. The list of correlates reported in Table 2 stresses relevant key traits that are theoretically related to each other (e.g., vividness, fantasy, and absorption). It also draws attention to the importance of major social psychological influences on hypnotizability—factors such as rapport, demand characteristics, and setting constraints.

Looking at the implications of Tables 1 and 2 as a whole, the data associated with the measures and variables that are listed emphasize, for the most part, the importance of skill, the relevance of context, and the characteristics of the state of consciousness that we choose to label "hypnosis." The Model of hypnotic response that will inevitably embrace the full influence of imagery must be one that accentuates person attributes (incorporating attitudes, beliefs, skills, and abilities), setting features (involving expectancies, demand characteristics, and rapport), and processes related to state of consciousness (incorporating the effects of induction procedures). Figure 1 sketches the outline of such a model that attempts to draw some of the major parameters together. Three major groups of factors are categorized and arrows denote the hypothesized direction of influence of the different variables.

The evidence overall is very compelling that imagery ability is positively related to hypnotizability. The very notion of skill, for example, is reflected directly in the more modern concept of "fantasy-proneness" which has been researched extensively by Lynn et al. [28, 29] and Suita [30]. This concept has been linked to a range of relevant correlates that include level of hypnotizability,

Table 2. Major Correlates of Hypnotizability

Imagery
- Vividness of imagery
- Ease of imaging
- Control over imagery
- Imagic style

Fantasy
- Proneness to fantasy
- Ease of fantasizing
- Motivation for development

Absorption
- Attentional capacity
- Concentration on inner feelings and thoughts
- Effortless experiencing

Dissociation
- Involuntariness of response
- Dualistic thinking

Rapport
- Relationship with the hypnotist
- Interpersonal attraction
- Evaluation apprehension

Ease of Relaxation

Context
- Situational constraints
- Demand characteristics
- Attitudes and preconceptions
- Expectancies and beliefs

ability to hallucinate, and the subject's developmental history and psychological adjustment [28].

The major thrust of the data is that the relationship between hypnosis and imagery is essentially a nonlinear one in which high imagery ability does not predict hypnotizability quite as reliably as low imagery predicts insusceptibility. Some low susceptible subjects can and do utilize definite imagery skills in the hypnotic setting [31] and seem similar to Wilson and Barber's fantasy addicts in some aspects of their imaginative involvements [32]. A number of very susceptible subjects, on the other hand, who are high in imagery skills cannot

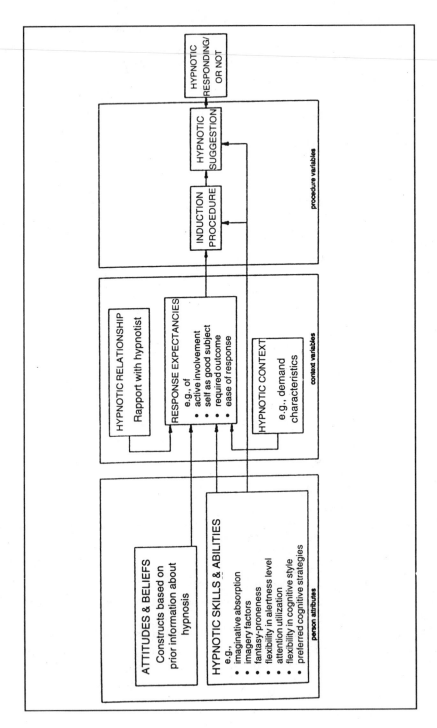

Figure 1. A model of hypnotic responding: Some major variables.

6

demonstrate aspects of fantasy proneness that other susceptible subjects will show. Most recently, Wallace has challenged us by the finding that 6.8 percent of his subjects were poor imagers but still highly susceptible to hypnosis, while a comparable proportion (6.6%) were vivid imagers but low in susceptibility to hypnosis [33]. The implications of the fact there is a nonlinear relationship between imagery and hypnosis [34] must be properly understood, for this will, in part, explain some of the apparent anomalies in the data. We need to understand why low susceptible subjects will evidence imagery capacity at times and make adaptive use of it while trying to do suggestion tasks.

Imagery and its related concepts, fantasy-proneness and absorption, are by no means pure predictors of hypnotizability, and high susceptible subjects may respond behaviorally just like low susceptible subjects but do so for different reasons. Co-determination of hypnotic effects occurs, but the variables contributing to the effects appear to combine differently for low and high susceptible subjects.

Let us consider by way of illustration some unpublished data gathered in the laboratory at the University of Queensland on the relationship between vividness of imagery, absorption, and hypnotic susceptibility. On the grounds that imagery and hypnosis are related, it seems plausible to argue that hypnotically-induced pseudomemory would be shown by subjects reporting more vivid imagery, greater absorption capacity and higher preference for an image cognitive style (see Table 1 for reference to relevant measures). Such a view draws support from the notion that pseudomemory is a distortion of what actually occurred and imagery inherently reflects what is unreal; commonality in both being counterfactual can be argued to determine the relationship. Research shows the opposite. Subjects who demonstrated pseudomemory, compared to those who did not, had significantly less (rather than more) vivid imagery, and indicated less of a preference for imagic cognitive style. (There were no significant differences between groups for absorption.) Table 3 illustrates the nature of the anomalous effect for imagic style. The relationship between imagery and level of susceptibility is in the expected direction, but there is a *reversal* of this relationship for pseudomemory response. The reasons for these data have been argued elsewhere [35] in terms of the overarching influence of cognitive style. Detail in the data, however, gives us a clue to the explanation of the effect. Subjects who were

Table 3. Mean Imagic Style Scores for Susceptibility Groups and for Categories of Pseudomemory Response

Level of Susceptibility		Pseudomemory Response	
High	12.45	Present	10.11
Medium	11.03	Absent	12.68
Low	10.89		

deluded about what was shown had appreciably less vivid imagery than those who showed pseudomemory motivated by compliance. It appears that imagery had less of a role to play in the occurrence of pseudomemory when subjects' belief systems were entirely consonant with what was suggested.

These data expose us to the interesting notion that imagery is important in hypnosis, but other variables like "belief" can achieve the same hypnotic outcomes and may do so at times in ways that diminish the apparent relevance of imagery. Obviously, because the relationship between hypnosis and imagery is nonlinear, it was overstepping the mark to argue that pseudomemory and imagery should be positively related. Data tell us it is the "believed-in" quality of the distortion in pseudomemory that could be its most distinguishing feature.

MEASURES OF IMAGERY: SOME CAVEATS

It must be recognized that the inconsistencies in the literature concerning the relationship between imagery and hypnosis may reflect not only the design of the correlation studies, as will be considered later in this chapter, but the idiosyncrasies of the measures being used and inherent problems in the methods of measurement. Concerning the measures themselves we can ask some basic questions which would yield revealing answers:

1. Is each test valid?—Is there an underlying construct, and if so, is it measured accurately by the test?
2. Are test results consistent?—Is there evidence of reliability of response and stability of construct?
3. Do the tests discriminate well between imagers?
4. Is there evidence of contextual contamination?—Do the social-psychological surroundings make a difference to results?
5. What is being measured and what is not being measured?—Do the measured constructs adequately specify the important characteristics of imagery in relation to hypnosis?

According to Sheehan, Ashton, and White who reviewed the assessment of mental imagery, the accuracy of what the tests in Table 1 measure is more debatable than the consistency of test scores [36]. They cite a number of self-report tests [36, p. 202] designed to overcome problems in the standard tests, but subsequent research continues to operate with a focus on the older tests. Factor analyses of tests (e.g., Visual Elaboration Scale, Vividness of Movement Imagery, Gordon's Test of Visual Imagery Control, Betts QMI, and Marks VVIQ) have all illustrated a variety of factors [37-39]. Conclusions based on these analyses have not always been favorable concerning the validities of the test concerned [38, 40, 41]. Work on the convergence of scores from different types of tests [42] is perhaps most promising in this regard.

The reliability of the scores on vividness of imagery tests has emerged as more of an issue after the publishing of work showing some instability of the construct being measured. Furthermore, there is evidence that ultradian rhythms [43, 44] and different physical states [45] produce fluctuations in the vividness (and amount) of imagery generated.

Kihlstrom et al. point out the lack of discriminability of the tests of vividness and control of imagery used in their study [39]. The items were found to be relatively insensitive to individual differences in ability. This lack of variation in response reduces the power of the test to differentiate between imagers and hence the utility of such tests in research.

Ahsen has further demonstrated that the VVIQ is limited by its content stimuli [46, 47]. By replacing the prevailing car image with that of a parent, he demonstrated dynamic components of imagery in operation. These were components previously untested whose influence was unrecognized.

This brief review leads us to address the final question of the adequacy and relevance of the factors measured by tests in Table 1. Even taken as a whole, the tests of imagery traditionally used in the literature appear to cover only a part of the range of all the aspects of imagery generation and maintenance. Thus, there may be room for testing other aspects important in hypnotic imagery.

What is this range? Integrating the work of experimenters in applied and allied fields of psychology [46-48] with experimental work on imagery [33] should give us a better idea of these factors involved in visual imagery perception, and which may be important in the generation of internal imagery. First, consider the image attributes: these include the spatial relationships between parts of the image, the clarity of the boundaries, the color, and the points of maximum information. Then there are the more dynamic qualities of percepts: those produced outside the person (e.g., the movement of some parts relative to the whole) and those arising from the movement and focusing of the eyes (e.g., the making up of a whole from the parts by learned scanning strategies, the patterning of generated perceptions by expectancies and beliefs based on memory modified by motivation). But what of hypnotic imagery? Which aspects of perceptual imagery might we reasonably suppose will be important in hypnotic responding? Are there other characteristics of internally produced imagery which are not relevant to external stimulus-produced imagery?

Traditionally, experimenters have focused on the vividness and controllability of imagery arising from internal sources (see Tables 1 and 2) as well as the autobiographical accounts of absorption in imagery and fantasy. Evidence is now gathering, however, that these imagery factors are not the only important indicators of successful hypnotic imagery. Research has been reported on temporal aspects of imagery production and degeneration [49], scanning strategies [50-53], the ability to dissociate information from semantic memory and somatic responses [54], the automaticity of information encoding [55], attentional flexibility [56], and the "thinness" of personal boundaries [57]. Research appears to be moving in an increasingly psychophysiological direction and one of the prime tasks of future research is to find which are the relevant dependent and which are the relevant independent factors.

Returning to the problems inherent in the methods of measurement themselves, one notices a move away from the studies using many subjects with the easily administered paper and pencil tests, to the more involving, performance tests which are perhaps the most demanding of the experimenter's resources. We would suggest that there is a need for a greater degree of in-depth research into imagery measurement, and more clarity of factors measured is required as well as more accuracy of measurement. Phenomenological studies offer a further methodological alternative [58-60].

Other Determinants of Hypnotic Responsivity

Upon close analysis of data-sets across a range of hypnotic phenomena, results point very firmly to the view that the association between imagery and hypnosis is multidimensional in character. Perhaps the most persuasive reason for pursuing cognate variables that pattern the data (such as absorption, attentional capacity, imagic style, and effortless experiencing) as well as indirectly related variables such as contextual constraints, motivations, and expectancies (see Figure 1) lies in the fact that the positive relationships that have been observed between imagery and hypnotizability are not just anomalous; they are also only moderate in strength. As asserted elsewhere, tests of imagery ability rarely account for more than 40 percent of the variance of subjects' scores on hypnotic test scales [61]. A link is evident, but only in part, and it is necessary to appeal to multiple dimensions at work. We believe one process (like delusion, for example) can "do the work," as it were, that makes another (like imagery, for example) redundant at times. Further, process variables measuring similar things like an imagic cognitive style and absorption may at other times jointly operate to determine hypnotic responsiveness. The latter notion we can easily accept; the former notion as yet is probably still foreign to the literature debates.

Before addressing some of the theoretical implications of this hypothesis of multidimensionality, we will comment briefly on the situational components of hypnosis. They represent an imposing category of influence.

IMAGERY AND THE INFLUENCE OF HYPNOTIC CONTEXT

The hypnotic setting itself emphasizes strongly the relevance of imagery. The susceptible subject brings particular cognitive skills to a specific test situation during which imagery responses are encouraged by the hypnotist's manner and procedures and the types of suggestions that the subject receives. Typical standard instructions for hypnosis request that subjects imagine suggested events just as they are happening; and hypnotic-test items themselves, more often than not, either suggest specific images that the subjects should evoke (e.g., "your hand and arm feel as if a heavy object is weighing it down"), or urge the subject to arouse imagery of his or her own choosing (e.g., "you are back at school now. Tell me what you see."). Response in hypnosis, then, as it reflects imagery and related processes of imaginative absorption is the result of behaving in a situation where, more often than not, there are explicit cues for responding in a make-believe, unreal, and fanciful way.

The lure of the hypnotic patter is so strong that it is not surprising that hypnotized subjects talk about images as if them really exist and are objects to be scrutinized. One is reminded immediately of Binet and Fere's remark that in every image there is the germ of an hallucination. If some theorists would have their way, we might even wish to argue that in every hallucination there is evidence of disguised imagination at work—with permission to the subject to speak in the "language of reality."

Discussion of the influence of setting in this chapter emphasizes the common understanding that context has a pervasive effect across the full range of hypnotic phenomena. Context may shape, modify, and define the nature of subjects' imagery responses as well, and this influence is highlighted most sharply by the data of Council, Kirsch, and Hafner [62] in their analysis of expectancy (vs. absorption) in the prediction of hypnotic responding which have been analyzed in more detail recently by Woody et al. [63].

Council et al. found that imaginative absorption was associated with hypnotic response expectancies more strongly than with actual hypnotic outcomes. They found that absorption was appreciably associated with measures of hypnotic response when the test of absorption occurred just prior to the induction of hypnosis, rather than when the test of absorption was administered previously in a context not associated with hypnosis. Council argued that absorption is related to hypnotic responsiveness through the mediation of hypnotic response expectancies—a challenging observation to many of the conclusions of workers in the field. The results of Council et al. constitute strong evidence for the relevance of context of testing to the observed relationship between imaginative absorption and hypnotic susceptibility. Although the debate is not yet entirely resolved—the effect has replicated for females, but not for males, for example [64], the issue continues to be strongly argued [65], and it is obvious that hypnotic subjects are highly sensitive to the effects of contextual cues and their expectations of being hypnotized.

The data gathered by Council et al. are entirely consistent with the wider point of view expressed by Lynn that a rich variety of variables moderates the relationships between scales that tap imaginative involvement and variables hypothetically related to fantasy proneness [28]. To quote, "Scales that measure absorption and fantasy proneness rely on subjects' interpretations of their experiences and abilities, and self-reports are notoriously sensitive to social-desirability biases, demand characteristics, and context and expectancy effects" [29, p. 42]. Evidence suggests as well that the direction of contextual influence is two-way [66]. Context effects operate by affecting hypnotic behavior when the hypnosis scales are administered first and when they are administered after tests of imagination.

THE MULTIDIMENSIONALITY OF THE RELATIONSHIP BETWEEN IMAGERY AND HYPNOSIS

There are by now a host of implications in the hypnotic literature that the observed relationship between imagery and hypnotizability is multifactorial in character (with consequent implications for the strength of the relationship between single variables), but still too frequently theories are proposed on the basis of the prediction that the degree of association is uncontentiously strong. One such view is that proposed by Wilson and Barber who talk of particular persons as "fantasy addicts" and "fantasy proneness" as a unitary entity [32, 67]. This has profound implications for our understanding of hypnosis. The viewpoint they espouse appeals to the primary influence of proneness to fantasy and imagination among excellent hypnotic subjects. This approach, analyzed elsewhere in detail by Lynn attempts to isolate a fundamental personality variable defined in terms of fantasy proneness that underlies hypnotic susceptibility [28].

One can argue, however, that imaginative involvement or fantasy proneness is only one of many possible expressions of a higher order imagery factor which also underlies hypnotic susceptibility—along with (for example) altered states of consciousness, aesthetic experiences, and other processes such as effortless experiencing [68]. Data supporting such a view have been reported by Jamieson [56] who conducted extensive analysis of subjects' responses on Tellegen's Absorption Scale [69] and examined the sensitivity of this test for differentiating subjects in terms of the level of their hypnotic susceptibility. His data supported a model where hypnosis, imagination, and several other variables can be viewed legitimately as expressions of a single underlying human capacity. Hypnosis and imagination were related to this underlying variable as primary factors to a higher order factor and not as the elements of a simple, single ability measure. Several candidates were canvassed for the identity of the higher order variable and imagination was rejected by Jamieson as inadequate to explain all of its manifestations. Flexibility in the ability to selectively shift between different patterns in the deployment of attention was regarded as the most plausible link between the factors of imaginative absorption and ability to respond to hypnotic suggestions. Other studies reflecting a similar theme focus on the flexibility in cognitive functioning or style found in high susceptible subjects [70]; the "thinness" of personal boundaries in high absorbers and hypnotizables [57]; and the competence of highs in developing efficient cognitive strategies [53]. This flexibility expresses what Sheehan [61] and Radar and Tellegen [70] have argued elsewhere—theorizing about the role of imagery must take account of the joint influence on response of both person and situation variables.

CONCLUSION

In conclusion, it is plausible to argue that examination of the role and functions of imagery in hypnosis has been dominated too much up to this point in time by concern about unidimensional processes of influence. The view prevalent in the literature that imagery is an altogether reliable and valid correlate of the hypnotizable personality is very likely incorrect.

Contemporary research has highlighted, in particular, that we need to give much more attention to the role context plays in shaping the imagery effects that have been observed, and the relationship existing between imagery and hypnosis is clearly of a character that attitudinal and/or expectancy variables have a much stronger influence than we have hitherto considered. Variables like dissociation—assumed originally to be relatively unrelated to imagery—are now being linked back to imaginative involvement (and ultimately to hypnosis) in theoretically provocative ways [54, 63].

Finally, there are paths in common to hypnosis among several separately named variables, and it is tempting to suggest (as supported by the data in Table 3) that process-related variables like imagery and delusion may at times provide alternative routes in the determination of hypnotic outcomes. Indeed, it may even be the case that some of the variables we study facilitate well-known outcomes or are the vehicle of them, but are not the substance of the effects.

ACKNOWLEDGMENTS

Research for this chapter was supported in part by a program grant from the Australian Research Council. The authors wish to thank especially Scott Ferguson for his help in that work.

REFERENCES

1. R. A. Finke, Theories Relating Mental Imagery to Perception, *Psychological Bulletin, 8,* pp. 236-259, 1985.
2. S. M. Kosslyn, *Image and Mind,* Harvard University Press, Cambridge, Massachusetts, 1980.
3. S. Pinker and R. A. Finke, Emergent Two-dimensional Patterns in Images Rotated in Depth, *Journal of Experimental Psychology: Human Perception and Performance, 6,* pp. 244-264, 1980.
4. R. N. Shepard and L. A. Cooper, *Mental Images and Their Transformations,* MIT Press, Cambridge, Massachusetts, 1982.
5. R. A. Finke, Mental Imagery and the Visual System, *Scientific American, 254,* pp. 88-95, 1986.
6. U. Neisser, *Cognition and Reality,* Freeman, San Francisco, California, 1976.

7. C. W. Perky, An Experimental Study of Imagination, *American Journal of Psychology, 21*, pp. 422-452, 1910.
8. R. A. Finke and M. J. Schmidt, Orientation-specific Color Aftereffects following Imagination, *Journal of Experimental Psychology: Human Perception and Performance, 3,*pp. 599-606, 1977.
9. A. Reeves, Visual Imagery in Backward Masking, *Perception and Psychophysics, 28,* pp. 118-124, 1980.
10. R. Rosenthal, *Experimenter Effects in Behavioral Research,* Halsted, New York, 1976.
11. Z. W. Pylyshyn, The Imagery Debate: Analogue Media versus Tacit Knowledge, *Psychological Review, 88,* pp. 16-45, 1981.
12. P. Q. Carpenter and M. A. Just, Eye Fixations during Mental Rotation, in *Eye Movements and the Higher Psychological Functions,* J. W. Senders, D. F. Fisher, and R. A. Monty (eds.), Erlbaum, Hillsdale, New Jersey, pp. 115-133, 1978.
13. J. P. Sutcliffe, "Credulous" and "Skeptical" Views of Hypnotic Phenomena: Experiments in Esthesia, Hallucination, and Delusion, *Journal of Abnormal and Social Psychology, 62,* pp. 189-200, 1961.
14. B. Wallace, M. W. Persanyi, and B. Gerboc, Imagery, Hypnosis, and the Creation of Subjective Contours, *Journal of Mental Imagery, 13,* pp. 139-152, 1989.
15. J. Broerse and B. Crassini, Misinterpretation of Imagery-induced McCollough Effects: A Reply to Finke, *Perception and Psychophysics, 30,* pp. 96-98, 1981.
16. D. Chambers and D. Reisberg, Can Mental Images by Ambiguous?, *Journal of Experimental Psychology: Human Perception and Performance, 11,* pp. 317-328, 1985.
17. J. Predebon and P. I. Wenderoth, Imagined Stimuli: Imaginery Effects?, *Bulletin of the Psychonomic Society, 23,* pp. 215-216, 1985.
18. M. T. Orne, On the Social Psychology of the Psychology Experiment: With Particular Reference to Demand Characteristics and Their Implications, *American Psychologist, 17,* pp. 776-783, 1962.
19. M. M. Farah, Is Visual Imagery Really Visual? Overlooked Evidence from Neuropsychology, *Psychological Review, 95,* pp. 307-317, 1988.
20. R. A. Finke, Levels of Equivalence in Imagery and Perception, *Psychological Review, 87,* pp. 113-132, 1980.
21. R. N. Shepard, Kinematics of Perceiving, Imagining, Thinking, and Dreaming, *Psychological Review, 91,* pp. 417-447, 1984.
22. Z. W. Pylyshyn, *Computation and Cognition,* MIT Press, Cambridge, Massachusetts, 1984.
23. S. M. Kosslyn, J. D. Holtzman, M. J. Farah, and M. S. Gazzaniga, A Computational Analysis of Mental Image Generation: Evidence from Functional Dissociations in Split-brain Patients, *Journal of Experimental Psychology: General, 114,* pp. 311-341, 1985.
24. S. M. Kosslyn, A. B. Koenig, A. Barrett, C. B. Cave, J. Tang, and J. D. E. Gabrieli, Evidence of Two Types of Spatial Representations: Hemispheric Specialization for Categorical and Coordinate Relations, in *Journal of Experimental Psychology: Human Perception and Performance, 15,* K. S. Pope and J. L. Singer (eds.), pp. 723-735, 1989.
25. P. W. Sheehan, *Imagery, Hypnosis and the Search for Meaning in the Relationship,* paper presented to the International Congress of Psychology, Sydney, August 1989.
26. S. P. Kahn, E. Fromm, L. S. Lombard, and M. Sossi, The Relation of Self-reports of Hypnotic Depth in Self-hypnosis to Hypnotizability and Imagery Production, *International Journal of Clinical and Experimental Hypnosis, 37,* pp. 290-304, 1989.

27. L. S. Lombard, S. P. Kahn, and E. Fromm, The Role of Imagery in Self-hypnosis: Its Relationship to Personality Characteristics and Gender, *International Journal of Clinical and Experimental Hypnosis, 38,* pp. 25-38, 1990.

28. S. J. Lynn, Fantasy Proneness: Hypnosis, Developmental Antecedents, and Psycho-pathology, *American Psychologist, 43,* pp. 35-44, 1988.

29. S. J. Lynn and J. W. Rhue, Hypnosis, Imagination, and Fantasy, *Journal of Mental Imagery, 11,* pp. 101-112, 1987.

30. J. Suita, Fantasy-proneness: Towards Cross-cultural Comparisons, *British Journal of Experimental and Clinical Hypnosis, 7,* pp. 93-101, 1990.

31. J. Jackson, *Imagining Capacity and Individual Differences in Hypnotic Response,* unpublished Masters dissertation, University of Queensland, Australia, 1984.

32. S. C. Wilson and T. X. Barber, The fantasy-prone personality: Implications for Understanding Imagery, Hypnosis and Parapsychological Phenomena, in *Imagery: Current Theory, Research, and Application,* A. A. Sheikh (ed.), Wiley, New York, pp. 340-390, 1983.

33. B. Wallace, Hypnotic Susceptibility, Imaging Ability, and Information Processing: An Integrative Look, in *Mental Imagery,* R. G. Kunzendorf (ed.), Plenum Press, New York, pp. 89-100, 1990.

34. W. Cross and N. P. Spanos, The Effects of Imagery Vividness and Receptivity on Skill Training Induced Enhancement in Hypnotic Susceptibility, *Imagination, Cognition and Personality, 8,* pp. 89-103, 1988-89.

35. D. J. Statham, *The Relationship between Imagery Ability, Absorption and Pseudo-memory Effects,* paper presented at the South Pacific Congress of Hypnosis, Melbourne, 1989.

36. P. W. Sheehan, R. Ashton, and K. White, Assessment of Mental Imagery, in *Imagery Current Theory, Research and Application,* A. A Sheikh (ed.), John Wiley and Sons, New York, pp. 189-221, 1983.

37. A. Campos and J. Perez, A Factor Analytic Study of Two Measures of Mental Imagery, *Perceptual and Motor Skills, 71,* pp. 995-1001, 1990.

38. J. Glicksohn, Cutting the "Gordonian Knot" Using Absorption and Dream Recall, *Journal of Mental Imagery, 15,* pp. 49-54, 1991.

39. J. F. Kihlstrom, M. L. Glisky, M. A. Peterson, E. M. Harvey, and P. M. Rose, Vividness and Control of Mental Imagery: A Psychometric Analysis, *Journal of Mental Imagery, 15,* pp. 133-142, 1991.

40. P. J. Chara, Jr., and D. A. Harim, An Enquiry into the Construct Validity of the Vividness of Visual Imagery Questionnaire, *Perceptual and Motor Skills, 69,* pp. 127-136, 1989.

41. S. J. McKelvie, The Vividness of Visual Imagery Questionnaire: Commentary in the Marks-Chara Debate, *Perceptual and Motor Skills, 70,* pp. 551-560, 1990.

42. K. Hasegawa, *Factorial Relationships between Self-rating Methods and Objective Tests in the Measurement of Mental Imagery Potential,* Bulletin No. 31, Department of Psychology, Aoyama Gakuin University, Shibuya, Tokyo, Japan, 1989.

43. D. F. Kripke and D. Sonnenschein, A Biologic Rhythm in Waking Fantasy, *The Stream of Consciousness,* Plenum, New York, pp. 321-334, 1978.

44. B. Wallace and A. Kokoszka, *Ultradian Rhythms and Imaging Ability,* paper read at the meetings of the Midwestern Psychological Association, Chicago, 1990.

45. R. J. Pekala, C. F. Wenger, and R. L. Levine, Individual Differences in Phenomenological Experience: States of Consciousness as a Function of Absorption, Journal of Personality and Social Psychology, 48, pp. 125-132, 1985.

46. A. Ahsen, AA-VVIQ and Imagery Paradigm: Vividness and Unvividness Issue in VVIQ Research Programs, *Journal of Mental Imagery, 14,* pp. 1-58, 1990.

47. A. Ahsen, A Second Report on AA-VVIQ: Role of Vivid and Unvivid Imagers in Consciousness Research, *Journal of Mental Imagery, 15*, pp. 1-32, 1991.
48. A. Baddeley, *Human Memory: Theory and Practice,* Laurence Erlbaum, Hove, England, 1990.
49. M. Cocude and M. Denis, Measuring the Temporal Characteristics of Visual Images, *Journal of Mental Imagery, 12*, pp. 89-102, 1988.
50. H. J. Crawford, Hypnotic Susceptibility as Related to Gestalt Closure Tasks, *Journal of Personality and Social Psychology, 40*, pp. 376-383, 1981.
51. H. J. Crawford and S. N. Allen, Enhanced Visual Memory during Hypnosis as Mediated by Hypnotic Responsiveness and Cognitive Strategies, *Journal of Experimental Psychology: General, 112*, pp. 662-685, 1983.
52. B. Wallace, Hypnotic Susceptibility and Proofreading Accuracy, *American Journal of Psychology, 100*, pp. 289-294, 1987.
53. B. Wallace, Imaging Ability and Performance in a Proof-reading Task, *Journal of Mental Imagery, 15*, pp. 177-188, 1991.
54. D. Barrett, Deep Trance Subjects: A Schema of Two Distinct Subgroups, in *Mental Imagery*, R. G. Kunzendorf (ed.), Plenum Press, New York, pp. 101-112, 1991.
55. M. Dixon, A. Brunet, and J. R. Laurence, Hypnotizability and Automaticity: Toward a Parallel Distributed Processing Model of Hypnotic Responding, *Journal of Abnormal Psychology, 99*, pp. 336-343, 1990.
56. G. Jamieson, *The Structure and Meaning of Absorption,* unpublished Masters dissertation, University of Queensland, Australia, 1987.
57. E. Hartmann, Thin and Thick Boundaries: Personality, Dreams and Imagination, in *Mental Imagery*, R. G. Kunzendorf (ed.), Plenum Press, New York, pp. 71-78, 1990.
58. R. J. Pekala, Hypnotic Types: Evidence from a Cluster Analysis of Phenomenal Experience, *Contemporary Hypnosis, 8*, pp. 95-104, 1991.
59. K. M. McConkey, M. L. Glisky, and J. F. Kihlstrom, Individual Differences among Hypnotic Vituosos: A Case Comparison, *Australian Journal of Clinical and Experimental Hypnosis, 17*, pp. 131-140, 1989.
60. P. W. Sheehan and K. M. McConkey, *Hypnosis and Experience: The Exploration of Phenomena and Process,* Lawrence Erlbaum, Hillsdale New Jersey, 1982.
61. P. W. Sheehan, Imagery and Hypnosis—Forging a Link, at Least in Part, Research Communications in Psychology, *Psychiatry and Behavior, 7*, pp. 257-272, 1982.
62. J. R. Council, I. Kirsch, and L. P. Hafner, Expectancy versus Absorption in the Prediction of Hypnotic Responding, *Journal of Personality and Social Psychology, 50*, pp. 182-189, 1986.
63. E. Z. Woody, K. S. Bowers, and J. M. Oakman, *Absorption and Dissociation as Correlates of Hypnotic Ability: Implications of Context Effects,* paper presented at 41st Annual Meeting of the Society for Clinical and Experimental Hypnosis, Tucson, Arizona, October 1990.
64. H. P. De Groot, M. I. Gwynn, and N. P. Spanos, The Effects of Contextual Information and Gender on the Prediction of Hypnotic Susceptibility, *Journal of Personality and Social Psychology, 54*, pp. 1049-1053, 1988.
65. N. P. Spanos, Empirical Support for an Ethogenic Perspective on Hypnotic Responding: A Reply to Kroger, *New Ideas in Psychology, 6*, pp. 67-73, 1988.
66. D. Marks, Visual Imagery Differences in the Recall of Pictures, *British Journal of Psychology, 64*, pp. 17-24, 1973.
67. S. C. Wilson and T. X. Barber, Vivid Fantasy and Hallucinatory Abilities in the Life Histories of Excellent Hypnotic Subjects ("Somnambules"): Preliminary Report with Female Subjects, in *Imagery, Vol. 2: Concepts, Results and Applications,* E. Klinger (ed.), Plenum Press, New York, pp. 133-149, 1981.

68. P. G. Bowers, Hypnotizability, Creativity and the Role of Effortless Experiencing, *International Journal of Clinical and Experimental Hypnosis, 26,* pp. 184-202, 1978.
69. A. Tellegen and G. Atkinson, Openness to Absorbing and Self-altering Experiences ("Absorption"), a Trait Related to Hypnotic Susceptibility, *Journal of Abnormal Psychology, 83,* pp. 268-277, 1974.
70. C. M. Radar and H. Tellegen, An Investigation of Synaesthesia, *Journal of Personality and Social Psychology, 52,* pp. 981-987, 1987.
71. G. H. Betts, *The Distributions and Functions of Mental Imagery,* Teachers College Contributions to Education, University of Columbia, New York, No. 26, 1909.
72. S. C. Wilson and T. X. Barber, The Creative Imagination Scale as a Measure of Hypnotic Responsiveness: Applications to Experimental and Clinical Hypnosis, *American Journal of Clinical Hypnosis, 20,* pp. 235-249, 1978.
73. R. Gordon, An Investigation into Some of the Factors that Favour the Formation of Stereotyped Images, *British Journal of Psychology, 39,* pp. 156-167, 1949.
74. J. S. Singer and J. S. Antrobus, Daydreaming, Imaginal Processes, and Personality: A Normative Study, in *The Function and Nature of Imagery,* P. W. Sheehan (ed.), Academic Press, New York, pp. 175-202, 1972.
75. A. Pavio, *Imagery and Verbal Processes,* Holt, Rinehart and Winston, New York, 1971.
76. S. C. Wilson and T. X. Barber, *The Inventory of Childhood Memories and Imaginings (ICMI),* Cushing Hospital, Framington, Massachusetts, 1983.
77. R. J. Pekala and R. L. Levine, Mapping Consciousness: Development of an Empirical Phenomenological Approach, *Imagination, Cognition and Personality, 1,* pp. 29-47, 1981-82.
78. P. Isaacs, *Hypnotic Responsiveness and the Dimensions of Imagery and Thinking Style,* unpublished doctoral dissertation, University of Waterloo, Waterloo, Ontario, Canada, 1982.
79. G. W. Farthing, S. W. Brown, and M. Venturino, Involuntariness of Response on the Harvard Group Scale of Hypnotic Susceptibility, *International Journal of Clinical and Experimental Hypnosis, 31,* pp. 170-181, 1983.
80. P. W. Sheehan, A Shortened Form of Bett's Questionnaire Upon Mental Imagery, *Journal of Clinical Psychology, 23,* pp. 386-389, 1967.
81. A. Richardson, Verbalizer-visualizer: A Cognitive Style Dimension, *Journal of Mental Imagery, 1* pp. 109-126, 1977.
82. J. Slee, *The Perceptual Nature of Visual Imagery,* unpublished doctoral dissertation, Australian National University, Canberra, Australia, 1976.

CHAPTER 2

Compliance and Imagination in Hypnosis

GRAHAM F. WAGSTAFF

IMAGINATION AND THE HYPNOTIC STATE

A continuing controversy in modern hypnosis research is the "state versus non-state" debate [1, 2]. According to the traditional state view, hypnosis is best conceptualized as an altered state of consciousness with various depths, such that the deeper one experiences the hypnotic state, or "condition," the more profoundly hypnotic phenomena will be experienced [3, 4]. However, a number of theorists have rejected this view of hypnosis as inaccurate and misleading; they argue that hypnotic phenomena are more readily explicable in terms of more mundane psychological concepts, such as, attitudes, expectancies, beliefs, compliance, attention, concentration, distraction, and relaxation [5-17].

In the mid 1970s there seemed to be some hope that the protagonists in this debate might be reaching some important points of agreement; the most important of which was an emphasis on the role of imagination. For example, in his 1975 review, E. R. Hilgard concludes, "there is a convergence of all investigators upon the role played by the subject's imaginative and fantasy reproductions" [18, p. 19]. Also, in 1974 Spanos and Barber suggested that the major theoreticians were converging on the conclusion that hypnotic behavior involves two factors, a willingness to cooperate with suggestions, and a shift in cognitive orientation to one of imaginative involvement [19]. This proposed convergence was influenced greatly by the appearance, in 1970, of J. R. Hilgard's book *Personality and Hypnosis: A Study of Imaginative Involvement* [20]. In this she reports that the capacity to become involved in imaginings in everyday life is a significant predictor of hypnotic susceptibility. Sarbin had for many years stressed the role of imagining in hypnotic performance, and his classic work with Coe, published in 1972, emphasized the importance of imaginative involvement in the enactment of the hypnotic role [7]. Also influential at this time was the appearance in 1974 of Tellegen and Atkinson's "absorption" measure [21], which seemed to correlate with hypnotic susceptibility. Optimism about a convergence of views seemed to mount further when one of the most ardent opponents of the state position, T. X. Barber et al., began to place increasing stress on the relationship between creative imagination and fantasy production, and hypnotic susceptibility [6, 22, 23].

Nevertheless, any optimism about imagination as a concept capable of playing a fundamental unifying role seems to have been short lived; the state-nonstate controversy is still very much alive, and sides in this debate seem to be as far apart as ever [1, 2, 24]. What happened?

One important factor preventing agreement was, and still is, a dispute as to *why* involvement in imaginings relates to hypnotic responding. Central to this disagreement is E. R. Hilgard's revival of the notion of hypnosis as a state in which dissociations occur. According to Hilgard's neo-dissociation theory, there exist multiple cognitive structures, or control systems, that are not all conscious at the same time [4, 25]. Normally these structures are under the influence of a central control structure, or "executive ego," but when subjects enter the hypnotic state they surrender to the hypnotist much of their capacity to control and monitor the various cognitive structures that are involved in behavior and experience. Thus, for example, in response to an arm lowering suggestion, subjects may be aware that they are moving their arms downwards, but not be unaware of, or unable to monitor, the cognitive structure (or "part of the mind") that is controlling the movement; hence the movement is experienced as involuntary. Hilgard's neo-dissociation theory is now very popular among state theorists, and this has important implications for the role of imagination in hypnosis. For instance, from a state perspective, Bowers argues that at the heart of hypnotic responding is dissociation, and it is the capacity to dissociate that facilitates imaginative involvement [26]. In other words, the relationship between hypnotic responding and imaginative involvement is, at least partly, a by-product of the relationship between hypnotic responding and the capacity to dissociate. This is rather different from the original non-state emphasis of those such as Barber and his colleagues who implied that, providing other factors are present, such as positive attitudes and appropriate expectancies, involvement in imaginings and fantasy per se can facilitate successful hypnotic responding; for example, by constructing a "goal-directed fantasy," such as imagining rocks tied to their arms, subjects more readily respond to the arm lowering suggestion and experience the movement as involuntary [6, 27].

It is perhaps understandable that state theorists should have become wary of emphasizing the role of imagination in hypnotic responding; for if hypnotic phenomena can mainly be accounted in terms of mundane imagination, along with appropriate attitudes and expectancies, why do we need to postulate an extra hypnotic state or special dissociative process? To counter this difficulty, some supporters of the dissociation position have tended to look for evidence that imaginative involvement alone cannot account for hypnotic responding. For example, Hilgard and Hilgard have argued that while imagination can account for some degree of pain reduction, imagination alone cannot account for the dramatic degree of pain reduction shown by some hypnotized subjects; to account for profound hypnotic analgesia we need to postulate an extra component, profound dissociation, available only in the hypnotic state [28]. Similarly, Zamansky [29] and Zamansky and Clark [30] have challenged the view that absorption in imaginings can account for responsiveness to suggestions. Subjects were instructed to imagine themselves performing behaviors counter to suggestions; for example, when it was suggested to subjects that their arms were rigid, they were told to imagine themselves bending their arms. The imagination instructions had little effect on hypnotic performance; instead, subjects responded in the direction of the suggestion. Zamansky and Zamansky and Clark thus conclude that there is more to hypnotic responding that imaginative involvement, and argue that it is possible that some dissociative process is at work.

Nevertheless, some state theorists seem to be reluctant to dismiss the concept of imaginative involvement entirely, because if measures of imaginative involvement are assumed to be indirect indices of dissociative capacity, then reliable correlations between imaginative involvement and hypnotic susceptibility can be used as evidence for a stable trait of hypnotic susceptibility, which in turn, would appear to contradict any non-state view that hypnotic responding results from subjects' interpretations of situational demands (i.e., subjects doing what they think they "ought to do" because of the pressures of, or cues conveyed by, the immediate context [3, 26]. Some non-state theorists, however, dispute the idea that hypnotic susceptibility is a stable trait and have reported evidence to suggest that the correlations between measures of imaginative involvement an hypnotic susceptibility may be, to some degree, context specific or are, at best, fairly modest [31-34]. However, if as Barber and other non-state theorists had argued previously, imaginative involvement is of fundamental significance in the production of hypnotic responses, then perhaps ironically, failures to find high and consistent relationships between hypnotic susceptibility and imaginative involvement could be deemed more problematical for the non-state view than the state view. Indeed, from a state theory perspective, it could be argued that, if it is dissociation, not imaginative involvement per se, that ultimately accounts for hypnotic responding, then failures to find high and consistent correlations between hypnotic susceptibility and imaginative involvement are not actually critical.

IMAGINATION AND THE MODIFICATION
OF HYPNOTIC SUSCEPTIBILITY

So if, from a non-state view, hypnotic phenomena are linked with the use of imagination or fantasy, why the poor or inconsistent relationship between hypnotic susceptibility and measures of involvement in imaginings? To answer this question, non-state theorists have tended to search for mediating factors, in particular, attitudes and expectancies toward hypnosis; the assumption being that, even if some subjects do have a high proclivity for imaginative involvement, if they have negative attitudes toward, or expectancies about, hypnosis, this will reduce their susceptibility and lower the overall correlations between imaginative involvement and hypnotic susceptibility. However, while some moderate success has been achieved in improving the relationship between imaginative involvement and hypnotic susceptibility by controlling for attitudes and expectancies, the improvements are extremely modest, and the proportion of variance in hypnotic susceptibility scores accounted for by a combination of these factors remains very small [32]. Something else must be involved. But what? To state theorists the answer is obvious; it is the capacity to enter the hypnotic state and experience dissociations. To non-state theorists, on the other hand, there has to be another explanation.

According to Spanos, who rejects the state view of hypnosis, subjects with negative attitudes and/or scoring low on measures of imaginal ability rarely, if ever, score high on hypnotic susceptibility; hence positive attitudes toward hypnosis, and a willingness and ability to construct and become involved in imaginings may be necessary to respond to hypnotic suggestions [10, 12]. However, these factors are not sufficient to guarantee high responsiveness to hypnotic suggestions, as some subjects with positive attitudes and scoring high on imaginal ability still score low on hypnotic susceptibility. Spanos argues that, to respond to hypnotic suggestions, what subjects need in addition are appropriate sets to interpret the suggestions; that is, they need to know what exactly it is they have to do to respond to a suggestion. Most important, they need to know that it is essential to become actively involved in suggestions, and not passively "wait for something to happen"; thus, for example, if subjects actively try to imagine that their arms are hollow, then when they raise their arms, the movement may be experienced as involuntary; and if when challenged to bend their arms, they actively imagine their elbows to be in a vice, subjects may feel they cannot bend their arms. Significantly, if this is the case, then it might be possible to modify hypnotic susceptibility; and Spanos and his colleagues have indeed reported success in increasing hypnotic susceptibility by means of the Carleton Skills Training Package (CSTP). The CSTP provides information to produce positive attitudes and motivations toward hypnotic responding, places emphasis on the importance of absorption in imagining "make-believe" situations, and provides details about how to interpret different suggestions [10, 35, 36].

Some state theorists are, however, understandably skeptical about claims that hypnotic susceptibility can be modified in this way, as the CSTP appears to make no attempt to modify what they believe to be a relatively stable capacity to enter the hypnotic state and experience dissociations [3]. Critics argue that the hypnotic susceptibility gains reported by Spanos et al. result from behavioral compliance; that is, to please the experimenter, subjects carry out the instructions but do not have appropriate subjective experiences; for instance in response to an arm movement suggestion subjects may deliberately move their arms without actually

experiencing involuntary movement; so when they do report involuntary movement, they are really lying. To support this view, critics report that gains using the
CSTP are small and short lived; this contrasts with conventional measures of
hypnotic susceptibility which tend to be relatively stable over time [3, 37]. In
reply, however, Spanos has argued that gains using the CSTP cannot be accounted
for solely in terms of compliance, and that susceptibility gains using the CSTP are
substantial and are stable over time [38].

It seems, therefore, that the role of imagination in hypnotic susceptibility is
controversial and far from clear. To some contemporary non-state theorists,
although a propensity to become involved in imaginings is certainly not the only
component in hypnotic responding, it is nevertheless important, and may even be
necessary; whereas to some state theorists, a capacity to become involved in
imaginings is secondary to, and possibly even a by-product of, the ability to enter
a condition or state whereby dissociations are experienced, and it is the latter that
accounts for the most profound hypnotic phenomena.

Perhaps some of the most compelling evidence state theorists would appear
to have against the idea that imagination alone is responsible for hypnotic
phenomena, is that some phenomena simply do not appear to lend themselves to
explanation in terms of mundane imagination. For example, it is difficult to see
how, no matter how positive one's attitudes or expectations, by the exercise or
ordinary imagination, in response to a suggestion, one could see a non-existent
person or object such that the person or object is perceived "as real as real"; or,
with one's eyes open, selectively blot out some part of the visual field to produce
a negative hallucination, so that, for example, one fails to see a number clearly
presented before one's eyes, or sees people walking around the room without their
heads and feet. It is difficult to see also how, by means of simple imagination, a
hypnotist could talk to another part of someone's consciousness in such a way that
the different parts of consciousness are not aware of each other; or enable a subject
to have a hand writing coherently away in a box while the subject remains
oblivious to what the hand is doing or what is being written. Yet all these
phenomena have been accepted at some time by state theorists [14, 25, 28, 39].

In the remainder of this chapter, however, I intend to argue that discussion about
the role of imagination in hypnotic responding has been hampered by a tendency
for theorists of both persuasions to underestimate and misunderstand the possible
role of compliance in *all* areas of hypnotic responding; that is, not just in hypnotic
susceptibility modification procedures.

To assess the role of compliance hypnotic responding it is first necessary to
define what exactly is meant by the term and its nature in social interaction.

THE NATURE OF COMPLIANCE

In everyday usage the term "compliance" can refer to the performance
of any behavior that accords with the directions or wishes of another. Hence

compliance can mean simply "doing what someone asks or demands." However, within social psychology, compliance usually refers to a particular form of conformity [40, 41]. It normally refers to overt behavior that is performed to accord with what others show or expect, *but runs counter to private convictions.* However, it can be useful to further divide behavior that runs counter to private convictions into two subsidiary categories: these are, 1) behavior that is contrary to the wishes or beliefs of the actor, and 2) behavior that is contrary to the beliefs or experiences of the actor, *and is intended to deceive others.*

Compliance of the first type would include, for example, the reluctant performance of antisocial acts because of social pressures to do so; as when, for example, Sheridan and King induced subjects to give harmful doses of electric shock to a live puppy [42]. If we assume that the obedient subjects would not have delivered these shocks had they not felt pressured by the experimental situation, then their behavior could be described as compliant; it ran counter to their private feelings or convictions about harming animals. Compliance of the second type would occur when, for example, to conform with the wishes or expectations of others, subjects say something they know or believe to be untrue, or do something they know will create an erroneous impression; for instance, in a classic set of studies Asch demonstrated that many subjects would give erroneous responses in judgments of the lengths of lines which confronted with the judgments of others who had, unknown to the subjects, been briefed by the experimenter to give incorrect responses [43]. If, as it is generally assumed, Asch's subjects knew that their responses were incorrect, then their responses were compliant; they overtly conformed to the behavior of the majority, but did not privately accept the judgments they had made.

Of course, these categories of compliance are not mutually exclusive; when subjects comply in the second sense (by, for example, telling a lie), frequently they may be complying in the first sense also (they may feel pressured to tell a lie, against their moral convictions); thus the processes that give rise to the compliance can be identical in both cases. For example, in one experiment, Calverley and Barber directed nursing students to sign slanderous statements about their hospital assistant superintendent [5]. The results indicated that when the directions were non-emphatic, only one student signed the statements. However, although about one-third of the subjects subsequently stated they had felt apprehensive and guilty about signing the statements, almost all of these subjects signed the statements when emphatically directed to do so. As, when not pressured, these subjects were unwilling do behave antisocially, then their behavior in response to the emphatic demands could be described as compliant in both senses; they were, against their wishes or convictions, signing statements they believed to be exaggerated or untrue. However, it is also possible to comply in the second sense (by, for example, telling a lie to impress or please others), without complying in the first sense (the actor might conceivably enjoy the deception and experience little conflict).

There seems to be little doubt that compliance, of both types, can be a powerful influence in experimental situations. In one particularly dramatic demonstration, Levy showed that a majority of subjects would deliberately lie about having previous knowledge of a verbal learning experiment if they thought such knowledge would ruin the experiment [44]. Levy concludes, "to rely upon the subject as an expert witness would be to betray as much naivete of the experimenter as that which he hopes exists in his subject" [44, p. 369]. But why should a majority of presumably otherwise honest individuals lie in this way? There is considerable evidence to suggest that subjects in experiments perceive their role as one of behaving like "good," cooperative subjects, and fulfilling the experimenter's expectations. So motivating is this perception that, in response to the commands of the experimenter, a majority of subjects are apparently willing to carry out ridiculous tasks for hours on end [45], as well as deliver (or at least give the impression they are delivering) painful and possibly lethal doses of electric shock to an innocent human victim [46]. According to writers such as Frank [47], Orne [45], and Milgram [46], such behavior occurs because, when they enter an experimental situation, subjects make a tacit agreement to do what is expected of them in terms of fulfilling the experimental hypothesis; and to break this agreement is to commit a severe social impropriety.

Given these considerations, it seems inappropriate to question the integrity of the subjects who, in such situations, comply by not being truthful. Normal, socialized individuals, placed in experimental, and indeed many other, situations, may sometimes unwittingly find themselves put in a genuine moral dilemma, and may feel that the most acceptable solution is some kind of deception. However, compliant behavior can, of course, be motivated by less noble concerns than wanting to appear cooperative and to "please the experimenter"; in the case of deception, people can comply for fun, as an attention seeking device, or as a way of satisfying their curiosity by ensuring their continued participation in a study [14].

Compliance in Hypnosis

If we apply compliance to hypnosis, then, as I have suggested previously [14-16], two broad categories of hypnotic response can be especially identified as illustrating "compliance only." The first is that in which an act is supposed to reflect an underlying subjective experience that is not present; for example, in response to an analgesia suggestion, a subject may claim pain is not felt, when actually pain is experienced, or, in response to a hallucination suggestion, a subject may move a hand as if brushing away a "hallucinated fly" that is not actually experienced. The second involves the conscious or deliberate performance of acts that are supposed (either explicitly or implicitly) to be performed involuntarily. For instance, in response to an arm levitation or lowering suggestion, the subject may deliberately move his or her arm without experiencing the movement as involuntary.

Given the potential for the operation of compliance in experimental situations it would not be surprising if it were to operate in hypnotic contexts. Indeed, the a priori likelihood of compliance operating in hypnotic situations would seem to be particularly high, for not only is the hypnotic situation one in which there are strong demands to fulfill, the hypnotist's expectations, but also, out of curiosity, subjects may be strongly motivated initially to "go along" with suggestions by overtly enacting them, even if they fail privately to experience them, in the hope that "something might happen" later. As a result they may fall victim to what social psychologists call the "foot in the door effect" [48], and the "low ball tactic" [49]; that is, having first committed themselves to respond in a particular way, even if minimally, subjects may find it difficult to "back out" in the face of more extreme demands.

There are some classic examples of compliance in the hypnosis literature. One of the first is Mark Twain's account of the miseries he went through pretending to experience suggested analgesia [7]. In a further famous case, a woman who claimed hypnotic uniocular blindness was eventually found not to be blind [50]. Subsequently, she admitted that she had employed tricks or devices to give the appearance of being blind, including practicing being blind at home with a friend. In another example, Barber, Spanos, and Chaves recount how, when some subjects are given a suggestion for hypnotic deafness and are then asked, "Can you hear me," they reply "No, I can't hear you" [6]. (In this latter example, an ardent dissociationist might wish to argue that the experimenter is asking questions of a dissociated "part of the mind" that can hear; but if this were so, surely the reply would be, "Yes, I can hear you"!)

Nevertheless, most state theorists, and even some non-state theorists have tended to deny that compliance is very influential in hypnotic responding. For example, in Hilgard and Hilgard's classic book *Hypnosis in the Relief of Pain* we are told that "deliberate 'faking' . . . is very rare and unimportant" [38, p. 16]; and there is indeed some evidence apparently against the idea that compliance is influential in hypnotic responding. For example, a time honored way of testing for compliance in hypnosis has been to compare "real" hypnotic subjects with others instructed to simulate or "fake" hypnosis, and although there is much evidence to suggest that a large number of hypnotic phenomena are readily exhibited by subjects instructed to simulate or "fake" hypnosis, nevertheless, sometimes differences do occur between simulators and so-called "real subjects" [26]. It has also been claimed that, contrary to a compliance hypothesis, posthypnotic responses persist outside the experiential setting [51], and demands for honesty have little effect on reports of hypnotic responding [24]. However, studies such as these have been subject criticized for a number of reasons [14-16]. For example, although differences do sometimes occur between simulators and so-called "real subjects," such differences can often be explained, without necessarily ruling out the influence of compliance, simply by reference to the fact that "reals" and "simulators" undergo different selection procedures and operate under different instructions [13, 14]. Early claims that posthypnotic responses persist outside the experimental setting have been criticized for failing to divorce the tester sufficiently from the experimental context; and there are a number of difficulties with the method of "demanding honesty" from subjects. The main difficulty with the honesty demands approach is that if subjects by their previous behavior have shown themselves committed to the role of presenting themselves as "hypnotized," to admit that they were faking could constitute a considerable loss of face, and so it would be unlikely that a simple demand for honesty would be effective. To demonstrate the full influence of compliance, therefore, paradigms must either place considerable pressure on subjects to "own up," or enable them to "own up" or "give themselves away" in a face-saving manner.

Now, with the advent of more appropriate paradigms, there is mounting evidence to support the view that compliance can be a powerful factor in hypnotic responding. For instance, it has been shown that, for a majority of subjects, hypnotic amnesia can be breached or eliminated by asking them to be honest, rigging them up to a lie detector, and showing them a videotape of their performance [52]. Also, hypnotic amnesia can be eliminated completely if subjects are given a "face-saving" opportunity to say they were "role-playing" rather than in a "trance" [53]. The possible influence of compliance in posthypnotic responding is illustrated by the finding of Spanos et al. that when subjects are tested for posthypnotic responses using a tester who ostensibly has nothing whatsoever to do with the experiment, the posthypnotic responses disappear entirely [54]. Compliance has also been shown to operate with negative hallucinations. In one study, Spanos et al. presented subjects with a highly visible figure "8" and suggested to them that they would see nothing; in response some subjects did indeed claim to have seen nothing [55]. However, these "negative hallucinators" were then told that deeply hypnotized subjects, unlike fakers, actually see the figure initially, and only then does it fade. When then asked what they had seen initially, all but one subject managed to produce a figure "8," even though they had not been told that "8" had been used as a stimulus.

Considerable additional support for the idea that compliance is implicated in hypnotic responding has come recently from another paradigm devised by Spanos [56]. In this, subjects are first given a stimulus and tested with no preceding suggestions (trial 1); then they are given hypnotic suggestions, followed by a stimulus and a second test (trial 2); and finally the suggestions are cancelled, the stimulus is given again and subjects are tested again, but after the stimulus and before the final test, half of the subjects receive a statement designed to induce compliance (trial 3). The compliance statement suggests that the subjects may have spontaneously "drifted back into hypnosis" during the third stimulus trial. If compliance operates, then hypnotically susceptible subjects receiving the compliance instruction should report a greater suggestion effect on trial 3 than those not receiving the instruction, and will report a suggestion effect equivalent to their trial 2 responses. Using this paradigm Spanos and his associates have found strong evidence for the influence of compliance in both reports of hypnotic analgesia, blindness, and deafness; moreover, those reporting the most profound hypnotic experiences on trial 2 (i.e., were most hypnotically susceptible), were those most likely to exhibit evidence of compliance on trial 3 [56-58].

THE EXPECTATION, STRATEGY, COMPLIANCE (ESC) PROCESS

If we accept the proposition that compliance may be very influential in hypnotic responding, then it may not be necessary to postulate some specialized dissociative process to account for hypnotic phenomena which appear to be beyond the powers of imagination or other mundane processes, for when, for example, hypnotic subjects claim not to see an object presented in front of them, claim to see an hallucinated person "as real as real," claim total amnesia for recent events, and claim not to know what their left hand is writing inside a box, the explanation could be very simple; their reports are not entirely truthful. But if compliance is influential in hypnotic responding, and imaginative involvement is not just a by-product of, or adjunct to, special states or dissociative processes, what exactly is the role of imagination in hypnosis? To establish a role for imagination we need to examine briefly some of the processes that may be involved in enacting the role of a "hypnotized" person.

Elsewhere, I have proposed that it is unhelpful and misleading to view hypnosis as a special state in which profound dissociations are experienced [14-16]. Instead, hypnotic responding may be more usefully viewed in terms of two main concepts, compliance and belief. According to this view, whether it be to please the hypnotist, to appease their curiosity, to enhance their self-esteem, or some combination of such factors, subjects who respond to hypnotic suggestions are strongly motivated to give the appearance of being "hypnotized." So strong is this motivation, that subjects involve themselves in strategic attempts to respond to suggestions in such a way that their experiences accurately reflect what is explicitly or implicitly required in the suggestions given to them; that is, they try to make sure their responses are "genuine" or "believable." However, very importantly, if such strategies are not deemed appropriate, simply not available, or are unsuccessful in generating the required experiences, "good" hypnotic subjects comply; that is, they verbally state, or behaviorally give the impression, that they are having experiences which, in reality, they are not.

I have also argued that it is pointless looking for some single explanation for all hypnotic phenomena, whether it be imagination, dissociation, or anything else; different phenomena may require different kinds of explanations, and, different subjects may employ different strategies to produce different effects [14, 16]. In fact, non-state theorists have proposed a variety of different strategies that might facilitate responding to hypnotic suggestions. For example, to experience a "genuine" or "believable" degree of hypnotic "amnesia" some subjects may find it helpful to distract themselves in some way so they will find it difficult to remember [52]; to achieve genuine pain relief, it can be helpful for subjects not only to distract themselves, but also to relax, and change their attitudes so as not to catastrophize about their sensations [37, 59]; to achieve a sensation of involuntary arm levitation, it may be useful to construct a "goal directed fantasy" [27]; to achieve greater strength or endurance in an hypnotic situation, subjects may motivate themselves more in the hypnotic situation [14, 60], and to experience a state of profound relaxation, sitting quietly and breathing deeply will obviously help. However, subjects may employ other strategies, including simple compliance, when responding to suggestions for some or all to the above, and some responses, such as total negative hallucinations, complete amnesia for recent events, total analgesia, and reports of "as real as real" hallucinations, can perhaps only be accounted for by compliance.

From this perspective, hypnotic responding is best conceptualized as a three-stage process, which I have called the "ESC" (expectation, strategy, compliance) process [15, 16, 61]; thus when subjects respond in an hypnotic situation, they do the following.

1. They try to work out what is appropriate to the hypnotic role, or what is expected of them.
2. They apply "normal" cognitive strategies or activities in response to suggestions to make the experiences veridical or "believable," in line with their previous expectations and what is explicitly or implicitly demanded of them in the general context.
3. If the application of "normal" strategies fails to evoke the appropriate subjective experiences, or such strategies are unavailable to the subject, or deemed inappropriate in the context, subjects behaviorally comply or "sham."

How subjects operate the ESC process may differ, and differences in the operation of the scheme will be reflected in differences in hypnotic susceptibility; for example, some subjects may go through the stages as defined, while others may skip stage 2, and comply to everything; others may apply stages 2 and 3 simultaneously (as will be discussed shortly), and still others may stop at stage 2, and fail to respond further if the stage 2 strategies fail to produce the desired effects.

COMPLIANCE AND IMAGINATION IN THE ESC PROCESS

Within the context of the ESC process, we can now see a possible role for imagination. In fact, imaginative involvement can play a dual role. First, it can facilitate the use of strategies to enable responses to specific suggestions to be experienced as "genuine" or "believable"; and second, it can influence attitudes and strategies that facilitate compliant responses.

As regards the first role, if we look at the strategies that have been identified by non-state theorists as helping subjects successfully experience hypnotic suggestions, it seems clear that many of these strategies would benefit from the exercise of vivid imagination. For example, one does not necessarily need to have a vivid imagination to distract oneself while responding to an amnesia suggestion, or enduring a painful stimulus so that less pain will be experienced, but an ability to visualize distractive scenes would seem to be of obvious benefit in both cases. Similarly, imagination may not be necessary for relaxation during an induction procedure, but an ability to visualize relaxing scenes might prove useful in this respect. Also any kind of distractive strategy might serve to enable a subject to interpret an arm movement as involuntary, but an ability to devise "goal directed imaginings" might be especially beneficial. Imagination would seem to come really into its own in the case of so-called hypnotic hallucinations; Spanos reports that many subjects, prefer to say that their suggested "hallucinations" were "imagined" rather than "seen"; so if, when subjects say they have "seen" an hallucinated object, what they really mean is they "imagined" it, "in their minds' eye," as it were, then it would be impossible to say this truthfully without the exercise of imagination.

However, if the ESC process is indeed at work in hypnotic responding, an obvious prediction can be made; if no "mundane" strategy, and no amount of creative imagery, would be likely to enable a subject to genuinely experience a suggestion, then any positive response would represent pure compliance; that is, there would be no necessity to predict a relationship between responsiveness and the degree to which imaginative and other strategies are used to produce the effect. And, indeed, in the case of negative hallucinations, Spanos et al. found no relationship between the degree of reported "blindness" and the degree of strategy use [57].

Nevertheless, this does not mean that compliance and imaginative involvement are necessarily unrelated; on the contrary, as well as helping subjects to subjectively experience hypnotic effects, imaginative involvement may play a second role, it may *facilitate compliance*. Almost all subjects in hypnotic situations are, at some stage, likely to experience some pressure to comply, and a capacity for imaginative involvement could be influential in affecting the confidence to carry out the role. Thus if, for instance, a subject is going to pretend that he or she has actually seen or heard something "as real as real," the pretense is going to be more effective, and the subject more confident in his or her ability to "carry it off," if the object concerned can be imagined in a vivid and detailed way. Similarly, subjects feigning amnesia, catatonia, analgesia, negative hallucinations, or regression to childhood, for example, may benefit from an ability to imagine what it would be like to experience such things. Compliant hypnotic responding requires what

Sarbin terms, "role-skills," and a willingness or capacity to become involved in imaginings would seem to be beneficial as part of a compliant responder's role-skill repertoire. Also, subjects with a propensity to involve themselves in imaginings might be more likely to attempt and experience hypnotic suggestions in the first place; by doing so they could be more likely to commit themselves early to responding, even if only to the induction procedure, and having committed themselves they would be susceptible to the "foot in the door" effect, and find it difficult to refrain from responding to suggestions that can only be enacted compliantly.

COMPLIANCE, IMAGINATION, AND INDIVIDUAL DIFFERENCES

If the analysis presented here is valid, then any findings of stability in hypnotic responding, and significant correlations between hypnotic responding and imaginative involvement, would certainly not, in themselves, rule out explanations of hypnotic responding in terms of compliance. There are two main reasons for this. First, although compliance may be influenced by the pressures of the immediate situation, nevertheless, in the absence of attempts to manipulate it, there is no reason why compliant responding should necessarily be unstable *within the hypnotic context*. It is important to note, for example, that Spanos and his colleagues found, using the compliance paradigm described earlier, that those exhibiting evidence of compliance turned out to be highly susceptible "hypnotic virtuosos" on a standard hypnotic susceptibility measure, and compliance generalized across different suggestions [56]. Second, as just mentioned, a proclivity to become involved in imaginings may in itself facilitate compliant performance, for compliant hypnotic responding will be maximized among subjects who not only feel a special motivation to perform according to the hypnotist's expectations, but also feel able or sufficiently competent to "get away with deception"; and having a capacity or liking for imaginative involvement, or playing "make-believe," could profoundly affect this perception of competence. Perhaps relevant here, is the finding that dramaturgic or acting skills correlate significantly with hypnotic susceptibility [7]. Also of potential interest here is the work of Wilson and Barber [23] on the "fantasy prone personality" [23].

Wilson and Barber argue that excellent hypnotic subjects derive from a small percentage of the normal population whom they have termed "fantasy-prone personalities," denoting a profound fantasy life. These subjects report particularly vivid sensory experiences, such as voluntary "as real as real" hallucinations, frequently claim abilities as "healers," and report numerous paranormal psychic experiences [23]. More recent studies suggest that the correlations between fantasy proneness and hypnotic susceptibility are somewhat modest [33], nevertheless, the relationship seems to be fairly reliable. Significantly, Wilson and Barber suggest that, compared to a control group, fantasizers were more likely to have experienced four childhood life patterns: they had 1) been encouraged to fantasize by significant adults, 2) fantasized because they felt lonely or isolated, 3) fantasized as an escape from a stressful or abusive environment, or 4) been involved in an early life situation that encouraged fantasy (such as the intensive study of piano, ballet, or dramatic acting at the ages of 2, 3, or 4 years). Wilson and Barber report that at least 70 percent of fantasizers showed two or more of these patterns in their lives. In the present context, an examination of these life patterns may be useful, not simply because the patterns provide possible explanations as to how and why certain people might become prone to using their imaginations, but also because of what they suggest to us about the capacity of such individuals for compliance in the hypnotic situation.

Many of Wilson and Barber's fantasizers reported that, as children, they felt lonely, isolated, and were sometimes even openly abused (one could also perhaps suggest that intensive ballet or piano studies at the age of 2, 3, or 4, hardly reflect an easy-going environment). In brief, fantasizers often report a history of deprivation and/or abuse of some kind; this fits well with Hilgard's observation that high hypnotic susceptibility is significantly related to severe punishment in childhood [62]. More recently, Rhue and Lynn have also reported a relationship between fantasy-proneness and greater frequency and severity of physical punishment during childhood (i.e., punishment producing bruises, and bleeding, or broken noses), and also sexual abuse [63]. This may be important, in that, even in their adult lives, survivors of childhood abuse may, as a result of their abuse, be prone to using a number of coping mechanisms, one of which is deception [64]. Indeed, Wilson and Barber themselves note how some of their fantasizers said they enjoyed deceiving strangers into thinking they are someone else; for instance, while riding on a bus just the day before the interview, one of Wilson and Barber's subjects who had lived in New York all her life introduced herself as an Eskimo to the person sitting next to her, and then proceeded to tell the stranger all about her (fantasized) life in Alaska. Many fantasizers may therefore feel confident of their abilities to use imagination skills to deceive others, and may even have found such deception rewarding in the past, either as an attention seeking device when they felt isolated or ignored, and/or a means of avoiding punishment and distress.

The childhood experiences reported by fantasizers may be significant for another reason. According to Bass and Davies, a further characteristic reported by some survivors of abuse is that, as children, they continually felt alone and powerless, and found themselves unable or unwilling to resist the demands of others [64]. Subsequently, as adults, survivors can still be very prone to do what others ask of them, and can generally find it difficult to say "no." If the same is true of fantasizers, then it could be the case that some "fantasy-prones" not only possess the confidence and skill to act out fantasies to deceive others, and may even enjoy it in some cases, but also are especially keen to do the bidding of, and try to please others. Such factors might especially predispose such individuals to please the experimenter in the hypnotic situation; it is of interest to note here that Graham and Green found a significant relationship between hypnotic susceptibility and alumni giving [65].

It should be emphasized again, however, that according to the present analysis, a general or initial desire to please or impress others is not the only reason why someone might comply when responding to hypnotic suggestions. Both Wilson and Barber [23] and Rhue and Lynn [63] note that fantasizers often report that they were actively encouraged by adults to use fantasy activities. This could not only result in fantasizers being especially prone to attempt to please an authority figure in a situation apparently demanding fantasy activity, but it could also make them extra prone to use fantasy to respond initially to suggestions in the hypnotic situation, simply out of interest or curiosity. This might then lead to a situation in which, when eventually confronted with "impossible" suggestions, they feel obliged to comply.

In view of these considerations, it is perhaps not unreasonable to suggest that "fantasy-prone" individuals possess a combination of characteristics making them particularly sensitive to compliance pressures in hypnosis. However, any proposed relationship between fantasy-proneness and compliance in hypnosis is at this time, of course, only speculative, and it is important not to oversimplify the nature of any relationship between hypnotic susceptibility, imagination and fantasy involvement, and compliance in general. As has been pointed out, the relationship between involvement in imagination and fantasy, and hypnotic susceptibility, is not as strong as was once thought, and may be, to a certain extent, context dependent. Also, the issue of whether high hypnotically susceptible subjects are, in general, more compliant than low susceptibles, is contentious; for example, Shames [66] found a significant relationship between hypnotic susceptibility and compliance in the Asch conformity paradigm, whereas, Spanos [56], using his compliance paradigm, found that low susceptibles receiving nonhypnotic suggestions were as likely to show reporting biases as high susceptibles given hypnotic suggestions. Thus, inasmuch as compliance operates in hypnotic responding, it may be to a large degree, situationally specific to the hypnosis context. This is perhaps not really surprising; for example, as has been pointed out, compliance in hypnosis would seem to require certain role-skills, and these would seem to include an ability or willingness to display imagination and fantasy in acting out suggestions and generally taking on the hypnotic role. It is therefore possible that some subjects who feel they are lacking in, or who are reticent about employing, such skills, might feel reluctant to comply in the hypnotic situation. The same subjects might, however, exhibit a propensity for compliance in situations where such skills are less critical. The proposal that certain individuals may feel doubtful about their capacity to fake hypnosis is supported by the finding that, when subjects are asked to fake hypnosis, but are given no assurance that they will be able to handle the task successfully, there is considerable heterogeneity in responsiveness to simulation instructions. However, when given some assurance that they can be successful, simulators exhibit greater homogeneity in, and generally higher, responsiveness [67].

The issue of whether "fantasy-prones," or others who score high on measures of imaginative involvement, are in some sense superior to others in their general ability to use imagination, or whether they are simply more willing to use imagination in specific contexts, has yet to be fully addressed in the research literature. Indeed, we have yet to explore thoroughly the extent to which scales of imaginative involvement themselves could be biased by compliance. Also, imagery paradigms are very vulnerable to demand characteristic effects [68]. Thus, at this point, I am making no assumptions about whether the "capacity" for imaginative involvement in the hypnotic situation is in any sense fixed or difficult to modify; though if we accept Spanos' view [10, 12] that hypnotic susceptibility is modifiable, and that, in part, this is achieved by increasing imaginative involvement in hypnotic responding, then it may be that a willingness to employ imagination is more important than any relatively enduring capacity for imaginative involvement.

Nevertheless, the main conclusion I wish to draw here is that, in principle at least, the finding that a propensity to become involved in imaginings and fantasy correlates with hypnotic susceptibility is certainly not at variance with the idea that compliance may be strongly implicated in hypnotic responding; in fact it may complement it.

COMPLIANCE, EXPECTATION, IMAGINATION, AND "GENUINE" RESPONDING

According to the view expressed so far in this chapter, imagination can facilitate both compliant and "genuine" hypnotic behavior. However, it is important to recognize that, from the present perspective, what essentially distinguishes a compliant response from a "genuine response" is not the nature or degree of imaginative involvement employed, but whether subjects' overt actions and subjective experiences are in line with their *expectations* as to what constitutes a "genuine" response.

Compliance occurs when overt behavior is discrepant with private experience or conviction. In the case of many hypnotic behaviors, it is not difficult to conceptualize a compliant response; a man who deliberately raises his arm and claims it "rose by itself," is acting compliantly; similarly, a woman who claims she cannot see an object before her, when she can see it as clear as day, is acting compliantly. However, compliance can vary depending on subjects' expectations [16]. For instance, inasmuch as subjects believe or expect that it is legitimate to interpret an amnesia suggestion as an invitation to attend away from the target, then if an imaginative strategy that diverts attention is effective in disrupting recall, such subjects are not necessarily acting compliantly, at least not in the sense I am using here, for their overt verbal reports of "forgetting" and their private convictions about what passes for "forgetting" might coincide. Similarly, if subjects interpret an hallucination suggestion as an invitation to imagine and describe an imaginary object, in "their mind's eye," and believe this to be a legitimate response, then if, in response to the suggestion, they describe their imagined object, this is not strictly compliance either. This interpretation may have implications for research methodology; for example, one implication is that, with regard to some suggestions, it may be naive to think that simple requests for honesty, even if effective, would necessarily enable experimenters to distinguish between the hypnotic experiences of so-called "fakers" and "genuine" subjects; for those admitting dishonesty and those claiming honesty could actually be employing similar strategies and having similar experiences, but holding different expectancies. The only difference might be that those labeled "fakers" would "own up" because they think that their strategies and experiences are not legitimate in the context, and constitute faking, whereas so-called "genuine" subjects would not "own-up," because they believe that the *same* strategies and experiences are legitimate, and do not constitute faking.

A simple division of responses into "genuine" and "compliant" on the basis of the degree or nature of imaginative involvement may also be precluded by the possibility that, even in response to a single suggestion, subjects may use imaginative strategies to evoke appropriate subjective experiences and yet still, at some stage, exhibit compliance while responding to the suggestion. For example, some degree of compliance may actually be necessary for the performance of certain hypnotic suggestions if those suggestions are to be experienced as "genuine." Some subjects in our laboratory at Liverpool have noted how, no matter what imaginative strategy they use, they cannot subsequently experience arm levitation and lowering as "involuntary" unless, at first, they deliberately initiate the movement (see also [69, p. 104]). In line with this view is the finding that an important factor differentiating low from high susceptibles is that, even when they involve themselves in appropriate imaginings, lows still fail to respond to suggestions [33]; Lynn and Rhue propose that this occurs because lows "fail for the most part, to perceive or construct a connection between their suggestion related imaginings and moving in response to the suggestion . . . they wait passively for suggested events to occur" [33, p. 424]. This fits well with the hypothesis that highs, at least initially, perform some active, deliberate, very "voluntary," movement when responding to ideomotor suggestions. Thus when highs claim their responses were "effortless" or "involuntary," it is possible that such statements could be partly valid and partly false. The movement could have started off as compliance and ended up as "genuine." Of course, one interesting corollary of all this is the possibility that, for some suggestions, unless a subject is prepared to exhibit some degree of compliance, he or she may never actually be able to experience the suggestion as "genuine."

There are other possible instances of an interaction between imaginative involvement, expectation, and compliance. For example, as noted earlier,

Zamansky found that when subjects were told to employ an imaginative strategy appropriate to one response (such as, to imagine their arm bending), but at the same time were given a suggestion for an opposite response ("you cannot bend your arm"), they tended to perform the latter suggested response [29, 30]. Moreover, all subjects insisted that they *were* actually imagining as instructed. Zamansky and Clark concluded that these results show that absorption in imaginings is inadequate as an explanation of hypnotic responding, and, as one interpretation, suggest that some dissociative process may be at work [30]. However, an alternative and perhaps more parsimonious explanation could be that, in accordance with what they thought was expected of them, subjects deliberately ignored the instruction to engage in imaginings of one kind, and used a different imaginative strategy to produce experiences in line with the suggested effect. In other words they were complying by falsely claiming to have used one kind of imaginative involvement, yet using another kind of involvement to experience the response as genuine! Of course they could also have simply ignored the instruction to use the imaginative strategy and deliberately carried out the suggestion with full volition, but either way, given that subjects insisted afterwards they were imagining in the instructed direction, compliance is implicated.

CONCLUSION

According to the non-state view I have presented here, imagination may play an important role in hypnotic responding, but if we are to understand the nature of that role we must examine the significance of other factors, particularly compliance, in the hypnotic situation. My position can be summarized briefly as follows.

Responsiveness to the majority of hypnotic suggestions requires the active deliberate participation by subjects. Moreover, different suggestions may require different strategies to "pass" them; some (such as "involuntary" arm lowering, and some degree of forgetting) may, at least at some point, be experienced as "genuine," so long as subjects know what strategies to adopt and how to interpret their experiences; while others can only be "passed" by employing pure compliance (these include "real as real" hallucinations, total negative hallucinations, and profound hypnotic deafness). So, if subjects are to respond to a full range of suggestions, the following factors must be present: 1) they must have positive attitudes toward hypnosis (for instance, they must not be extremely afraid or totally unwilling to actively participate); 2) they must have appropriate expectancies (for instance, they have to realize that they must actively try to respond by adopting a range of strategies, and not passively wait for something to happen; and they must accept such action as "legitimate" if they are to experience certain phenomena as "genuine"); 3) they must have the capacity to devise the appropriate strategies; and very importantly, 4) subjects must have a willingness or capacity to comply in the hypnotic situation. Perhaps it is not necessary to add a *high* general propensity for imaginative involvement as an extra requirement, nevertheless, it seems reasonable to assume that all these conditions are more likely to be fulfilled if subjects have some minimal capacity for, and certainly willingness to employ, imaginative involvement.

REFERENCES

1. B. J. Fellows, Current Theories of Hypnosis: A Critical Overview, *British Journal of Experimental and Clinical Hypnosis, 7,* pp. 81-92, 1990.
2. I. Kirsch, Current Theories of Hypnosis: An Addendum, *Contemporary Hypnosis, 8,* pp. 105-108, 1992.
3. K. S. Bowers and T. M. Davidson, A Neo-dissociative Critique of Spanos's Social-Psychological Model of Hypnosis, in *Theories of Hypnosis: Current Models and Perspectives,* S. J. Lynn and J. W. Rhue (eds.), Guilford Press, New York, pp. 105-143, 1991.
4. E. R. Hilgard, A Neodissociation Interpretation of Hypnosis, in *Theories of Hypnosis: Current Models and Perspectives,* S. J. Lynn and J. W. Rhue (eds.), Guilford Press, New York, pp. 83-104, 1991.
5. T. X. Barber, *Hypnosis: A Scientific Approach,* Van Nostrand, New York, 1969.
6. T. X. Barber, N. P. Spanos, and J. F. Chaves, *Hypnosis, Imagination, and Human Potentialities,* Pergamon Press, Elmsford, New York, 1974.
7. T. R. Sarbin and W. C. Coe, *Hypnosis: A Social Psychological Analysis of Influence Communication,* Holt, Rinehart and Winston, New York, 1972.
8. N. P. Spanos, A Social Psychological Approach to Hypnotic Behavior, in *Integrations of Clinical and Social Psychology,* G. Weary and H. L. Mirels (eds.), Oxford University Press, Oxford, pp. 231-271, 1982.
9. N. P. Spanos, Hypnotic Behavior: A Cognitive and Social Psychological Perspective, *Research Communications in Psychology, Psychiatry and Behavior, 7,* pp. 199-213, 1982.
10. N. P. Spanos, Hypnosis and the Modification of Hypnotic Susceptibility: A Social Psychological Perspective, in *What is Hypnosis? Current Theories and Research,* P. L. N. Naish (ed.), Open University Press, Philadelphia, pp. 85-120, 1986.
11. N. P. Spanos, Hypnotic Behavior: A Social Psychological Interpretation of Amnesia, Analgesia and Trance Logic, *Behavioral and Brain Sciences, 9,* pp. 449-467, 1986.
12. N. P. Spanos, A Sociocognitive Approach to Hypnosis, in *Theories of Hypnosis: Current Models and Perspectives,* S. J. Lynn and J. W. Rhue (eds.), Guilford Press, New York, pp. 324-362, 1991.
13. G. F. Wagstaff, The Problem of Compliance in Hypnosis: A Social Psychological Viewpoint, *Bulletin of the British Society of Experimental and Clinical Hypnosis, 2,* pp. 3-5, 1979.
14. G. F. Wagstaff, *Hypnosis, Compliance, and Belief,* Harvester Press, Brighton, 1981.
15. G. F. Wagstaff, Hypnosis as Compliance and Belief, in *What is Hypnosis: Current Theories and Research,* P. L. N Naish (ed.), Open University Press, Milton Keynes and Philadelphia, pp. 59-84, 1986.
16. G. F. Wagstaff, Compliance, Belief and Semantics in Hypnosis: A Non-state Sociocognitive Perspective, in *Theories of Hypnosis: Current Models and Perspectives,* S. J. Lynn and J. W. Rhue (eds.), Guilford Press, New York, pp. 362-396, 1991.
17. G. F. Wagstaff and D. Benson, Exploring Hypnotic Processes with the Cognitive-Simulator Comparison Group, *British Journal of Experimental and Clinical Hypnosis, 4,* pp. 83-91, 1987.

18. E. R. Hilgard, Hypnosis, *Annual Review of Psychology, 26,* pp. 19-44, 1975.
19. N. P. Spanos and T. X. Barber, Toward a Convergence in Hypnosis Research, *American Psychologist, 29,* pp. 500-511, 1974.
20. J. R. Hilgard, *Personality and Hypnosis,* University of Chicago Press, Chicago, 1970.
21. A. Tellegen and G. Atkinson, Openness to Absorbing and Self-altering Experiences ("Absorption"), a Trait Related to Hypnotic Susceptibility, *Journal of Abnormal Psychology, 83,* pp. 268-277, 1974.
22. T. X. Barber and S. C. Wilson, Hypnosis, Suggestions and Altered States of Consciousness: Experimental Evaluation of the New Cognitive-Behavioral Theory and the Traditional Trance-State Theory of "Hypnosis," *Annals of the New York Academy of Sciences, 296,* pp. 34-47, 1977.
23. S. C. Wilson and T. X. Barber, The Fantasy Prone Personality: Implications for Understanding Imagery, Hypnosis and Parapsychological Phenomena, in *Imagery: Current Theory, Research and Application,* A. A Sheikh (ed.), Wiley, New York, pp. 340-387, 1982.
24. S. J. Lynn and J. W. Rhue (eds.), *Theories of Hypnosis: Current Models and Perspectives,* Guilford Press, New York, 1991.
25. E. R. Hilgard, *Divided Consciousness: Multiple Controls in Human Thought and Action* (Expanded Edition), Wiley, New York, 1986.
26. K. S. Bowers, Hypnosis for the Seriously Curious, *Norton,* New York, 1986.
27. N. P. Spanos, Goal-directed Phantasy and the Performance of Hypnotic Test Suggestions, *Psychiatry, 34,* pp. 86-96, 1971.
28. E. R. Hilgard and J. R. Hilgard, *Hypnosis in the Relief of Pain,* William Kaufmann, Los Altos, California, 1983.
29. H. S. Zamansky, Suggestion and Countersuggestion in Hypnotic Behavior, *Journal of Abnormal Psychology, 86,* pp. 346-351, 1977.
30. H. S. Zamansky and L. E. Clark, Cognitive Competition and Hypnotic Behavior: Whither Absorption?, *International Journal of Clinical and Experimental Hypnosis, 34,* pp. 205-214, 1986.
31. J. R. Council, I. Kirsch, and L. P. Hafner, Expectancy versus Absorption in the Prediction of Hypnotic Responding, *Journal of Personality and Social Psychology, 50,* pp. 182-189, 1986.
32. M. M. de Groh, Correlates of Hypnotic Susceptibility, in *Hypnosis: The Cognitive-Behavioral Perspective,* N. P. Spanos and J. F. Chaves (eds.), Prometheus Books, Buffalo, New York, pp. 32-62, 1989.
33. S. J. Lynn and J. W. Rhue, An Integrative Model of Hypnosis, in *Theories of Hypnosis: Current Models and Perspectives,* S. J. Lynn and J. W. Rhue (eds.), Guilford Press, New York, pp. 397-438, 1991.
34. A. H. Perlini, A. Lee, and N. P. Spanos, The Relationship between Imaginal Ability and Hypnotic Susceptibility: Does Context Matter?, *Contemporary Hypnosis, 9,* pp. 35-41, 1992.
35. L. D. Bertrand, The Assessment and Modification of Hypnotic Susceptibility, in *Hypnosis: The Cognitive-Behavioural Perspective,* N. P. Spanos and J. F. Chaves (eds.), Prometheus Books, Buffalo, New York, pp. 18-31, 1989.
36. N. P. Spanos, W. P. Cross, E. P. Menary, and M. de Groh, Attitudinal and Imaginability Predictors of Social Cognitive Skill Training for the Enhancement of Hypnotic Susceptibility, *Personality and Social Psychology Bulletin, 13,* pp. 379-398, 1987.
37. B. Bates, R. J. Miller, H. J. Cross, and T. A. Brigham, Modifying Hypnotic Suggestibility with the Carleton Skills Training Program, *Journal of Personality and Social Psychology, 55,* pp. 120-126, 1988.

38. N. P. Spanos, Experimental Research on Hypnotic Analgesia, in *Hypnosis: The Cognitive-Behavioural Perspective*, N. P. Spanos and J. F. Chaves (eds.), Prometheus Books, Buffalo, New York, pp. 206-241, 1989.
39. H. S. Zamansky and S. P. Bartis, The Dissociation of an Experience: The Hidden Observer Observed, *Journal of Abnormal Psychology, 94,* pp. 243-248, 1985.
40. C. A. Kiesler and S. B. Kiesler, *Conformity,* Addison-Wesley, Reading, Massachusetts, 1970.
41. J. T. Tedeschi, S. Lindskold, and P. Rosenfeld, *Introduction to Social Psychology,* West, St. Paul, Minnesota, 1985.
42. C. L. Sheridan and R. G. King, Obedience to Authority with an Authentic Victim, *Proceedings of the 80th Convention of the American Psychological Association, 7,* pp. 165-166, 1972.
43. S. E. Asch, Studies of Independence and Conformity: A Minority of One Against a Unanimous Majority, *Psychological Monographs, 70* (9, Whole No. 416), 1956.
44. L. H. Levy, Awareness Learning and the Beneficent Subject as Expert Witness, *Journal of Personality and Social Psychology, 6,* pp. 365-370, 1967.
45. M. T. Orne, On the Social Psychology of the Psychological Experiment: With Particular Reference to Demand Characteristics and Their Implications, *American Psychologist, 17,* pp. 776-783, 1962.
46. S. Milgram, *Obedience to Authority,* Tavistock, London, 1974.
47. D. P. Frank, Experimental Studies of Personal Pressure and Resistance: 1. Experimental Production of Resistance, *Journal of General Psychology, 30,* pp. 23-41, 1944.
48. J. L. Freedman, and S. C. Fraser, Compliance Without Pressure: The Foot in the Door Technique, *Journal of Personality and Social Psychology, 7,* pp. 117-124, 1966.
49. R. B. Cialdini, J. T. Cacioppo, R. Bassett, and J. A. Miller, Low-ball Procedure for Producing Compliance: Commitment Then Cost, *Journal of Personality and Social Psychology, 36,* pp. 463-476, 1978.
50. F. A. Pattie, A Report of Attempts to Produce Uniocular Blindness by Hypnotic Suggestion, *British Journal of Medical Psychology, 15,* pp. 230-241, 1935.
51. M. T. Orne, P. W. Sheehan, and F. J. Evans, Occurrence of Posthypnotic Behavior Outside the Experimental Setting, *Journal of Personality and Social Psychology, 9,* pp. 189-196, 1968.
52. W. C. Coe, Post-hypnotic Amnesia: Theory and Research, in *Hypnosis: The Cognitive-Behavioral Perspective,* N. P. Spanos and J. F. Chaves (eds.), Prometheus Books, Buffalo, New York, pp. 110-148, 1989.
53. G. F. Wagstaff, An Experimental Study of Compliance and Post-hypnotic Amnesia, *British Journal of Social and Clinical Psychology, 16,* pp. 225-228, 1977.
54. N. P. Spanos, E. Menary, P. J. Brett, W. Cross, and Q. Ahmed, Failure of Posthypnotic Responding to Occur Outside the Experimental Setting, *Journal of Abnormal Psychology, 96,* pp. 52-57, 1987.
55. N. P. Spanos, D. M. Flynn, and N. Gabora, Suggested Negative Visual Hallucinations in Hypnotic Subjects: When No Means Yes, *British Journal of Experimental and Clinical Hypnosis, 6,* pp. 63-67, 1989.
56. N. P. Spanos, Compliance and Reinterpretation in Hypnotic Responding, *Contemporary Hypnosis, 9,* pp. 7-14, 1992.
57. N. P. Spanos, C. A. Burgess, and C. A. Perlini, Compliance and Suggested Deafness in Hypnotic and Nonhypnotic Subjects, *Imagination, Cognition and Personality, 11,* pp. 211-223, 1992.
58. N. P. Spanos, A. H. Perlini, L. Patrick, S. Bell, and M. I. Gwynn, The Role of Compliance in Hypnotic and Nonhypnotic Analgesia, *Journal of Research in Personality, 24,* pp. 433-453, 1990.

59. J. F. Chaves, Hypnotic Control of Clinical Pain, in *Hypnosis: The Cognitive-Behavioral Perspective*, N. P. Spanos and J. F. Chaves (eds.), Prometheus Books, Buffalo, New York, pp. 242-271, 1989.

60. W. P. Morgan, *Ergogenic Aids and Muscular Performance*, Academic Press, New York, 1972.

61. G. F. Wagstaff, A Comment on McConkey's Challenging Hypnotic Effects: The Impact of Conflicting Influences in Response to Hypnotic Suggestions, *British Journal of Experimental and Clinical Hypnosis, 1,* pp. 11-15, 1983.

62. J. R. Hilgard, Imaginative Involvement: Some Characteristics of the Highly Hypnotizable and Nonhypnotizable, *International Journal of Clinical and Experimental Hypnosis, 22,* pp. 238-256, 1974.

63. J. W. Rhue and S. J. Lynn, Fantasy Proneness, Hypnotizability, and Multiple Personality Disorder, in *Human Suggestibility,* J. F. Schumaker (ed.), Routledge, London, pp. 200-218, 1991.

64. E. Bass and L. Davis, *The Courage to Heal: A Guide for Women Survivors of Child Sexual Abuse,* Cedar, London, 1991.

65. K. R. Graham and L. D. Green, Hypnotic Susceptibility Related to an Independent Measure of Compliance—Annual Alumni Giving, *International Journal of Clinical and Experimental Hypnosis, 29,* pp. 351-354, 1981.

66. M. L. Shames, Hypnotic Susceptibility and Conformity: On the Mediational Mechanism of Suggestibility, *Psychological Reports, 49,* pp. 563-565, 1981.

67. P. W. Sheehan and C. W. Perry, *Methodologies of Hypnosis: A Critical Appraisal of Contemporary Paradigms of Hypnosis,* Lawrence Erlbaum, Hillsdale, New Jersey, 1976.

68. M. J. Intons-Peterson, Imagery Paradigms: How Vulnerable are They to Experimenters' Expectations?, *Journal of Experimental Psychology: Human Perception and Performance, 9,* pp. 394-412, 1983.

69. E. Cardena and D. Spiegel, Suggestibility, Absorption and Dissociation: An Integrative Model of Hypnosis, in *Human Suggestibility,* J. F. Schumaker (ed.), Routledge, London, pp. 93-107, 1991.

CHAPTER 3

Imagination, Expectancy, and Hypnotic Responding*

JAMES R. COUNCIL, IRVING KIRSCH, AND DEBORA L. GRANT

Throughout the history of hypnosis, imagination and expectancy have been intertwined as explanatory constructs. When the French Royal Commission of 1784 concluded that mesmerism operated through "the imagination," they did so on the basis of placebo-controlled studies. In addition to exposing subjects to bona fide mesmeric procedures, Franklin and his colleagues used sham procedures to manipulate expectancy. For example, subjects became mesmerized when exposed to ordinary objects that they mistakenly believed had been magnetized.

Concluding that mesmerism was due to the imagination was tantamount to dismissing it as unreal, just as drug effects are dismissed today if duplicated by placebos. However, as Charles D'Eslon noted at the time,

> If Mesmer had no secret than that he has been able to make the imagination exert an influence upon health, would he not still be a wonder doctor? If treatment by the use of imagination is the best treatment, why do we not make use of it? (quoted in Gravitz [1]).

Contemporary scholars also view hypnotic phenomena as imaginative productions (see [2]). Ironically, this view now enhances the credibility of hypnosis, since imagination falls in the purview of mainstream personality and cognitive psychology.

The situation differs for expectancy. Although acknowledging its importance, theorists view expectancy as an artifact that obscures the essence of hypnosis [3]. That is, expectancy is just one of many "social psychological" factors that may account for relatively easy ideomotor responses, but cannot explain virtuoso responses like hallucination, age regression, or amnesia [4].

*The preparation of this chapter, and some of the new research reported herein, were supported by grant SES-9123378 from the National Science Foundation to James R. Council.

Paradoxically, the potency of expectancy in pharmacological research is responsible for its status as an artifact. Physicians have long known that the curative powers of "wonder drugs" wear off with their novelty [5]. Through most of recorded history, however, placebos were regarded as medications that might placate troublesome patients, but that certainly could not cure them. This is reflected in the term itself, which is Latin for "I shall please."

It was not until the 1950s that the power of placebos to produce genuine changes became widely recognized. Subsequent research has shown that patients' beliefs about placebo drugs influence their responses to a wide range of physiological and self-report measures (see [6]). However, this research has been conducted to determine the pharmacological action of drugs by controlling for expectancy. Placebo effects were viewed as nuisance factors to be ruled out.

Placebo controls soon were extended to psychotherapy research, and a spate of outcome studies compared the effects of "bona fide" and "placebo" psychotherapies. However, the extension of placebo controls to psychotherapy was founded on a conceptual error. The function of placebos in medical research was to control for psychological effects. But the effects of psychotherapy are intended to be psychological. We do not need research to establish that they are not due to the chemical properties of the treatment. Instead, placebo controlled psychotherapy research addresses the question of the degree to which a treatment's effects are due to a particular class of psychological variables (expectancies) as opposed to other psychological variables.

Expectancies are artifact variables in medical research because all psychological factors are artifacts when one's aim is to establish pharmacological efficacy. But there is no reason to consider them any less legitimate than other psychological variables. Expectancy has the same logical status as *abreaction, unconditional positive regard,* and *contingent reinforcement.* It is one hypothesized mechanism of treatment effectiveness, and the degree to which the effects of a psychological treatment are due to this mechanism does not diminish its legitimacy or efficacy.

Some contemporary theorists have acknowledged the power and legitimacy of expectancy effects in psychotherapy, but they have been the exceptions rather than the rule. Frank argued that negative expectations are primary causes and cures of psychological distress [7]. Fish prescribed methods of expectancy modification in his facetiously titled book, *Placebo Therapy* [8], and Coe stressed the importance of expectancies in hypnotherapy [9]. In *Changing Expectations: A Key to Effective Psychotherapy,* Kirsch presented a systematic explanation of expectancy effects in hypnosis and psychotherapy [6].

Kirsch [6, 10] distinguished *response expectancy* from other expectancy constructs and integrated it with Rotter's Social Learning Theory [11]. Response expectancies influence nonvolitional responses, which are not completely under direct conscious control and can include both psychological and physiological effects. Kirsch proposed that response expectancies can have direct effects; that is, they can affect responses with no mediation by other psychological variables. We have hypothesized that response expectancy is an essential (as opposed to arti-factual) component of hypnosis [12]. However, response expectancy theory does not hold expectancy to be the only factor influencing hypnotic experiences or other nonvolitional responses.

In sum, imagination and expectancy have parallel histories. Both were initially regarded as artifacts, and their effects were suspect. Subsequently, both have been recognized (though not universally) as legitimate psychological variables. Finally, both constructs have been used to explain hypnotic phenomena. In this chapter, we explore the interaction of expectancy and imagination in determining hypnotic experiences and behaviors.

EXPECTANCY AND HYPNOSIS

Hypnotic Inductions

Hypnotic inductions are as nonspecific as psychological procedures can be. Subjects can be told to relax or exercise, sleep or stay alert, to actively generate responses or just let them happen [12]. They can be stroked, poked, or dosed with sugar pills. When presented as "hypnotic" drugs, placebo pills have effects that seem indistinguishable from verbal inductions [13, 14]. A false biofeedback procedure has produced results on a par with traditional hypnotic inductions and imaginative skill training [15]. Furthermore, nonhypnotic procedures like guided imagery and relaxation training seem to differ from hypnosis only by their labels. As Sheehan and Perry note, "it is not the procedural conditions per se that are important (for inducing trance) but whether or not the subject perceives them as part of a context that is 'appropriate' for displaying hypnotic behavior" [16, p. 72].

The nonspecific nature of hypnotic inductions is recognized, but its implications are not acknowledged. If no specific chemicals are needed to duplicate a drug effect, the effect is attributed to expectancy. Since hypnotic inductions do not require any specific procedures, they are best understood as expectancy manipula-tions and their effects as expectancy effects. This does not mean that the effects are not real or important. In fact, the response expectancy hypothesis is com-patible even with altered state conceptions of hypnosis, since consciousness can be altered by response expectancies.

Hypnotic Responses

Expectancies determine not only the occurrence of hypnotic responses, but their very nature. Following a hypnotic induction, subjects report alterations in awareness that conform to their preconceptions about hypnosis [17]. Similarly, depending on their preconceptions or on information provided by experimenters, good hypnotic subjects may or may not show spontaneous arm catalepsy [3] and spontaneous amnesia [18]. A variety of other effects are influenced by expectations, including resistance to suggestions, breaching amnesia, and the "hidden observer" [19-22].

These data should come as no surprise, since culturally-based expectations have figured significantly in the history of hypnosis. In the eighteenth century, mesmerized subjects followed the example of Mesmer's first patient by routinely displaying violent convulsions. After the Marquis de Puysegur discovered artificial somnambulism, convulsions faded from subjects' repertoire of responses. Toward the end of the nineteenth century, some hypnotic subjects displayed three distinct stages of hypnotic behavior—lethargy, catalepsy, and somnambulism—but only if they were patients at the Salpêtrière hospital, where this had become the norm. Today, some good subjects display a hidden observer, but only when instructed to do so.

In sum, hypnotic experiences and behaviors appear to be as nonspecific as the procedures that elicit them. Not only does expectancy determine when hypnotic responses occur—it also determines what subjects experience and how they behave in hypnotic situations.

Hypnotizability

Expectancy determines the circumstances in which hypnotic phenomena are displayed, as well as their specific characteristics. But what determines the degree to which a subject responds? Does expectancy interact with some preexisting level of hypnotic susceptibility, or could expectancy itself underlie hypnotic susceptibility?

Expectancy is one of the few stable correlates of hypnotizability (see review [23]). Most correlations between expectancy and suggestibility are moderate, accounting for approximately 10 percent of the variance in responding. However, substantially higher correlations have been reported in some studies. Very high correlations with expectancy are obtained when waking suggestibility is measured, or when expectancy is assessed after the provision of a hypnotic induction (but before the administration of test suggestions). The nature of the expectancy measure can also make a difference. Higher correlations are obtained when expectancies for responding to specific suggestions are assessed, as opposed to merely obtaining a global estimate of future responsiveness. Stronger associations are also found when expectancies for each suggestion are assessed on Likert scales, rather than dichotomously. Also, subjects' predictions of their subjective experiences are better than behavioral response expectancies in predicting both behavioral and subjective hypnotic responsiveness [23]. Finally, the confidence with which the expectations are held can make a difference in their accuracy. Confidently held expectancies are strongly related to subsequent responding, whereas mere guesses are not [6, 24].

Still, correlation does not establish causality. It is possible that expectancy is an epiphenomenon rather than a cause. More convincing evidence is provided by studies in which manipulated expectancies produced changes in responsiveness to suggestion [12, 24-28]. These studies indicated that manipulated expectancies account for more variance in subsequent hypnotic suggestibility than trait hypnotizability (i.e., pre-manipulation responsiveness). Furthermore, the prediction of altered hypnotizability was supported even when pre-manipulation hypnotizability and expectancies were statistically controlled.

These data provide strong evidence for a causal relation between expectancy and hypnotizability, but they still leave some variance in responsiveness unexplained. It is possible that expectancy is the sole proximal determinant of hypnotizability and that the residual variance is a result of measurement error. Conversely, as is commonly supposed, the unexplained variance may be due to a talent or personality characteristic, the nature of which is yet to be established.

Expectancy and Compliance

Good hypnotic subjects report unlikely experiences (e.g., claiming to see something that is not present) that arouse the suspicion of faking. The term *compliance* is typically used in place of *faking,* but the latter term is more accurate. All cooperative subjects comply with hypnotic instructions. When asked to, they stare at a target at the beginning of an induction, extend their arms in preparation for an arm lowering suggestion, clasp their hands in preparation for a finger lock suggestion, and so on. The question is whether they also fake subsequent responding by lowering their arms even if they do not feel heavy or keeping their hands clasped together despite not feeling them stuck together.

The relation of expectancy to hypnosis can easily be explained by the so-called compliance hypothesis. However, there are data indicating that hypnotized subjects are not simply faking. Highly responsive subjects are as responsive when they think they are alone as they are when an observer is present [29]. In contrast, subjects instructed to fake high levels of hypnotizability drop the pretense when they think they are alone.

Although Kirsch et al. [29] established that hypnotic responding cannot be completely explained as faking, Wagstaff [30, 31] has proposed a more sophisticated compliance hypothesis that has yet to be disconfirmed. Consistent with the social learning model of hypnosis [6, 12, 23], Wagstaff hypothesizes that subjects are motivated to experience suggested hypnotic phenomena and that they actively try to generate those experiences. However, if they are unable to generate the requisite experience, Wagstaff supposes that they fake the behavior in order to fulfil the role of "good" subjects. It follows that there would be less faking in response to relatively easy suggestions (e.g., arm heaviness) and more in response to difficult suggestions (e.g., negative hallucinations). Indeed, Wagstaff suspects that the more difficult responses may entirely be due to faking [31]. In contrast, trait theorists like Balthazard and Woody argue that imaginative abilities become progressively more important as the difficulty of suggestions increases [32].

It is important to note that the test used in the Kirsch study was composed largely of relatively easy suggestions (hand lowering, moving hands, finger lock, and eye catalepsy) and only one rather difficult item (posthypnotic suggestion) [29]. These are precisely the suggestions that may not require sham behavior according to Wagstaff [31].

Spanos and his colleagues have reported data that support Wagstaff's hypothesis [33, 34]. Following the cancellation of a deafness or analgesia suggestion and the termination of hypnosis, subjects were informed that people tend to drift back into hypnosis and that they have probably displayed deafness or analgesia in posthypnotic trials. Subjects exposed to this manipulation reported a reduction in the loudness or painfulness of posthypnotic test stimuli. Because the manipulation occurred after the auditory or pain stimulus had been presented, it could not have affected subjects' perceptions of the stimulus. Therefore, Spanos and colleagues concluded that their data strongly supported Wagstaff's compliance hypothesis.

There is, however, another rather straightforward explanation of these so-called compliance data. As Spanos and his associates have cogently noted elsewhere, "human memory is reconstructive and strongly influenced by expectations concerning what should have occurred as well as by what actually happened" [35]. Rather than inducing subjects to fake, the so-called compliance instruction may simply have altered subjects' memory of the experience. Rather than biasing their reports, subjects may have honestly reported the levels of sound or pain that they clearly, but mistakenly, remembered. Since the instruction implied that it was linked to hypnosis, it is unsurprising that the effect was correlated with expected and actual responsiveness to the initial suggestion. Spanos's data are not inconsistent with the compliance hypothesis, but neither do they provide strong evidence for it.

In sum, the hypothesis that more difficult responses are generally faked remains untested. Nevertheless, response levels that are characteristic of the vast majority of the population seem fully explicable without resort to the compliance hypothesis [29]. Their nature and the situations in which they occur can be fully explained by the response expectancy hypothesis. Levels of responsiveness are also influenced by expectancy, but may be affected by other subject variables as well.

IMAGINAL ABILITY AND HYPNOSIS

The notion that hypnotic responses are imaginative productions has been so widely accepted that for a while it seemed to provide a point of convergence between warring theoretical factions in the hypnosis community. Psychoanalytic theorists noted a shift toward primary process thinking following hypnotic inductions [36, 37], cognitive-behavioral theorists hypothesized that hypnotic responses were produced by involvement in goal-directed fantasies [38], and almost everyone agreed that hypnotizability was associated with a personality trait or ability to become engrossed in imaginative productions [39-41]. Although there is now less consensus on the importance of imaginative ability than there was ten years ago, this view continues to typify the majority of researchers and clinicians.

There are two compatible hypotheses about the relation of imaginal variables and hypnosis. One views imaginative activity as a cognitive strategy (goal-directed fantasy) which produces or enhances hypnotic responding. The second views imaginative ability as a personality trait (e.g., imaginative involvement or absorption) which underlies hypnotizability.

Goal-Directed Fantasy

Goal-directed fantasies (GDFs) are images of situations that might produce the suggested response. For example, a subject responding to an arm levitation suggestion might imagine a helium-filled balloon attached to his or her wrist. There are three sorts of evidence linking fantasies of this sort to hypnotic responding. The first involves the effect of including goal-directed fantasies in the wording of suggestions, the second involves training subjects to produce these fantasies, and the third consists of assessing the degree to which responsive subjects intentionally generate goal-directed fantasies.

Instructions to generate goal-directed fantasies are contained in many hypnotic suggestions. In the Harvard Group Scale of Hypnotic Susceptibility, for example, subjects are instructed to intentionally imagine a force pulling their hands together [42]. The effects of including instructions for goal-directed imagining in the wording of suggestions as been evaluated in a number of studies reviewed in Lynn and Sivec, [43]. In general, these studies indicate that GDF instructions facilitate responding, although the effect may not be significant for all suggestions or all measures of response (e.g., behavioral vs. reports of involuntariness). Similar results have been reported in studies assessing the relationship between spontaneously occurring GDFs and successful responding to suggestions [43]; however, see Silva and Kirsch [44]. Overall, the size of the effect is generally modest, and inconsistencies in the reported results may be due to insufficient power in many of the studies.

Training subjects to use GDFs as a way of generating hypnotic responses is the cornerstone of a number of hypnotizability modification programs [15, 45-49] all of which have produced small to moderate increases in responsiveness. More substantial increases have been reported using the Carleton Skill Training Program, in which subjects are instructed to enact the behavioral components of the response while using GDFs to make the response feel involuntary [50]. These enactment instructions have generally been credited with the impressive effects of the CSTP [51, 52]. However, Gearan, Schoenberger, and Kirsch [53] reported that a modified version of the CSTP, in which enactment instructions had been eliminated, was as effective as the original program in enhancing hypnotizability.

Trait Measures of Imaginal Involvement

Although hypnotizability is trait-like in its consistency and stability, it does not seem to be predicted by self-report personality scales [23]. This lack of correlates has been problematic for theories which anchor hypnotic ability in some broader dimension of personality or cognition. The saving exception has been a consistent positive correlation between self-reported imaginative ability and hypnotizability. In particular, the Tellegen Absorption Scale (TAS) has been a robust predictor of scores on standardized hypnotic susceptibility scales [54, 55]. Findings with this scale have become central to trait conceptions of hypnotizability. Comprehensive reviews on the TAS and its relation to hypnotizability may be found in de Groh [56], Kirsch and Council [23], and Roche and McConkey [57]. Although most writers have focused on the imaginative content of the TAS, Roche and McConkey define absorption more broadly as a willingness to experience a wide range of cognitive and affective states, and relate it to the "Big Five" factor, *openness to experience.*

Other trait measures of imaginal variables include Hilgard's interview and questionnaire assessing *imaginative involvement* [39], and Wilson and Barber's Inventory of Childhood Memories and Imaginings (ICMI), which measures *fantasy-proneness* [41, 58]. De Groh has also reviewed research on scales measuring imagery vividness, which some consider to be a stable individual difference variable [56]. Overall, these measures seem to overlap considerably with absorption and with each other [23, 56, 57], and predict hypnotizability at significant but low-to-moderate levels. However, the validity of these relationships has been called into doubt by research on context effects [59], which will be discussed later in this chapter.

There are other reasons besides context effects to question the validity of self-report imagination/imagery measures as predictors of hypnotic performance. For example, although reports of vivid hallucinatory and other hypnotic-like experiences are necessary to obtain high scores on the ICMI, two studies have failed to show that the scale can discriminate between high and average hypnotizability [60, 61]. Furthermore, a number of studies indicate that self-report measures of imaginal ability do not relate to actual performance on imagery tests [62-66]. Council, Chambers, Jundt, and Good [66] used the ICMI and the Vividness of Visual Imagery Questionnaire [67] to select subjects whose mental imagery should have been "as real as real," according to their self-reports. These subjects were then presented with a difficult visual imagery problem requiring picture-like mental images for solution. The results indicated that subjects scoring extremely high on fantasy-proneness and imagery vividness were no more likely to pass the test than those reporting average levels. Such findings question whether self-report imagination scales actually measure imaginative ability, and whether some non-imaginal components, like acquiescence and response bias, are responsible for their relation to hypnotizability [23].

IMAGERY AND EXPECTANCY

Extending Arnold's [68] ideomotor action hypothesis, Barber, Spanos, and Chaves [38] maintained that thinking about and imagining an event produces corresponding overt behaviors, subjective experiences, and physiological changes. From this perspective, positive expectancies enhance hypnotic responding because they "give rise to a willingness to think and imagine with the themes that are suggested" [38]. Because the placebo literature indicates that expectancies can produce changes in experience independently of imagery [10], we began researching hypnosis with a different assumption. We assumed that expectancy and imagination contributed independently to hypnotic responding.

However, our own data, as well as those of other researchers, have led us to question that assumption. Although involvement in goal-directed imagery may enhance responsiveness, the causal link between imagery and expectancy appears to be contrary to that proposed by Barber and his colleagues. The data suggest that goal-directed imagery enhances responsiveness by virtue of its effects on expectancy. Similarly, the relation between trait measures of hypnotizability and imagery involvement may be at least partially mediated by expectancy or may be partly artifactual.

Response Expectancy and Goal-Directed Fantasy

Evidence about the relation between imagery and expectancy as determinants of hypnotic response can be found in a series of five studies in which these variables were pitted against each other. Lynn, Nash, Rhue, Frauman, and Sweeny [19] and Spanos, Cobb, and Gorassini [20] found that when provided with information leading them to believe that they would be able to do so, highly hypnotizable subjects resisted complying with suggested effects while simultaneously becoming absorbed in imagining those effects. Conversely, Zamansky [69] and Spanos, Weekes, and de Groh [70] reported that when given appropriate instructions, highly hypnotizable subjects could experience a suggested effect while actively imagining conflicting events. Finally, Kirsch, Council, and Mobayed demonstrated that these effects are generalizable to moderately hypnotizable subjects as well [25].

The clearest evidence of the relation between expectancy and goal-directed fantasy as determinants of hypnotic responding was provided by Lynn, Snodgrass, Rhue, and Hardaway [71]. They reported that when instructed to do so, low hypnotizable subjects were able to generate just as many fantasies as their highly hypnotizable counterparts, and they were able to become every bit as much involved and absorbed in these fantasies. Nevertheless, they were not as responsive behaviorally. Unlike highly responsive subjects, the low hypnotizable subjects did not believe that imagination produces hypnotic responses, an expectancy that was very strongly related to behavioral responding ($r = .64$).

Expectancy and Trait Measures of Imagination

Although expectancy and imagination appear to be entirely different constructs, studies using both types of measures to predict hypnotizability report that they are significantly intercorrelated [15, 44, 72]. In fact, relations between expectancy and imagination have typically been stronger than relations between imagination and hypnotizability. In studies with both the TAS [15, 72] and the ICMI [44], regression analyses indicated that hypnotic response expectancies mediated the relation between imagination and hypnotizability. Also, Silva and Kirsch reported that expectancy accounted for most of the variance in the relation between fantasy proneness and hypnotizability [44].

Council, Kirsch, and colleagues proposed two hypotheses about how expectancies might mediate the relation between hypnotizability and trait measures of imaginative experiences [15, 72]. First, instruments like the TAS might sample the kinds of experiences that are the basis for subjects' expectations about their responsiveness. Second, these instruments might influence hypnotic response expectancies when administered in the context of a hypnosis study. Since the measure is undisguised and positively keyed, answering "true" to many items would imply that one is highly imaginative and will therefore be a good hypnotic subject. Conversely, nonendorsement of TAS items would lead to the judgment that one will probably not respond to hypnotic suggestions.

The reactivity hypothesis should apply to virtually all self-report imagination scales, since their content is as obvious as that of the TAS. This explanation accounts for both the positive correlation of absorption and expectancy, and for the relation between absorption and hypnotizability. However, it also implies that significant correlations are dependent on subjects perceiving a connection between the TAS and the hypnotizability assessment.

Absorption, Hypnotizability, and Context Effects

In more general terms, the apparent relation of absorption to hypnotizability may be due to a context effect [23, 59, 72]. Context effects may occur when criterion variables and their predictors are assessed in the same research setting [59]. In this situation, subjects may infer relationships among the measures based on available situational information.

Subjects' inferences about personality measures and their relationships often affect correlations among predictor and criterion measures. For example, subjects may bias their responses toward greater consistency between predictor and criterion measures or try to confirm the research hypothesis as they perceive it. To explain the absorption-hypnotizability connection, we proposed that subjects infer their hypnotic ability from their TAS responses [72]. Since our 1986 report, context effects have been shown to affect a variety of relations within the domain of hypnosis [23, 59]. More recent studies have indicated that context effects are robust and general within personality research, affecting relationships across a wide range of variables [59].

The most intensely studied context effect in personality research involves the relationship between absorption and hypnotizability [59]. Below, we review the twelve studies to date on context effects, absorption, and hypnotizability.

Council, Kirsch, and Hafner [72] tested the context effects hypothesis by having one sample complete the TAS in a nonhypnotic context. These subjects were later recruited for an apparently unrelated assessment of hypnotizability. Other subjects received the TAS just prior to hypnosis in the usual manner. The results supported the reactivity hypothesis. Correlations between absorption and all measures of hypnotic responsivity were significant only when the TAS had been completed just prior to hypnosis. When the TAS was administered outside the hypnotic setting, the correlations were nonsignificant and sometimes even negative.

Our initial investigation of context effects was not definitive. Problems included our use of a nonstandard hypnosis scale, and a failure to demonstrate significant differences in correlations on all measures. There were also different intervals between the absorption and hypnotizability assessments in each condition, introducing a potential time confound. Thus, further research was required to determine the validity of the context effects hypothesis.

Subsequent research on context effects has either replicated our original between-subjects design or has tested the context effects hypothesis using within-subjects designs. Since the two approaches have led to seemingly discrepant findings, we will consider them separately. For convenience, we discuss the studies in the order of their citation dates, although this will not conform exactly to the order in which the studies were conducted. We will start with between-subjects designs.

De Groot, Gwynn, and Spanos [73] argued that our subjects' prior beliefs about hypnosis might have influenced their responses to the TAS, since those assessed in the hypnotic context knew they would be hypnotized when they completed the TAS. These investigators exposed subjects to three different information manipulations. In one condition, subjects were informed about the hypnosis assessment before completing questionnaires. Subjects in the second condition initially completed the questionnaires, and were then told the study involved an assessment of hypnotizability. In the third condition, subjects were not informed of any connection between the questionnaires and a subsequent test of hypnotizability.

Context effects could not be examined for males, since there was no significant relation of absorption to hypnotizability in any condition. However, a context effect was found with females, for whom the relation between absorption and hypnotizability was significant only when subjects knew it was being studied. De Groot et al. concluded that their findings were congruent with our report of a context-dependent relation between hypnotic responsivity and absorption [73]. Furthermore, since TAS responses in the "told after" condition could not have been influenced by the hypnotic context, the results supported our hypothesis that subjects base inferences about their hypnotic ability on their TAS responses.

Rhue, Lynn, and Jaquith [74] administered the TAS either with no title, as the "Inventory of Hypnotic Experiences," or as the "Inventory of Unusual Experiences." Subjects were later recruited for an apparently independent study involving hypnosis. They then received either the "Pre-Hypnosis Inventory," which had no content related to imagination, or the "Hypnosis and Imagination Inventory," designed to facilitate an association between imagination and hypnosis. Correlations between the TAS and HGSHS were significant when the title was associated with hypnosis or unusual experiences, and the HGSHS was preceded by the "Hypnosis and Imagination" questionnaire. In contrast, when the non-imaginative "Pre-Hypnosis Inventory" preceded the HGSHS, correlations were not significant.

Woody, Bowers, and Oakman [75] administered the TAS to one group of subjects, and later assessed their hypnotizability with no mention of the prior absorption measure. The other group was first tested for hypnotizability, and later completed the TAS at a separate session. This group filled out the questionnaires after hearing instructions which linked them to the earlier hypnosis measure. The correlation of the TAS with hypnotizability was around zero in the non-hypnotic context, but was highly significant in the hypnotic context. The significant same-context correlation could not have been due to an effect of the TAS on hypnotic responses, since the scale was administered after hypnosis.

Drake, Nash, and Cawood [76] had subjects complete both the TAS and measures from Hilgard's research on imaginative involvement [39]. One group of subjects completed the imagination measures immediately prior to hypnosis, and two other groups completed them two to three days prior to hypnosis. Subjects in one of the delayed hypnosis conditions were told that they were completing the imagination questionnaires as part of a hypnosis experiment. In the other, no mention was made of hypnosis, and subjects were later recruited by another experimenter for an apparently independent study on hypnosis. In contrast to other studies, which used group measures to assess hypnotizability, this study used the individually administered SHSS: C [77]. Only the same-session data yielded significant correlations, despite telling subjects in one delayed hypnosis condition that the questionnaires were related to hypnosis. Significant correlations were obtained between all three imagination measures and the SHSS: C when they were completed in the same session, but there were no significant correlations with hypnotizability in either separate administration group. The authors proposed that temporal contiguity could account for findings from previous studies on context effects.

Green, Kvaal, Lynn, Mare, and Sandberg [78] administered the TAS along with other measures which had correlated significantly with hypnotic responsivity. Hypnotizability was assessed either following those measures in the same session, or in a later, apparently independent, study. In the same context, correlations of absorption with hypnotizability were all significant. None of the out-of-context correlations were significant.

Spanos, Arango, and de Groot [79] administered the TAS to subjects who had previously been assessed for hypnotizability, while manipulating information about its association with hypnotizability. In-context subjects were told that the TAS would be related to their hypnotizability scores from the previous assessment. The TAS assessment was described to out-of-context subjects as "personality research," and no mention was made of the earlier hypnotic testing. Spanos et al. reported that absorption did not correlate with hypnotizability in the out-of-context condition [79]. Both subjective and behavioral indices of hypnotizability were significantly correlated with the TAS when tested in the hypnotic context.

The seven studies described above all presented hypnosis and absorption measures to some subjects in the same context, and to others in different contexts. Beyond that, there was considerable variation in methods and measures, indicating the robustness of context effects in hypnosis. It can be noted here that these studies also demonstrated context effects with measures of mysticism, daydreaming frequency, beliefs in paranormal phenomena, temporal lobe dysfunction, and several different dissociation scales.

Some investigations of context effects have employed *within-subjects* designs, administering the TAS first in a nonhypnotic context and later in conjunction with hypnosis. These studies have been described as "mixed" designs, since they included conditions to replicate Council et al.'s [72] between-subjects analyses.

Nadon, Hoyt, Register, and Kihlstrom [80] conducted two studies in which subjects completed the TAS along with other measures in large groups. In the first study, the same subjects were later recruited for an apparently independent study on hypnosis, where they completed the TAS prior to the Harvard Group Scale of Hypnotic Susceptibility (HGSHS) [42]. In the second study, one group of subjects did not receive the second hypnotic-context administration of the TAS, allowing a between-subjects analysis.

The primary statistical procedure was "regressed change" analysis, in which the hypnotic context TAS score was the criterion variable. Absorption scores from the initial group testing were entered first into the regression equation, removing variance shared by the scales across contexts. Then, the HGSHS score was entered. Nadon et al. proposed that a context effect would be indicated only if hypnotizability predicted additional variance in the residualized hypnotic context absorption scores [80].

Nadon et al. reported that absorption scores from the same-context (hypnosis research) condition significantly predicted hypnotic responsivity when variance shared by the absorption scores across contexts was partialed out [80]. Although their analyses indicated significant context effects, they were minor, relative to the overall relationship of absorption to hypnotizability. However, it should be noted that there was no significant relationship between absorption and subjective hypnotizability scores ($r = .05$) for subjects who only received the TAS during initial testing. Nadon concluded that any effects of context on the relation of absorption to hypnotizability were inconsequential, and that future studies need not exert special controls for context effects [80].

Perlini, Lee, and Spanos [81] replicated Nadon et al. [80] while testing alternative explanations for context effects. In three out of four conditions, subjects completed the TAS and a self-report imagery scale during a group testing procedure which was not associated with hypnosis. Subjects in the first condition were initially tested for hypnotizability and later completed the TAS and imagery scale in the nonhypnotic group testing context. Subjects in the second condition initially completed the self-report scales in group testing, and were assessed at a later session for hypnotizability. The third condition was similar to Nadon et al.'s [80] procedure, in that the self-report measures were administered twice—once in group testing and then later immediately before the hypnosis assessment. In the fourth condition, subjects completed the imaginal scales a single time immediately before the hypnosis scale.

The results are difficult to interpret. Imagery generally failed to correlate with hypnotizability. Correlations of the TAS with hypnotizability were significant, but *only* when the TAS had been completed in the nonhypnotic context. In contrast, correlations were *non*significant when the TAS was completed *only* in conjunction with hypnosis. However, when the TAS was administered to the same subjects in both contexts, correlations were greater in the hypnotic context. The only significant correlation occurred in the hypnotic context and involved the TAS and subjective hypnotizability scores. Regressed change analyses indicated a significant context effect on this relation.

Perlini, Lee, and Spanos's findings offer mixed support for the context effects hypothesis [81]. The within-subjects analysis was supportive, since hypnotic-context correlations were larger than those from the initial group testing. The only significant context effect was found with subjective hypnotizability scores. The between-groups comparisons failed to support the context-effects hypothesis, since significant correlations were mainly found when the TAS was administered in non-hypnotic contexts.

De Groh [82] followed up on questions raised by the two previous studies. All of her subjects completed the TAS in group testing. Later, with no mention of the earlier assessment, subjects were recruited for a "hypnosis testing session." During this session, subjects completed the TAS, attitude, and imagery measures either before or after assessment of hypnotic responsivity. The design allowed both between- and within-subjects analyses.

As with other studies using this design, within-subjects analyses supported the context effects hypothesis, while between-groups analyses did not. Within-subjects analyses were performed separately for groups which had received the hypnotic context TAS before versus after hypnosis. Results of these analyses indicated that the scale by context interaction was significant for subjects who completed the TAS before, but not after, hypnosis. The between-subjects analyses contrasted TAS scores obtained immediately before hypnosis with scores from the group-administered TAS in the remainder of subjects who completed the hypnotic context TAS after hypnosis. The regressions, which followed those of Council et al., showed no significant context effects, although the hypnotic context correlations were higher [72].

Finally, *Council, Grant, Frigen, Forseen, and Jensen* [83] have reported preliminary data from a large scale study designed to resolve discrepancies in the results of between- versus within-subjects research on context effects. The initial assessment of absorption used Tellegen's Multidimensional Personality Questionnaire (MPQ) [54], which imbeds TAS items in a 300-item omnibus personality questionnaire. Subjects were later recruited for an apparently independent study involving hypnosis.

The first group received the 34-item TAS, followed by the HGSHS, and a 34-item dummy questionnaire consisting of non-absorption items randomly selected from the MPQ. With the exception of the dummy questionnaire, this condition duplicated Nadon et al.'s design [80]. A second group received the dummy questionnaire, the HGSHS and the TAS in that order. Two other groups received the HGSHS only during the second assessment session. In one of these groups, the HGSHS assessment was associated with the same experimenter who had earlier administered the MPQ. In the other group, great care was taken to eliminate any association between the two assessments.

When the second TAS assessment preceded the assessment of hypnotizability, correlations of both the TAS and MPQ absorption scores with the HGSHS were highly significant. However, when the dummy questionnaire preceded the HGSHS, the MPQ absorption score was not significantly related to hypnotizability. This result indicates that when Nadon et al. reassessed absorption along with hypnotizability, they provided a contextual link between the HGSHS and the initial TAS [80].

For the two groups that received only the HGSHS in the second session, correlations were dramatically different, depending on whether or not the assessment contexts were completely separated. With the common presence of the experimenter across contexts, correlations between hypnotizability and the MPQ absorption score were highly significant. However, with no common cues across contexts, correlations were around zero. These results indicate that very subtle cues may be sufficient to establish a contextual linkage between absorption and hypnotizability assessments.

A Meta-Analysis of Context Effects

At first, the research on context effects seems confusing and contradictory. Significant context effects have been found in some studies, but not in others. When testing contexts are separated, significant correlations between absorption and hypnotizability are occasionally found. Sometimes, significant correlations between hypnotizability and absorption are not found even when both variables are assessed in the same context. The confusion has been compounded by periodic pronouncements that the context effects hypothesis is dead and buried [80, 84, 85].

Inconsistent results are not uncommon when actual effects are relatively small and when statistical power is often low. In this situation, box scores of studies reporting significant findings versus those reporting insignificant findings can be misleading. Meta-analysis provides a more reliable alternative. Twelve studies with almost 4000 subjects have been conducted, providing sufficient data for definitive conclusions. The results of these studies are summarized in Table 1. Estimates of the population correlations were calculated according to the method described by Hedges and Olkin, which adjusts for differences in sample size [86]. Comparisons of these correlations followed procedures recommended by Rosenthal [87].

These data address two separate issues. First, is the magnitude of the correlations between the TAS and hypnotizability affected by assessment context? Second, is there a valid relationship between hypnotizability and absorption? Our meta-analysis provides definitive answers to both questions.

First, the correlations from data collected in separate contexts were significantly ($p < .01$) and substantially smaller than those obtained in other testing situations. This was true for both behavioral and subjective measures of hypnotizability, and it was true whether the hypnotic context was established before or after TAS administration. In fact, about 75 percent of the variance in same-context correlations appears to be a context mediated artifact.

Second, the TAS appears to be significantly related to both behavioral and subjective measures of hypnotizability even when both variables are measured in separate contexts. However, this effect is very small. It is even smaller than the context effect and accounts for only about 1 percent of the variance.

We have classified some correlations as deriving from hypnotic contexts although they were originally described as nonhypnotic. This is because the basic within-subjects design inadvertently establishes a hypnotic context for the initial TAS assessment. TAS items are distinctive, and debriefing data from Council et al. [83] indicate that the majority of subjects recognize them upon retesting. Since Nadon used the undisguised TAS for both initial and hypnotic assessments, it seems certain that subjects recognized items from previous testing [80]. Far from being context free, the initial TAS was strongly linked to the HGSHS when the TAS was readministered in the hypnotic context. If our interpretation is correct, only one condition in one of Nadon et al.'s two studies [80] yielded context-free correlations. Our conceptualization of context effects encompasses both between- and within-subjects designs, viewing the key correlation as that between *initial* absorption scores and the hypnotizability measure. Everything that happens in between, including additional TAS administrations, merely serves to enhance or diminish a contextual link between assessment sessions.

In fact, recent data question how "context-free" any of these correlations have been. For example, Rhue et al.'s [74] results indicate that the titles of scales can influence correlations across sessions, and our own data [83] suggest that the common presence of a specific experimenter can establish a contextual link. Published information is usually insufficient to determine whether precautions were taken to minimize contextual cues.

Ours is actually the second meta-analysis to examine context effects on the absorption-hypnotizability correlation. Lyons presented a meta-analysis which concluded that the relation between these variables was not affected by context [85]. However, Lyon's list of correlations, purportedly obtained with absorption and hypnotizability tested in separate contexts, actually contained some that were assessed in the same context. For example, Balthazard and Woody explicitly stated that although some subjects filled out the questionnaires in a nonhypnotic context, others "completed the absorption scale in the context of an experiment that did involve the use of hypnosis" [32, p. 26]. In Sweeny et al., the TAS and hypnosis administrations took place in separate sessions, but subjects were informed that they were parts of the same study [88]. Spanos et al. also informed their subjects that the TAS and hypnotizability assessment were parts of the same study [89]. Lyons failed to include Buckner and Coe [90] in the non-hypnotic context group, even though they administered the scales in separate contexts and found no significant correlation. Most significantly, Lyons failed to include six studies that employed valid controls for context effects [74, 75, 78, 79, 81, 82]. In our own meta-analysis, we included only studies which manipulated the assessment context. This ensured that the comparisons employed subjects drawn from the same populations, and tested for effects in both hypnotic and nonhypnotic assessment contexts.

Mechanisms: Expectancy, Consistency, or Both?

Our original formulation of context effects described a self-attributional process which affected hypnotic response expectancies. We proposed that as subjects completed the TAS, they used the content of their responses to infer their own levels of hypnotic ability. The content and format of the TAS lent credence to this explanation—the items are all positively worded and self-descriptive (e.g., "If I wish, I can imagine that my body is so heavy that I could not move it if I wanted to"). The True-False scoring should simplify and sharpen the process of forming subjective probabilities for responding to suggestions. It should be noted that

Table 1. Correlations between Absorption and Hypnotic Responsiveness as a Function of Testing Context

Hypnotic Context	N	Type of Hypnosis Measure	
		Behavioral	Subjective
Established Before Absorption Testing			
Council et al. [72]	64	.22	.31
de Groot et al. [73] (males)[a]	56	.14	.22
de Groot et al. [73] (females)	56	.27	.31
Drake et al. [76] (no delay)	48	.32	
Drake et al. [76] (delay)	43	.14	
Woody et al. [75]	42	.44	
Green et al. [78]	225	.16	.28
de Groh [56]	99	.25	.33
de Groh [56][b]	99	.21	.31
Nadon et al. [80] (study 1)	475	.17	.22
Nadon et al. [80] (study 2)	209	.24	.21
Perlini et al. [81] (group 4)	90	.09	.16
Perlini et al. [81] (group 3)	90	.16	.21
Council et al. [83] (group 1)[b]	65	.31	.33
Council et al. [83] (group 2)	112	.33	.29
Estimated Population Correlations		.21***	.25***
(total sample size)		(1773)	(1640)
Established After Absorption Testing			
de Groot et al. [73] (males)	61	.14	.13
de Groot et al. [73] (females)	56	.32	.37
Rhue et al. [74]	31	.49	
de Groh [56]	99	.14	.21
Nadon et al. [80] (study 1)	475	.14	.19
Nadon et al. [80] (study 2)	225	.25	.24
Perlini et al. [81] (group 3)	90	.01	.07
Spanos et al. [79]	76	.34	.40
Council et al. [83] (group 1)	65	.14	.12
Council et al. [83] (group 2)	112	.33	.29
Council et al. [83] (group 3)	46	.45	.51
Estimated Population Correlations		.21***	.23***
(total sample size)		(1336)	(1305)

Table 1. (Cont'd.)

Hypnotic Context	N	Type of Hypnosis Measure	
		Behavioral	Subjective
Kept Separate			
Council et al. [72]	64	-.03	-.14
de Groot et al. [73] (males)	52	.10	.04
de Groot et al. [73] (females)	52	-.16	-.15
Drake et al. [76]	43	.02	
Rhue et al. [74]	41	.10	
Woody et al. [75]	42	.04	
Green et al. [78]	240	.09	.07
de Groh [56]	99	.16	.26
Nadon et al. [80] (Study 2)	209	.18	.05
Perlini et al. [81] (group 1)	90	.27	.31
Perlini et al. [81] (group 2)	90	.19	.20
Spanos et al. [79]	75	.13	.09
Council et al. [83] (group 4)	97	.06	-.01
Estimated Population Correlations		.12***	.09**
(total sample size)		(1194)	(1068)

[a]Data not reported in published article.
[b]Hypnotizability assessed before absorption.
**$p < .01$
***$p < .001$

Nadon et al. altered the original TAS for continuous scoring in one study [80], which could account for the weak associations they found between hypnotizability and absorption.

However, further research on context effects has indicated that the best overall explanation involves the motivation to present one's self consistently across personality measures [59]. Research with nonhypnotic variables indicates that subjects strive for consistency across measures regardless of the order of scale presentation. Significantly, all three studies that administered the TAS after hypnosis reported correlations equivalent to those when the TAS was administered immediately before hypnosis [75, 82, 83]. The TAS could not have affected hypnotizability, but the correlation was inflated nonetheless. Thus, consistency may provide the best explanation of context effects on the absorption-hypnotizability correlation. Whether absorption or hypnotizability is assessed first, within the same research situation subjects should formulate self-appraisals based on their performance on the initial measure. Based on their understanding of the measures, they will strive to make performance on the second measure consistent with that on the first.

On the other hand, it is possible that experiences during hypnotizability testing could alter expectancies for hypnotic-like experiences in everyday life. Thus, expectancy could inflate correlations when the TAS is administered last. Expectancy and consistency are entirely compatible processes, and may work together in research on personality correlates of hypnotizability. Research is needed to address the relative contributions of consistency and expectancy in each order of scale administration.

CONCLUSIONS

Less than a decade has passed since response expectancy theory was proposed as an explanation of hypnotic experiences and behavior [10]. It has been an extremely fruitful source of research hypotheses, and an impressive body of research support has emerged during this time. The data suggest an alternative conception of the role of imaginal variables in the production of hypnotic behavior. Rather than being causal, imagination may be peripheral to the basic processes of hypnosis. This chapter reviewed research demonstrating that the power of both imaginative strategies and personality questionnaires to predict hypnotic responding is largely due to the mediation of situational or contextual factors. Conversely, expectancy appears to be an exceptionally robust predictor.

Whereas expectancy effects are considerably more substantial than most believe them to be, well-controlled studies reveal that imagery effects are surprisingly small. For example, the effects of imaginative strategies on hypnotic responding are easily overridden by information provided to subjects. In the domain of personality predictors, absorption is significantly associated with hypnotizability, even when testing contexts are kept separate. But the association is negligible, accounting for only 1 percent of the variance. The effects of context are also small, accounting for approximately 3 percent of the variance. However, these data also indicate that about 75 percent of the variance in hypnotizability/absorption correlations is due to contextual factors. Despite our advocacy of expectancy theory, we were surprised to see these data amass. Although response expectancy theory suggested that expectancies play an important role in hypnosis, it did not negate a similar role for imaginative variables.

It would be premature to announce that the relative roles of imagination and expectancy in determining hypnotic behavior have now been decided. However, the research evidence is clearly accumulating on the side of expectancy.

REFERENCES

1. M. A. Gravitz, Early Theories of Hypnosis: A Clinical Perspective, in *Theories of Hypnosis: Current Models and Perspectives*, S. J. Lynn and J. W. Rhue (eds.), Guilford Press, New York, pp. 19-42, 1991.
2. S. J. Lynn and J. W. Rhue (eds.), *Theories of Hypnosis: Current Models and Perspectives*, Guilford Press, New York, 1991.
3. M. T. Orne, The Nature of Hypnosis: Artifact and Essence, *Journal of Abnormal Psychology, 58*, pp. 277-299, 1959.
4. E. Z. Woody, K. S. Bowers, and J. M. Oakman, A Conceptual Analysis of Hypnotic Responsiveness, in *Contemporary Hypnosis Research*, E. Fromm and M. Nash (eds.), Guilford Press, New York, pp. 3-33, 1992.
5. A. K. Shapiro, A Contribution to the History of the Placebo Effect, *Behavioral Science, 5*, pp. 109-135, 1961.
6. I. Kirsch, *Changing Expectations: A Key to Effective Psychotherapy*, Brooks/Cole, Pacific Grove, California, 1990.
7. J. D. Frank, *Persuasion and Healing* (Revised Edition), Johns Hopkins, Baltimore, 1973.
8. J. M. Fish, *Placebo Therapy*, Jossey-Bass, San Francisco, 1973.
9. W. C. Coe, Expectations and Hypnotherapy, in *Handbook of Clinical Hypnosis*, J. W. Rhue, S. J. Lynn, and I. Kirsch (eds.), American Psychological Association Press, Washington, D.C., pp. 73-94, 1993.
10. I. Kirsch, Response Expectancy as a Determinant of Experience and Behavior, *American Psychologist, 40*, pp. 1189-1202, 1985.
11. J. B. Rotter, *Social Learning and Clinical Psychology*, Prentice Hall, Englewood Cliffs, New Jersey, 1954.
12. I. Kirsch and J. R. Council, Response Expectancy as a Determinant of Hypnotic Behavior, in *Hypnosis: The Cognitive-behavioral Perspective*, N. P. Spanos and J. F. Chaves (eds.), Prometheus Press, Buffalo, New York, pp. 360-379, 1989.
13. S. L. Baker and I. Kirsch, Hypnotic and Placebo Analgesia: Order Effects and the Placebo Label, *Contemporary Hypnosis*, in press.
14. L. B. Glass and T. X. Barber, A Note on Hypnotic Behavior, the Definition of the Situation, and the Placebo Effect, *Journal of Nervous and Mental Diseases, 132*, pp. 539-541, 1961.
15. J. Council, I. Kirsch, A. R. Vickery, and D. Carlson, "Trance" vs. "Skill" Hypnotic Inductions: The Effects of Credibility, Expectancy, and Experimenter Modeling, *Journal of Consulting and Clinical Psychology, 51*, pp. 432-440, 1983.
16. P. W. Sheehan and C. W. Perry, *Methodologies of Hypnosis*, Lawrence Erlbaum Associates, Hillsdale, New Jersey, 1976.
17. D. Henry, *Subjects' Expectancies and Subjective Experience of Hypnosis*, unpublished doctoral dissertation, University of Connecticut, 1985.
18. J. Young and L. M. Cooper, Hypnotic Recall Amnesia as a Function of Manipulated Expectancy, *Proceedings of the 80th Annual Convention of the American Psychological Association, 7*, pp. 857-858, 1972.
19. S. J. Lynn, M. R. Nash, J. W. Rhue, D. C. Frauman, and C. A. Sweeney, Nonvolition, Expectancies, and Hypnotic Rapport, *Journal of Abnormal Psychology, 93*, pp. 295-303, 1984.
20. N. P. Spanos, P. C. Cobb, and D. Gorassini, Failing to Resist Hypnotic Test Suggestions: A Strategy for Self-presenting as Deeply Hypnotized, *Psychiatry, 48*, pp. 282-292, 1985.

21. C. E. Silva and I. Kirsch, Breaching Amnesia by Manipulating Expectancy, *Journal of Abnormal Psychology, 96,* pp. 325-329, 1987.
22. N. P. Spanos and E. C. Hewitt, The Hidden Observer in Hypnotic Analgesia: Discovery or Experimental Creation?, *Journal of Personality and Social Psychology, 39,* pp. 1201-1214, 1980.
23. I. Kirsch and J. R. Council, Situational and Personality Correlates of Suggestibility, in *Contemporary Hypnosis Research,* E. Fromm and M. Nash (eds.), Guilford, New York, pp. 267-291, 1992.
24. C. Wickless and I. Kirsch, The Effects of Verbal and Experiential Expectancy Manipulations on Hypnotic Susceptibility, *Journal of Personality and Social Psychology, 57,* pp. 762-768, 1989.
25. I. Kirsch, J. R. Council, and C. Mobayed, Imagery and Response Expectancy as Determinants of Hypnotic Behavior, *British Journal of Experimental and Clinical Hypnosis, 4,* pp. 25-31, 1987.
26. A. R. Vickery and I. Kirsch, The Effects of Brief Expectancy Manipulations on Hypnotic Responsiveness, *Contemporary Hypnosis, 8,* pp. 167-171, 1991.
27. P. Gearan, N. Schoenberger, and I. Kirsch, *The Modification of Hypnotizability: A New Component Analysis,* paper presented at the Convention of the American Psychological Association, Washington, D.C., 1992.
28. P. Gearan and I. Kirsch, Response Expectancy as a Mediator of Hypnotizability Modification, *International Journal of Clinical and Experimental Hypnosis, 41,* pp. 84-91, 1993.
29. I. Kirsch, C. E. Silva, J. E. Carone, J. D. Johnston, and B. Simon, The Surreptitious Observation Design: An Experimental Paradigm for Distinguishing Artifact from Essence in Hypnosis, *Journal of Abnormal Psychology, 98,* pp. 132-136, 1989.
30. G. F. Wagstaff, *Hypnosis, Compliance and Belief,* St. Martin's Press, New York, 1981.
31. G. F. Wagstaff, Compliance, Belief, and Semantics in Hypnosis: A Nonstate Sociocognitive Perspective, in *Theories of Hypnosis: Current Models and Perspectives,* S. J. Lynn and J. W. Rhue (eds.), Guilford Press, New York, pp. 362-396, 1991.
32. C. G. Balthazard and E. Z. Woody, The Spectral Analysis of Hypnotic Performance with Respect to "Absorption," *International Journal of Clinical and Experimental Hypnosis, 40,* pp. 21-43, 1992.
33. N. P. Spanos, C. A. Burgess, P. A. Cross, and G. MacLeod, Hypnosis, Reporting Bias, and Suggested Negative Hallucinations, *Journal of Abnormal Psychology, 101,* pp. 192-199, 1992.
34. N. P. Spanos, A. H. Perlini, L. Patrick, S. Bell, and M. I. Gwynn, The Role of Compliance in Hypnotic and Nonhypnotic Analgesia, *Journal of Research in Personality, 24,* pp. 433-453, 1990.
35. N. P. Spanos, E. Menary, N. J. Gabora, S. C. DuBreuil, and B. Dewhirst, Secondary Identity Enactments during Hypnotic Past-life Regression: A Sociocognitive Perspective, *Journal of Personality and Social Psychology, 61,* pp. 308-320, 1991.
36. E. Fromm, An Ego-psychological Theory of Hypnosis, in *Contemporary Hypnosis Research,* E. Fromm and M. R. Nash (eds.), Guilford Press, New York, pp. 131-148, 1992.
37. M. Gill and M. Brenman, *Hypnosis and Related States: Psychoanalytic Studies in Regression,* International Universities Press, New York, 1959.
38. T. X. Barber, N. P. Spanos, and J. F. Chaves, *Hypnosis, Imagination, and Human Potentialities,* Pergamon Press, New York, 1974.
39. J. R. Hilgard, *Personality and Hypnosis: A Study of Imaginative Involvement* (2nd Edition), University of Chicago Press, Chicago, 1979.
40. N. P. Spanos and T. X. Barber, Toward a Convergence in Hypnosis Research, *American Psychologist, 29,* pp. 500-511, 1974.

41. S. C. Wilson and T. X. Barber, The Fantasy-prone Personality: Implications for Understanding Imagery, Hypnosis, and Parapsychological Phenomena, in *Imagery: Current Theory, Research, and Application,* A. A. Sheikh (ed.), Wiley, New York, pp. 340-387, 1983.
42. R. E. Shor and E. C. Orne, *Harvard Group Scale of Hypnotic Susceptibility, Form A,* Consulting Psychologists Press, Palo Alto, California, 1962.
43. S. J. Lynn and H. Sivec, The Hypnotizable Subject as Creative Problem Solving Agent, in *Contemporary Hypnosis Research,* E. Fromm and M. R. Nash (eds.), Guilford Press, New York, pp. 292-333, 1992.
44. C. E. Silva and I. Kirsch, Interpretive Sets, Expectancy, Fantasy Proneness, and Dissociation as Predictors of Hypnotic Response, *Journal of Personality and Social Psychology, 63,* pp. 847-856, 1992.
45. J. Comins, F. Fullam, and T. X. Barber, Effects of Experimenter Modeling, Demands for Honesty, and Initial Level of Suggestibility on Response to Hypnotic Suggestions, *Journal of Consulting and Clinical Psychology, 43,* pp. 668-675, 1975.
46. N. Katz, Hypnotic Inductions as Training in Self-control, *Cognitive Therapy and Research 2,* pp. 365-369, 1978.
47. N. Katz, Comparative Efficacy of Behavioral Training, Training Plus Relaxation, and a Sleep/Trance Induction in Increasing Hypnotic Susceptibility, *Journal of Consulting and Clinical Psychology, 47,* pp. 119-127, 1979.
48. L. B. Sachs and W. L. Anderson, Modification of Hypnotic Susceptibility, *International Journal of Clinical and Experimental Hypnosis, 37,* pp. 100-106, 1967.
49. M. J. Diamond, The Use of Observationally Presented Information to Modify Hypnotic Susceptibility, *Journal of Abnormal Psychology, 79,* pp. 174-180, 1972.
50. D. R. Gorassini and N. P. Spanos, A Social-Cognitive Skills Approach to the Successful Modification of Hypnotic Susceptibility, *Journal of Personality and Social Psychology, 50,* pp. 1004-1012, 1986.
51. B. L. Bates and T. A. Brigham, Modifying Hypnotizability with the Carleton Skill Training Program: A Partial Replication and Analysis of Components, *International Journal of Clinical and Experimental Hypnosis, 38,* pp. 183-195, 1990.
52. N. P. Spanos, L. A. Robertson, E. P. Menary, and P. J. Brett, Component Analysis of Cognitive Skill Training for the Enhancement of Hypnotic Susceptibility, *Journal of Abnormal Psychology, 95,* pp. 350-357, 1986.
53. P. Gearan, N. Schoenberger, and I. Kirsch, *The Modification of Hypnotizability: A New Component Analysis,* paper presented at the convention of the American Psychological Association, Washington, D.C., 1992.
54. A. Tellegen, *The Multidimensional Personality Questionnaire,* University of Minnesota, Minneapolis, 1982.
55. A. Tellegen and G. Atkinson, Openness to Absorbing and Self-altering Experience ("Absorption"), a Trait Related to Hypnotic Susceptibility, *Journal of Abnormal Psychology, 83,* pp. 268-277, 1974.
56. M. de Groh, *Absorption, Empathy and Interpersonal Orientation: Measurement Issues and Relationships,* unpublished doctoral dissertation, Carleton University, Ottawa, 1991.
57. S. M. Roche and K. M. McConkey, Absorption: Nature, Assessment, and Correlates, *Journal of Personality and Social Psychology, 59,* pp. 91-101, 1990.
58. S. C. Wilson and T. X. Barber, *Inventory of Childhood Memories and Imaginings,* Cushing Hospital, Framingham, Massachusetts, 1981.
59. J. R. Council, Context Effects in Personality Research, *Current Directions in Psychological Science, 2,* pp. 31-34, 1993.

60. J. R. Council and K. D. Huff, Hypnosis, Fantasy Activity, and Reports of Paranormal Experiences in High, Medium, and Low Fantasizers, *British Journal of Experimental and Clinical Psychology, 7*, pp. 9-15, 1990.
61. J. W. Rhue and S. J. Lynn, Fantasy-proneness, Hypnotizability, and Absorption: A Re-examination, *International Journal of Clinical and Experimental Hypnosis, 37*, pp. 100-106, 1989.
62. S. J. Lynn and J. Rhue, Fantasy Proneness: Hypnosis, Developmental Antecedents and Psychopathology, *American Psychologist, 43*, pp. 35-44, 1988.
63. C. H. Ernest, Imagery Ability and Cognition: A Critical Review, *Journal of Mental Imagery, 2*, pp. 181-216, 1977.
64. D. Reisberg, C. Culver, F. Heuer, and D. Fischman, Visual Memory: When Imagery Vividness Makes a Difference, *Journal of Mental Imagery, 4*, pp. 93-113, 1986.
65. K. White and R. Ashton, Visual Imagery Control: One Dimension or Four?, *Journal of Mental Imagery, 1*, pp. 245-252, 1977.
66. J. R. Council, D. Chambers, T. A. Jundt, and M. D. Good, Are the Mental Images of Fantasy-prone persons Really More "Real"?, *Imagination, Cognition and Personality, 10*, pp. 319-327, 1990-91.
67. D. F. Marks, Visual Imagery Differences in the Recall of Pictures, *British Journal of Psychology, 64*, pp. 17-24, 1973.
68. M. B. Arnold, On the Mechanisms of Suggestion and Hypnosis, *Journal of Abnormal Psychology, 41*, pp. 107-128, 1946.
69. H. S. Zamansky, Suggestion and Countersuggestion in Hypnotic Behavior, *Journal of Abnormal Psychology, 86*, pp. 346-351, 1977.
70. N. P. Spanos, J. R. Weekes, and M. de Groh, The "Involuntarily" Countering of Suggested Requests: A Test of the Ideomotor Hypothesis of Hypnotic Responsiveness, *British Journal of Experimental and Clinical Hypnosis, 1*, pp. 3-11, 1984.
71. S. J. Lynn, M. Snodgrass, J. W. Rhue, and R. Hardaway, Goal-directed Fantasy, Hypnotic Susceptibility, and Expectancies, *Journal of Personality and Social Psychology, 53*, pp. 933-938, 1987.
72. J. R. Council, I. Kirsch, and L. P. Hafner, Expectancy versus Absorption in the Prediction of Hypnotic Responding, *Journal of Personality and Social Psychology, 50*, pp. 182-189, 1986.
73. H. P. de Groot, M. T. Gwynn, and N. P. Spanos, The Effects of Contextual Information and Gender on the Prediction of Hypnotic Susceptibility, *Journal of Personality and Social Psychology, 54*, pp. 1049-1053, 1988.
74. J. W. Rhue, S. J. Lynn, and L. Jacquith, *Context Effects, Hypnosis, and Absorption: Effects of Labelling and Sensitization,* paper presented at the 97th Annual Meeting of the American Psychological Association, New Orleans, 1989.
75. E. Z. Woody, K. S. Bowers, and J. O. Oakman, *Absorption and Dissociation as Correlations of Hypnotic Ability: Implications of Context Effects,* paper presented at the meeting of the Society for Clinical and Experimental Hypnosis, Tucson, Arizona, 1990.
76. S. D. Drake, M. R. Nash, and G. N. Cawood, Imaginative Involvement and Hypnotic Susceptibility: A Re-examination of the Relationship, *Imagination, Cognition and Personality, 10*, pp. 141-155, 1990-91.
77. A. M. Weitzenhoffer and E. R. Hilgard, *Stanford Hypnotic Susceptibility Scale, Form C*, Consulting Psychologists Press, Palo Alto, 1962.
78. J. P. Green, S. Kvaal, S. J. Lynn, C. Mare, and M. S. Sandberg, *Dissociations, Fantasy Proneness, and Hypnotizability: A Test of Context Effects,* paper presented at the meeting of the American Psychological Association, San Francisco, 1991.

79. N. P. Spanos, M. Arango, and H. P. de Groot, Context as a Moderator in Relationships between Attribute Variables and Hypnotizability, *Personality and Social Psychology Bulletin,* in press.
80. R. Nadon, I. P. Hoyt, P. A. Register, and J. F. Kihlstrom, Absorption and Hypnotizability: Context Effects Re-examined, *Journal of Personality and Social Psychology, 60,* pp. 144-153, 1991.
81. A. H. Perlini, A. Lee, and N. P. Spanos, The Relationship between Imaginal Ability and Hypnotic Susceptibility: Does Context Matter?, *Contemporary Hypnosis, 9,* pp. 35-41, 1992.
82. M. de Groh, *Absorption, Empathy and Interpersonal Orientation: Measurement Issues and Relationships,* unpublished doctoral dissertation, Carleton University, Ottawa, 1991.
83. J. R. Council, D. L. Grant, K. Frigen, S. Forseen, and L. Jensen, *New Findings on the Moderating Effects of Context in Hypnosis Research,* paper presented at the meeting of the American Psychological Association, Toronto, 1993.
84. J. F. Kihlstrom, I. P. Hoyt, R. Nadon, and P. A. Register, *Cognitive Correlates of Hypnotizability: A Re-examination of Context Effects,* paper presented at the meeting of the American Psychological Association, New York, 1987.
85. L. C. Lyons, *A Quantitative Review of the Effects of Measuring Absorption in a Hypnotic Context,* paper presented at the meeting of the Society for Clinical and Experimental Hypnosis, Arlington, 1992.
86. L. V. Hedges and I. Olkin, *Statistical Methods for Meta-Analysis,* Academic Press, Orlando, 1985.
87. R. Rosenthal, *Meta-analytic Procedures for Social Research,* Sage, Newbury Park, California, 1991.
88. C. A. Sweeny, S. J. Lynn, and F. S. Bellezza, Hypnosis, Hypnotizability, and Imagery-mediated Learning, *International Journal of Clinical and Experimental Hypnosis, 34,* pp. 29-40, 1986.
89. N. P. Spanos, S. Steggles, H. Radtke-Bodorik, and S. Rivers, Nonanalytic Attending, Hypnotic Susceptibility, and Psychological Well-being in Trained Meditators and Nonmeditators, *Journal of Abnormal Psychology, 88,* pp. 85-87, 1979.
90. L. G. Buckner and W. C. Coe, Imaginative Skill, Wording of Suggestions, and Hypnotic Susceptibility, *International Journal of Clinical and Experimental Hypnosis, 25,* pp. 27-35, 1977.

CHAPTER 4

Daydreaming, Fantasy, and Psychopathology

STEVEN JAY LYNN, VICTOR NEUFELD,
JOSEPH P. GREEN, DAVID SANDBERG,
AND JUDITH RHUE

Much of our waking life is spent daydreaming and fantasizing. Our thoughts constantly vary with respect to whether they are reality based or fanciful. Daydreams and fantasies are so woven into the fabric of our mental activity that it is difficult to conceive of what life would be like absent the workings of the imagination. Daydreaming and fantasy play a pivotal role in many domains of experience and behavior. Our ability to imagine, to create vivid alternative realities, and to step into a future of possibility in our daydreams and fantasies, serves multiple adaptation-enhancing functions, not the least of which is what Sarbin has described as "muted role-taking" [1]. If imagination is not the mother of invention, it is at least an activity that facilitates planning for the future, problem solving, and creativity.

Fantasy and daydreams are, for the most part, viewed by the scientific community as adaptive and integral to healthy psychological functioning. And yet, at least in the public's eye, fantasy, daydreams, and imaginative activities are still associated with escapist activities, a retreat from reality, and the disturbing hallucinations and delusions of schizophrenia. Who has not been advised to, "not let our imagination run away," or "to get our heads out of the clouds?" Is there a darker side, a potentially less functional aspect of imaginative activities that is associated with negative thought content and affect, psychopathology, and poor adjustment? It is this question that we turn to after we examine definitions of the constructs central to our discussion, the evolution of scientific attitudes about fantasy and daydreaming, and the function of daydreaming and fantasy.

Mental images are the building blocks of daydreams and fantasies [2]. Richardson has defined mental imagery as quasi-sensory and quasi-perceptual experiences that people are aware of, but which are produced" . . . in the absence of those stimulus conditions that are known to produce their genuine sensory or perceptual counterparts [3, p. 15]. Fantasies and daydreams are the resultant product of the combination of mental images.

Singer defined daydreaming as,

> A shift of attention away from an ongoing physical or mental task or from a perceptual response to some internal stimulus. The inner processes usually considered are "pictures in the mind's eye," the unrolling of a sequence of events, memories, or creatively constructed images of future events of various degrees of probability of occurrence. Also included as objects of daydreaming are introspective awareness of bodily sensations, affects, or "monologues interieurs" [4, p. 3].

Starker defined daydreaming somewhat more succinctly, as ". . . any form of waking thought which is not goal-directed toward some immediate task in the environment" [5, p. 21]. Starter argued that the domain of daydreaming encompasses memories, "wishful flights, of fantasy, morbid obsessions, and paranoid suspicions." According to Starker and others, daydreams and fantasies are difficult to distinguish because they are part of a continuous flow of cognitive activity that range from planful problem-solving to uninhibited fantasy [5-7].

Segal, Huba, and Singer maintain that fantasy can be viewed as a subset of dreaming ". . . that usually involves somewhat greater speculation, somewhat more of a thrust toward future possibilities, or a juxtaposition of elements from long-range memory that may have much less probability of occurrence in the external life of the individual" [8, p. 37]. In everyday life these internal events are constantly changing, with boundaries and transitions that are difficult to mark.

Klinger and Cox proposed that daydreaming and fantasy are overlapping constructs [9]. They further identified three definitions of daydreaming that have played prominent roles in research and theory. According to one definition, fancifulness, or thought content that contains a significant departure from reality, is the hallmark of daydreaming. Another definition suggests that the key feature of daydreaming is its lack of relation or connection to the immediate environment; that is, its "stimulus-independence." A third definition of daydreaming emphasizes its respondent or unintentional and undirected nature, and contrasts daydreaming with operant or directed, intentional goal-directed thought.

Each of these definitions seems to capture an important aspect of daydreaming, yet in none of these definitions are daydreaming and fantasy clearly distinguished. Like other contemporary theoreticians, we will not make rigid distinctions between and among daydreaming, fantasy, and imagination. As Lynn and Sivec have noted, workers in the field have not drawn sharp boundaries around these constructs, which have been operationalized in a variety of ways [10]. In the review that follows our brief overview of historical attitudes about daydreaming and fantasy, and our discussion of the nature and function of fantasy, we will attempt to operationalize the constructs examined wherever possible.

In American psychology, early introspectionist psychologies, including those propounded by Titchener and Wundt, never achieved wide popularity, and were superceded by an emphasis on externally observable events that were more readily quantifiable than internal processes that were the subject of introspection. In America, psychology came to be defined as the "science of behavior"; the very existence of subjective experience itself was questioned. For example, Watson suggested that mental images were "ghosts" of sensations and may not actually exist [11]. Holt noted that subjectively experienced mental processes were "anathemized as mentalistic and cast into outer darkness" [12, p. 257]. And Klinger called attention to a "moratorium on inner experience" in the United States between 1920 and 1960 [6].

Not only was there an absence of interest during this period, but the subjects of imagery and fantasy were associated with pathology. Earlier, Freud characterized daydreaming as an inadequate substitute for "real" experience and a potential precursor to neurosis and psychosis [13]. Fantasy came to be implicated in the development of "neurotic dispositions" [14, p. 169] and hysteria, psychoses, and organic diseases [12, p. 255]. This orientation was reflected in the limited fantasy research that did occur during this period (e.g., studies of Rorschach and TAT responses), which focused on the relation between fantasy and psychopathology. In short, for a considerable period of time during the twentieth century, the study of the contents of consciousness languished, as the study of fantasy and imagination was tainted by its association with psychopathology.

The title of Holt's article, *The Return of the Ostracized—Imagery,* heralded the reversal of these trends [12]. Holt delineated developments in engineering psychology, neurophysiological research, biochemistry, cognition, memory, sleep, and creativity studies that suggested that imagery played a central role in psychology. Watkins outlined other developments that contributed to an increased interest in fantasy, consciousness, and inner experience [14]: the work of Penfield that established a physiological basis of imagery [16], Dement and Kleitman's discovery of the association between dreaming and rapid eye movements during sleep [17], Kris's discussion of the link between creativity and fantasy [18], and Foulkes et al. research that documented the relation between positive personality characteristics and imagery ability [19].

It is now widely believed that daydreams and fantasies are a normal occurrence in everyday life. According to Klinger, they reflect current concerns, regulate mood, provide self-relevant information and facilitate learning, and stimulate decision making [2]. The recent legitimatization of fantasy and daydreaming research, its "mainstreaming" into the scientific community, and the view that fantasy and daydreaming reflect positive psychological functioning, suggests that a careful examination of the relation between fantasy activity and psychopathology would be fruitful at this time.

THE FUNCTION OF DAYDREAMING

Freud viewed daydreaming as a vehicle for the discharge of impulses and wish gratification. He stated,

> I cannot pass over the relation of fantasies to dreams. Our nocturnal dreams are nothing but such fantasies, as we can make clear by interpreting them. Language, in its unrivaled wisdom, long ago decided the question of the essential nature of dreams by giving the name "daydreams" to the airy creations of fantasy. If the meaning of our dreams usually remains obscure in spite of this clue, it is because of the circumstance that at night wishes of which we are ashamed also become active in us, wishes which we have to hide from ourselves, which were consequently repressed and pushed back into the unconscious. Such repressed wishes and their derivatives can there-fore achieve expression only when almost completely disguised. When scien-tific work had succeeded in elucidating the distortion in dreams, it was no longer difficult to recognize that nocturnal dreams are fulfillments of desires in exactly the same way as daydreams are—those fantasies with which we are all so familiar [13, pp. 178-179].

Although Freud believed that fantasy and daydreaming were capable of provid-ing solutions to problems, he viewed this as an incidental effect, not a primary function of fantasy [6]. Implicit, if not always explicit, in Freud's writings was the idea that fantasy was a primitive, regressive activity, closely linked to the most basic sexual and aggressive instincts, and inferior to rational, reality-based cog-nitive activities subservient to more mature secondary process mental operations. Freud's ultimately pessimistic views of the role of imagination-based mental activities were revised by neo-Freudian theorists (e.g., [20-22]) who have empha-sized the adaptive nature of fantasy and the idea that fantasy can be used pro-ductively to modulate and channel a wide variety of impulses toward socially appropriate ends.

In recent years, investigators have proposed information processing models of fantasy and daydreaming. Like Freud, Klinger argued that fantasy is evident in such diverse activities as dreaming, play, and daydreaming [6]. However, Klinger proposed that fantasy was a ceaseless activity that humans engage in when not involved in scanning or acting on their environment [6]. He described this baseline mental activity as "respondent" or involuntary and automatic, as contrasted to "operant" or directed and deliberate activity. These respondent activities are partially unconscious, associated with affective arousal, and expressed as "inte-grated response sequences" responsive to feedback from the environment.

Klinger proposed that these fantasy sequences have the adaptive function of prioritizing, organizing, reorganizing, and continuously cycling through con-sciousness the enormous amount of information acquired over time that may be relevant to the sometimes creative solution of current problems [6]. Fantasy thus provides an opportunity to rehearse potential solutions to problems and provides continual reminders of current concerns.

Current concerns can be defined as, ". . . the internal state corresponding to an unmet goal, something the person was committed to making happen in his or her life but has not yet brought about and had not yet given up on, either" [23, p. 6]. When Gold and Reilly asked subjects to rank-order five important or significant current concerns, they found that the higher that individuals ranked a current concern, the more frequently it was represented as a daydream theme [7]. In fact, more than a third of the subjects' daydreams focused on the two most important current concerns. In keeping with Klinger's assertions, the authors concluded that current concerns have a major impact on thought and daydreaming content.

Singer has devised an information processing model of consciousness [24, 25], similar in many respects to Klinger's model. Singer suggested that fantasy is an ongoing private experience that functions to organize experience, construe the meaning of events, plan for the future, and, in general, guide individuals through their world and help them to achieve their goals [24].

Although Singer and Klinger's models of the function of daydreaming and fantasizing emphasize the positive, adaptation-enhancing value of these activities, it is conceivable that fantasy and daydreaming are nevertheless associated with psychological dysfunction and maladjustment. For example, various affective disturbances, behavioral problems, and psychological disorders have the potential to infiltrate a person's imaginal life. Golding and Singer [26] used Beck's [27] notion of schemas as knowledge structures that organize and regulate the flow of experience and information to hypothesize that the content of schemas is reflected in a person's daydreams and depressive behavior. Thus, if a person's schemas are negative and engender depression, then daydreams would be expected to be correspondingly negative in feeling tone. Not surprisingly, Golding and Singer found that depressed people reported fewer positively toned daydreams [26]. To the degree that negative schemas are stable structures that persist over time, they may be associated with particular styles of daydreaming and fantasy linked with negative affect.

It is also possible to extrapolate from Klinger's idea of current concerns to suggest that if a person feels unworthy of achieving a desired goal related to a current concern, or if the goal is appraised as beyond the person's grasp, then anxiety and depression would eventuate. This, in turn, could dampen motivation; diminish rewarding, goal-seeking behavior; and intensify negative affect in a recursive manner.

Another possibility is that the normal adaptive control of fantasy and daydreaming may be somehow disrupted so that failures in attention, concentration, and the regulation of emotion and behavior ensue. Rather being channeled or directed in a seamless, flexible manner to cope with life challenges, a person's thoughts, images, and fantasies may instead be rigid and obsessive in nature or chaotic, bizarre, and frightening in content.

Each of these possibilities suggests that there may be an association between affect, psychopathology, and adjustment and daydreaming and fantasy activities. Before we examine this possibility, we first present normative aspects of daydreaming and fantasy, and introduce the construct of fantasy style.

THE NATURE OF DAYDREAMING: NORMATIVE CONTENT AND PROCESS

Beginning in the early 1960s, Jerome Singer and his colleagues began collecting data about daydreaming in the normal population [4, 28, 29]. Starting with his clinical experience, research, and his own introspection, Singer created the General Daydreaming Questionnaire (GDQ) which was a compilation of daydreams that subjects were asked to rate in terms of frequency of occurrence [4]. Examples of the daydreams that were included are the following:

I suddenly find I can fly, to the amazement of passers-by.
I see myself participating with wild abandon at a Roman orgy.
I picture an atomic bombing of the town I live in.
I plan how to increase my income next year.
I see myself in the arms of a warm, loving person who satisfies all of my
    needs.

These daydreams were grouped into subscales that were designed to assess the content and structure of daydreams as well as attitudes toward daydreaming [5].

Data gathered with the GDQ on 240 normal adults aged nineteen to fifty revealed that 96 percent had daily daydreams; that visual imagery was the dominant mode of fantasy; and that daydreaming occurred most frequently when the respondents were alone and shortly before sleep, and was least frequent immediately upon awakening, during meals, and sexual activity [28]. Most of the subjects reported that they enjoyed their daydreams and that daydreaming was often related to future interpersonal behavior.

Common daydreaming themes included sexual satisfaction, altruistic attitudes, unusual good fortune, and various magical possibilities that have little likelihood of occurrence. A minority of subjects reported unconventional fantasies such as being the messiah, homosexual relationships, and murder of family members [30].

Singer [4] and Streissguth, Wagner, and Wechsler [30] found that daydreaming frequency was unrelated to gender or marital status. However, Giambra found that women reported higher levels of daydreaming frequency [32]. Furthermore, Giambra found that women, compared to men, reported more dreams of a problem-solving nature and more of an emotional response [32], whereas Streissguth et al. reported the opposite results [31]. These differences may be due to different instruments used to measure daydreaming.

Singer reviewed previous work on gender differences in daydreaming and noted that although gender differences do not account for much variance in the frequency of daydreaming, cultural stereotypes about sex roles are reflected in the content of daydreams [24]. Women reported more daydreams concerning relationships, they displayed less aggressiveness, and they reported more content related to fashion and their bodies, than did men. Men, on the other hand, had more fantasies related to heroic achievement and athletic feats.

Golding and Singer found that sex role differences accounted for more differences in daydreaming styles than did biological sex [26]. Androgyny, the capacity to blend both masculine and feminine sex roles, was associated with more positive daydreaming and with greater efficacy, one of the subscales of the Depressive Experiences Questionnaire [33] than either masculine or feminine sex role scores. Golding and Singer further interpreted their results as demonstrating that mind wandering was more problematical for men than for women, insofar as the relation between inefficacy, the inverse of efficacy scores, and mind wandering was stronger for men than for women [26].

Socio-cultural background and age differences have also been associated with daydreaming content differences. For example, Black Americans show a greater concern for material achievement in their daydreaming than do Anglo-Saxon subjects who are presumably more secure in their social status [24]. Frequency of daydreaming peaks in late adolescence then gradually declines with age [30]. Daydreaming containing guilt and fearful content gradually declines from grade five through high school, college, and young adulthood [34, 35]. Daydreaming continues to be reported by those in their eighties, and has patterns or structures similar to that of younger people. However, when compared with younger people, older people report more reminiscence, with reliving of past experience, and more affectively positive daydreams and fewer dreams with themes of guilt, aggression, and anxiety. Rosenfeld investigated daydreaming in young children and found patterns of daydreaming similar to those exhibited by adults [36].

Not only is daydreaming content associated with current concerns, as we have already noted, but it is also associated with personality variables. For instance, Brannigan, Hauk, and Guay found that subjects with an internal locus of control engaged in more achievement and fewer fear of failure daydreams than subjects with an external locus of control [37]. The research also demonstrated that men exhibited a greater frequency of these themes than women. Gold, Andrews, and Minor examined the relation between self concept, daydreams, and academic performance in college students [38]. Results indicated that subjects reporting five or more school-related daydreams had a lower self concept than the other subjects. The former group of subjects also had a higher average grade point average at the end of the semester. The fact that there are individual differences in daydreams, which vary as a function of personality variables, suggests that it may be worthwhile to consider differences in daydreaming styles and their potential link with maladjustment and psychopathology.

DAYDREAMING STYLES

Our discussion of the ubiquity of daydreaming in everyday life might suggest that it is a unitary construct. This, however, is not the case. Indeed, three distinct fantasy styles have been identified [29, 39, 40].

The 100-item General Daydreaming Questionnaire [4], alluded to above, evolved into the Imaginal Processes Inventory (IPI), a 400-item questionnaire consisting of twenty-nine subscales, twenty-two of which concern the content or structure of daydreaming and seven subscales that measure curiosity and attentional patterns [29]. An important outcome of the large sample data collections using various editions of the IPI was the finding that three second-order factors, representing different styles or types of daydreaming, consistently emerged, regardless of the nature of the sample [41].

These factors have been described as 1) Positive-constructive (PC), marked by pleasant feeling, positive attitudes toward daydreaming (e.g., worthwhile, solve problems, pleasant thoughts), and vivid visual and aural qualities; 2) Guilt-fear-of-failure (GFF), associated with themes of depression, guilt, fear, sadness, fear of failure, and achievement fantasies; and 3) Poor attentional control (PAC), involving anxiety, a tendency toward mind wandering, easy distractibility, and an inability to remain involved in a single task [29, 39].

The Short Imaginal Processes Inventory (SIPI) was developed to provide a brief, easily administered method of measuring the three daydreaming styles referred to above. It consists of forty-five items organized into three fifteen-item scales, each of which measures one of the daydreaming styles.

Tanaka and Huba examined the longitudinal stability of the three daydreaming styles with the SIPI, and found one month test-retest reliabilities of .59 for Positive-Constructive daydreaming, .73 for Guilt Fear of Failure, and .73 for Poor Attentional Control [42]. After testing the measurement of the three factors across the one-month interval with various mathematical models, they concluded that the factor structure remained relatively constant, that the three factors remained largely independent of one another, and that fantasy styles constitute cognitive predispositions and a measure of personality that is less variable across time than measures of depression.

Relation between Daydreaming Styles and Measures of Personality and Psychopathology

Singer and Antrobus [29] administered the IPI to 206 college students along with the Maudsley Personality Inventory [43], the Guilford-Zimmerman Temperament Survey [44], the California Psychological Inventory [45], and the Stein-Craik Activity Preference Inventory [46]. The factors that emerged from this research corresponded to the three daydreaming styles previously described.

The Guilt-Fear of Failure style was labeled Obsessional Neurotic, "a classic superego conflict pattern . . . much oriented to striving and achievement but also tormented by guilt, fears of failure, and hostile wishes" [29, p. 200]. A second factor that emerged from this study was labeled "Neuroticism-anxious absorption in daydreaming," approximately corresponding to the Poor Attentional Control style. Singer and Antrobus described this as similar to the "Anxiety-Hysteria syndrome . . . a personality style characterized by much anxiety, attempts at repression, fleeting and poorly organized intrusive thoughts, images from the past that haunt and distract one" [29, p. 200]. A third factor, described by Singer and Antrobus as a "happy daydreamer," corresponded to the Positive Constructive style.

This research indicated that the daydreaming styles identified by the IPI tend to correspond, to some extent, to personality constructs measured by traditional personality questionnaires. Certain styles of daydreaming were found to be associated with tendencies toward anxiety and neuroticism. This research suggests that frequency and absorption in daydreaming are manifested in individuals who were relatively conflict-free, and psychological healthy, as well as in those who evidence neurotic, dysfunctional characteristics.

This conclusion is consistent with research indicating that depression and daydreaming styles are related. Giambra and Traynor [47] administered the Beck Depression Inventory [48], the Zung Self-Rating Depression Scale [49], the Lubin Depression adjective checklists [50], and the IPI to a sample of college students and inmates. They found evidence for a positive relation between the IPI scales of Boredom, Distractibility, Mindwandering, Fear-of-Failure, Guilt and Hostility, and a negative relation between depression scores and Positive Reactions to Daydreams. Relatedly, Cundiff and Gold [51] reported a positive relationship between the Beck Depression Inventory [48] and the Fear of Failure Daydreams, Guilty Daydreams, and Boredom scales of the IPI. Golding and Singer [26] also found positive relationships between the Depressive Experiences Questionnaire [33] and the Guilt-Fear of Failure and Poor Attentional Control Scales of the SIPI. The relation between various measures of depression and the IPI and SIPI is congruent both with cognitive theories of depression that posit a relation between affect and thoughts, and with the view that fantasy functions as an integral part of cognitive and affective experience.

Daydreaming Styles and Psychiatric Patients

The above cited studies are limited by their general focus on college students and nonpathological populations. This methodological issue was addressed in Starker and Singer's studies of psychiatric patients. Starker and Singer examined the relation between a scale derived from the IPI and pathology with a sample of 113 male patients who were newly admitted to outpatient treatment at a Veterans Administration Hospital [52]. The patients reported a variety of problems, with common complaints involving "depression, anxiety, lack of relatedness, and alcoholism." Using factor analytic methods, the investigators found no relation between daydreaming and obsessiveness, compulsivity, and anxiety. However, positive relationships were found between depressive symptoms and the following daydream scales: distractibility, fear-of-failure, mindwandering, guilt, and visual imagery. When Starker and Singer specifically examined symptoms associated with psychosis (e.g., auditory and visual hallucinations, delusions, and bizarre behaviors), the daydream variables failed to discriminate psychotic and nonpsychotic patients. Thus, psychotic symptoms and daydreaming did not appear to be related.

In a follow-up investigation, Starker and Singer studied a sample of sixty of the original 113 patients who entered a day hospital program [53]. These patients, instead of receiving the standard IPI, received a modified version, in which they were asked about their most recent fantasy experience and about their level of relaxation during an experiential self-awareness group they participated in just prior to completing the IPI-based questionnaire. The forty-five group members who met the minimal criterion of providing fantasy reports on four different occasions, were also asked about whether they were aware of blocking or forgetting fantasy during introspection. Using this improved methodology, that relies on more contemporaneous fantasy reports rather than retrospective evaluation, the authors again failed to find a connection between fantasy reports and psychotic symptoms.

An interesting finding was that psychotic patients reported significantly greater difficulty in experiencing and reporting fantasy during introspection than did non-psychotic patients. Thus, some forms of pathology may interfere with daydreaming frequency or involvement in fantasy. Rather than supporting the myth that the psychotic person lives in a "fantasy world," Starker [53] concluded that ". . . psychosis involves the severe disruption of the rich, varied fantasy life that constitutes an important resource for healthy individuals" [54, p. 30]. In a later paper, Starker postulates ". . . some normal processes within the psychophysiologic organization of the brain that produces imagic thought and, when blocked, presses toward the experience of hallucination" [40, p. 28].

This speculation was also supported by a well-controlled study by Brett and Starker which compared hallucinatory (i.e., auditory) schizophrenics, nonhallucinatory schizophrenics, and medical patients tested on measures of imagery control and vividness [55]. Overall, the groups were equivalent in terms of daydreaming frequency and intensity. However, hallucinatory schizophrenics, alone, reacted with less auditory imagery when they generated emotional-interpersonal imagery in response to a task involving imagining sounds and modifying auditory images in accordance with instructions. What Starker concluded from this research was that the "basic image-forming apparatus" was preserved in hallucinatory schizophrenics, at least as far as neutral imagery is concerned; however, emotion-loaded imagery interrupts the normal flow of imagery that under "neutral" circumstances remains intact. The emotional content of the imagery process is hypothesized to "reappear in a more dissociated form as hallucination."

Starker [40] reported that when the sample of 113 patients was compared with a sample of 146 college students studied by Segal, Huba, and Singer [8], it was found that the patients' daydreams were less positive and visual, and more characterized by fear of failure than the college students' daydreams. These findings were consistent with research on college student samples [47] that also documented an association between fantasy styles and depression, and with research on a sample of sixty depressed, relatively well-diagnosed psychiatric patients [56]. In this later study, severity of depression and guilty, fearful, and hostile daydreams were related, and depression was negatively associated with positive daydreams. Associations between fantasy style and depression demonstrate that fantasy style is related to other constructs that are meaningful, and suggest that fantasy style constitutes an important dimension of thought and affect.

Daydreaming and Sleep Disturbances

Validity of the construct of daydreaming style could also be demonstrated by showing that fantasy activity is consistent, in many respects, across different contexts and states of consciousness. Klinger, for example, concluded that there is evidence for stylistic, structural, and functional correspondence between dreams and waking fantasy [6]. Klinger's theory assumes an ongoing "baseline" activity present at all times, interwoven with other mental activities [6]. Supportive of this concept, Webb's review of the nocturnal dream literature indicated that nocturnal dreams manifest important thematic and affective continuities with waking concerns and styles [58].

A number of studies have focused specifically on the relation between daydreaming styles and nocturnal dreams. Starker selected subjects on the basis of their rank order on the relevant IPI subscales, and assigned them to categories of positive daydreaming, negative daydreaming, and anxious-distractible daydreaming [59]. The nocturnal dreams of the top three scorers in each of the daydreaming categories were rated by judges on scales of length, emotion present in the dream, and bizarreness of dream content.

The positive daydreaming group showed less negative affect than the negative daydreaming group. The negative daydreaming group reported shorter dreams and less bizarre dreams than the anxious, distractible group, whereas the anxious distractible group had longer dreams and more negative affect, more aggression, fear, and bizarreness in their dream content than did the positive daydreaming group.

Starker extended the work described above by examining the nocturnal dream content a sample of eight subjects who represented each of the three fantasy styles described above (total $N = 24$) [60]. He found that the positive daydreamers manifested less negative affect in their dreams than the negative daydreaming group. The negative daydreamers, in turn, had shorter nocturnal dream reports and less bizarre dreams than did the anxious, distractible dreamers. Finally, the positive daydreamer's had shorter dreams, less negative affect, aggression, fear, gratification, and bizarreness than did the anxious distractible daydreamers in their nocturnal dreams.

In a study with the greatest clinical significance, Starker and Hasenfeld used another sample of ninety-nine male and female college students to explore the relation between sleep and IPI daydreaming styles [61]. A relation was found between the anxious distractible and the guilty-dysphoric failure styles and self-reports of insomnia and nightmares. Taken together, these studies support the construct validity of daydreaming styles, which can be manifested in sleep as well as in waking consciousness, as well as the relation between daydreaming styles and psychological symptoms (e.g., nightmares and sleep disturbance).

Daydreaming and Drug Use

Segal [62] and Segal et al. [8] investigated the relation between drug use in college students and fantasy orientation or characteristics. Segal found that he could predict 70 percent of the non-drug users and 67 percent of drug using students with fourteen subscales of the IPI [62]. Drug users had higher mean scores on all of the subscales, including absorption in daydreams, visual imagery in daydreams, bizarre improbable daydreams, and mindwandering, but had lower scores on hostile daydreams.

Segal et al. found that drug use was associated more with nonconformity and "thrill seeking" than with frequency of fantasy or interest in self-awareness [8]. However, differences emerged in terms of the type of drug used: alcohol users reported more guilty-dysphoric daydreams than marijuana users. Finally, D. Segal and Lynn [63] found that there was a tendency for guilty-dysphoric daydreams to be related to subjects' endorsement of items on an alcohol use scale [64]. In short, there appears to be evidence for a relation between daydreaming and the use of alcohol and drugs in a college student population.

Anastasi has suggested that agreement between alternative methods of measuring a construct provides evidence pertinent to the demonstration of construct validity [65]. In terms of fantasy style and psychopathology, most of the evidence to date has been derived from factorial analyses of self-report measures, and correlations between these measures and other constructs. These studies have contributed to the validation of daydreaming style, and to understanding the link between certain psychological symptoms and daydreaming style. However, studies that rely on alternate types of measurement, such as content analysis of daydreams and fantasies, would enhance the scope and utility of the daydreaming style construct and provide greater confidence in data pertinent to daydreaming and psychopathology.

FANTASY PRONENESS AND PSYCHOPATHOLOGY

Much of the research we have reviewed has examined the relation between different daydreaming or fantasy styles and psychopathology. This research indicates that fantasy activity by no means presupposes psychopathology, but that certain daydreaming or fantasy styles (e.g., guilt, fear of failure, and poor attentional control) are more likely to be correlated with maladaptive behavior and dysphoric affect than others (e.g., positive constructive).

The question that has not been addressed, so far, is whether a history of intense and vivid imagining and fantasizing is a risk factor in the development of psychopathology. Before we address this question, we first review research on the characteristics of persons who report such a history of fantasy proneness. Wilson and Barber identified a group of individuals whom they alternately termed "fantasy addicts," "fantasy-prone personalities," and "fantasizers" in the context of an intensive interview study of excellent hypnotic subjects [66, 67]. The authors described a syndrome estimated to be evident in as much as 4 percent of the population and to represent generally adaptive experiences, fantasy abilities, and personality traits organized around a deep, profound, and long-standing involvement in fantasy and imagination.

When compared with the twenty-five nonexcellent (poor, medium, and medium-high susceptible) hypnotic subjects they interviewed, Wilson and Barber found that the twenty-seven excellent hypnotic subjects reported 1) fantasizing much of their waking life; 2) the ability to hallucinate objects and fully experience what they fantasize "as real as real," including rich and vivid hypnagogic imagery, the achievement of orgasm in the absence of physical stimulation, physical manifestations and concomitants of observed violence on television (e.g., nausea, anxiety), and vivid recall of personal experiences; 3) psychic and out-of-body experiences; 4) occasional difficulty in differentiating fantasized events and persons from nonfantasized ones; 5) the belief in their ability to heal (e.g., "they feel a natural tendency to move toward injured or sick individuals while empathizing with them and touching them" [67, p. 363]); and finally, 6) a sense of social awareness along with a sensitivity to social norms that resulted in a secret fantasy life that few were privy to.

Research following Wilson and Barber's initial investigation has, in general, secured support for the construct of fantasy proneness. Lynn and Rhue [68], for example, selected subjects who scored in the upper 4 percent of college students on a measure (Inventory of Childhood Memories and Imaginings; ICMI of Wilson and Barber [66]) of fantasy-proneness, derived from Wilson and Barber's interview protocol, and compared high scoring subjects (fantasizers) with subjects who scored in the medium range and in the lowest 4 percent of the population (nonfantasizers). Fantasizers outscored less fantasy-prone subjects (medium range and low fantasy prone-lower 4%) on measures of hypnotizability, creativity, waking suggestion, and absorption.

Like Lynn and Rhue [68], Myers and Austrin [69] found that the ICMI and the absorption scale [70] were highly correlated ($r = .73$), supporting the similarity between the constructs of fantasy proneness and absorption, as conceptualized by Tellegen and Atkinson [71] as the capacity for absorbed and self-altering attention. Furthermore, the ICMI identified 3 percent of the population as fantasizers, a percentage that approximates the prevalence in the population estimated by Wilson and Barber [67]. Finally, fantasizers also reported more paranormal and out-of-body experiences than did the other subjects, consistent with Wilson and Barber's observations. This latter finding was also confirmed by Irwin's [72] research on the paranormal beliefs of Australian students who completed the ICMI, as well as by Council and Huff's [73] findings based on an American sample. Rhue and Lynn tested fantasizers and nonfantasizers on a clairvoyance task, and found that although fantasizers overestimated their success on the task and endorsed more items on a test of magical thinking, their actual ESP performance was indistinguishable from that of the nonfantasizers [74].

Along with Hilgard [75, 76], Wilson and Barber [66] identified two childhood developmental pathways to extreme fantasy proneness in later life: 1) encouragement to fantasize from a significant adult; and 2) fantasizing and involvement in imaginative activities as a means of coping with loneliness, isolation, and as an escape from an aversive environment. Rhue and Lynn likewise noted that these two distinct developmental trajectories were represented in their sample, and found that six of the twenty-one fantasizers they studied reported that they were physically abused as children (e.g., broken bones, bruises), whereas none of the nonfantasy prone persons reported a history of abuse [77]. Compared to their less fantasy prone counterparts (medium and nonfantasizers), fantasizers reported a greater frequency and severity of punishment, being hit more even if they were good, more thoughts of revenge toward the person who punished them, and greater loneliness.

In a later study, Rhue, Lynn, Boyd, Buhk, and Henry contrasted college students who reported being physically and sexually abused during childhood with students who reported the loss of a parent before age ten, and who reported they were from an intact family [78]. The students who reported a history of physical and sexual abuse scored higher on the fantasy proneness measure than did the nonabused students from parental loss and intact family backgrounds. Subjects who met the criteria for fantasy proneness (upper 4% of the population) reported some type of abuse.

In general, the findings summarized support Wilson and Barber's conception of fantasy proneness. Fantasy proneness can be described as an adaptive constellation of traits and abilities which, in times of emotional duress, can serve a useful, perhaps compensatory function. However, research has not been uniformly supportive of certain of Wilson and Barber's observations of fantasy prone subjects.

Wilson and Barber suggested that hypnotic-like experiences are a part of the fantasizer's normal behavioral repertoire, and are, therefore, quickly and easily accessed and utilized in a hypnotic context [67]. This contention has received only qualified support. As noted above, Lynn and Rhue found that fantasizers were more hypnotizable than both medium range subjects and nonfantasizers [79]. However, several subsequent studies revealed that fantasizers' and medium range subjects' hypnotizability scores were comparable [73, 80, 81]. Furthermore, across studies, the correlation between hypnotizability and fantasy proneness, although statistically significant, is consistently small (average $r = .23$), and in a recent study it was found that only 16.66 percent of hypnotic virtuosos (subjects who pass at least 11 of 12 suggestions on both the Harvard Group Scale and the Stanford Hypnotic Susceptibility Scale) scored in the fantasy prone range on the ICMI [82]. Interestingly, the lack of an impressive relation between imaginative involvement and hypnotizability has also been documented in several studies of children [83, 84]. In conclusion, although Wilson and Barber [72, 73] implied that hypnotizability and fantasy proneness are closely related, the general association between fantasy proneness and hypnotizability is weak. Nevertheless, up to 80 percent of fantasizers test as highly hypnotizable [68].

Research has also cast doubt on fantasizer's reports that their imagery is "as real as real." For instance, Council, Chambers, Jundt, and Good devised an experimental procedure in which subjects were shown a picture of a geometric design and then asked to rotate their image of it in memory [85]. Because nonfantasizers and fantasizers performed comparably on the task, fantasizers' imagery was no more realistic or lifelike than less fantasy prone subjects. In a study by Rhue and Lynn, most fantasizers were able to hallucinate a cup on demand, in contrast with less than half of the medium range subjects and only about a fifth of the nonfantasizers [80]. However, contrary to Wilson and Barber's observations, only about a quarter of the fantasizers who could visualize a second cup said that their image of the cup was lifelike. As a rule, the fantasizers' images were neither life-like, stable, nor elaborated with detail. Whether fantasizers have more realistic and elaborated hallucinatory experiences in response to self-directed fantasies that are intrinsically gratifying, reduce anxiety, or have some compensatory function is worth examining in future research [79].

We now turn to the question of whether Wilson and Barber were justified in claiming that fantasizers are, for the most part, well adjusted and capable of meeting the challenges of everyday life [67]. Wilson and Barber based their observations on a relatively high functioning group of women, many of whom were successful professionals with postgraduate degrees. Not only was their sample limited to women, but they also recruited the majority of subjects from the ranks of participants in workshops the authors conducted and from personal or professional relationships, such as therapy clients. It is therefore possible that Wilson and Barber might have located a very select, atypical, and non-representative sample of fantasy prone women. Fantasizers with personal relationships with the authors might have minimized their adjustment difficulties, while fantasizers in psychotherapy might have been particularly well-motivated to cope with their problems in living.

Whereas Wilson and Barber emphasized the adaptive qualities of fantasy involvement, they also noted that fantasizers exhibited signs of more regressed or primitive thought processes, as well as symptoms associated with diagnosed hysterics such as false pregnancies and physical concomitants of vivid fantasies and memories [67]. Rhue and Lynn conducted three studies to profile fantasizers' affect, ideation, and symptom report. In their first study (Study 1 [77]), Rhue and Lynn administered objective (MMPI) and projective (Rorschach) measures to fantasizers, medium fantasy prone subjects, and nonfantasizers. Subjects who were fantasizers appeared to use fantasy for defensive or adaptive purposes compared with others and produced eight ($T = 83.90$)/9 (77.95) modal code types on the MMPI. These relatively high elevations were interpreted as reflecting ideational productivity; a tolerance for unusual, atypical, unconventional and peculiar perceptions, experiences, and ideation; and perhaps greater alienation and preoccupation with an internal world of fantasy. A recent study by Johnson justifies this conservative interpretation of elevations on the MMPI Schizophrenia scale [86]. This research suggested that in the college student population, the scale appears to index an inward directedness and an emphasis on fantasizing.

Further evidence that it is inappropriate to emphasize psychopathological implications (e.g., schizophrenia, schizoid tendencies) of the 8/9 elevations derives from the fact that the fantasizers studied were generally successful in meeting the academic demands of college (e.g., indexed by official grade point average) and evidenced no indications of tangential thinking, looseness of associations, and inappropriate or bizarre ideation in the interviews Rhue and Lynn conducted [77]. Moreover, Rorschach test data confirmed the finding that fantasizers exhibit a great deal of imaginative ideation, but failed to reveal indications of morbid or pathological cognitive processes. In contrast, fantasizers' responses suggested an ability to recognize and conform to social norms, a rich affective and cognitive life, and an adequate balance between their inner life and the constraints of reality. Neither the MMPI nor the Rorschach data indicated that fantasy proneness was associated with depression, anxiety, or hysterical tendencies.

Our findings are consistent with the hypothesis that fantasy may serve an adaptive and perhaps compensatory function in relatively nondefensive individuals. As we have noted, instances of child abuse and lonely childhoods were overrepresented among the fantasizers. In addition to scoring higher than other subjects on an index of projected hostility on the Rorschach test, fantasizers reported using fantasy as an escape, as an outlet for anger, and as a means of regulating their internal life. Our results are consistent with Kris's [22] concept of adaptive regression and his hypothesis that some individuals (e.g., those who are fantasy-prone) may evidence pronounced tendencies to use fantasy adaptively to modulate and channel ego-dystonic impulses, using imagination and fantasy as an integral part of their everyday functioning.

In Rhue and Lynn's second study (Study 2 [77]) in which they assessed 50 high, 46 medium, and 33 low fantasy-prone persons on a variety of questionnaire measures pertinent to their adjustment and self-concept, the great majority of fantasizers did not report psychiatric hospitalizations, the use of psychotropic medications, or receipt of professional help from clergy, counselors, psychiatrists, or psychologists. Whereas the only three subjects who reported a history of psychiatric hospitalization and the use of medication for psychological problems were fantasizers, as a group fantasizers were indistinguishable from others on these measures.

If fantasizers were pathologically absorbed in their fantasy worlds, it would be expected that they would have fewer close friends than their less fantasy-prone counterparts. Contrary to this possibility, fantasizers reported having as many close friends as did subjects in the comparison groups. Although fantasizers reported more psychological problems, most fantasizers rated themselves in the range of extremely-to-moderately well-adjusted, and believed that others would rate them similarly. Furthermore, fantasizers' self-concepts were just as positive as those of their less fantasy-prone peers. Fantasizers are apparently able to incorporate the perception of having relatively more problems into their broader self-concept and identity as fantasy-prone persons. Indeed, fantasy proneness is adaptive in the sense that it may promote and preserve a positive self-concept.

One interesting finding that emerged from these two studies is a potential connection between abuse, fantasy proneness, and psychopathology. In their first study in this series, Rhue and Lynn [77] found that five of the twenty-three fantasizers' MMPI profiles conformed to the criteria of severe psychopathology delineated by Newmark et al. [87]. The common thread that runs through these fantasizers' backgrounds is a reported history of harsh childhood punishment and a frequency of physical punishment that averaged from thirteen to twenty-five instances per month.

In their second study, in response to the question of how others would rate their psychological functioning, only two of the fifty fantasizers gave ratings of 4 and 5 on a scale (4-5 representing disturbed end of the continuum, where 5 = many psychological problems/poorly adjusted) [77]. The one fantasizer who rated himself a 5 reported a history of severe abuse (i.e., broken bones, bad bruises, or scarring resulting from abuse). Additionally, the three fantasizers who reported histories of hospitalization and the use of medication for psychological problems rated their punishment as harsh during childhood and reported frequencies of physical punishment that averaged between thirteen and twenty-five instances per month. Eleven other subjects (3 fantasizers, 5 medium, and 3 low fantasy) rated their punishment as harsh or abusive.

Thus, the combination of fantasy proneness and a history of abuse may predispose some fantasizers to severe adjustment problems in adult life. In support of this possibility, Huff and Council found that fantasizers not only evidenced greater personality pathology, including being more likely to exhibit schizoid or borderline personality organization, but also reported more traumatic experiences during childhood [88]. Female fantasizers reported more childhood sexual abuse from nonfamily members than did either male fantasizers or medium or low fantasy-prone subjects. In a recent review of forty-five studies, Kendall-Tackett, Williams, and Finkelhor concluded that sexually-abused children had more symptoms than nonabused children, including fears, posttraumatic stress disorder, behavior problems, sexualized behaviors, and poor self-esteem [89]. In future research, it will be particularly important to tease apart the independent and interactive effects of a history of fantasy proneness and a history of physical or sexual abuse.

In a third study in this series, Lynn and Dudley [90] administered the ICMI screening instrument, the short-form MMPI (MMPI-168), the Magical Ideation Scale [91], and the Perceptual Aberration Scale [92] to nearly 300 students. The latter scales are measures of hypothetical psychosis proneness or schizotypy, where magical ideation is defined as the belief in conventionally invalid forms of causation, and perceptual aberration encompasses five kinds of schizophrenic body-image aberration.

Of the thirteen fantasizers identified in their sample, five scored more than two standard deviations above the mean on the combined Perceptual Aberration/ Magical-Ideation (PERMAG) scale of schizotypy or hypothetical psychosis-proneness. Furthermore, the scale of fantasy proneness and the PERMAG scale were found to share approximately 30 percent of their variance. Finally, the scale of fantasy proneness was a better predictor of scores on the measure of schizotypy than any of the scales of the MMPI-168 that were administered.

One interpretation of these findings is that overlap exists between relatively healthy imaginative tendencies and pathological ideational processes in the fantasy-prone population [90, 93]. This may be true. However, a recent study by Johnson suggests that magical ideation is, at heart, not psychopathological in nature, but rather indexes imaginative propensities [86]. This research indicated that although many psychopathology measures have an imaginal component, magical thinking is not related to measures of psychopathology when measures of absorption, role playing, and active imagination are statistically controlled. According to this research, magical ideation was more reliably associated with measures of imagination than measures of psychopathology.

Based on their first three studies, Lynn and Rhue [74] estimated that between 20 percent and 35 percent of fantasizers exhibit significant signs of maladjustment, psychopathology, or deviant ideation, and perhaps a smaller proportion of fantasizers can be aptly characterized as schizotypal or borderline personalities (see also Huff and Council [88].) However, these estimates were based on studies that, for the most part, used paper and pencil tests. This was also true of a recent study by Irwin which found that high fantasy-prone subjects exhibited more symptoms of psychopathology on Langer's Mental Health Scale than low fantasy-prone subjects [72].

In a recent study, Rhue, Lynn, and Sandberg [94] assessed the prevalence of personality disorders in the fantasy-prone population of college student subjects with the use of a structured diagnostic interview (SCID-II of Spitzer, Williams, and Gibbons [95]). The researchers compared the responses of twenty-four fantasizers (upper 4% of the population) and eighteen subjects who scored within half a standard deviation above and below the mean of the ICMI with respect to the SCID-II, which provided reliable diagnoses of the subjects tested. Fantasy-prone students reported more symptoms of personality disorders than did nonfantasy prone subjects. A quarter of the fantasy-prone sample was diagnosed as having a personality disorder (e.g., paranoid, hysteric, borderline), whereas none of the nonfantasy prone subjects was so diagnosed.

The results confirmed what Rhue and Lynn learned in their other studies of fantasy-prone college students: That the majority of fantasizers appear to be well adjusted, although a minority exhibit signs of psychopathology or maladjustment. At the same time, fantasy proneness does not appear to be secondary to or explicable in terms of long-standing character problems or personality disorders.

LIMITATIONS AND FUTURE DIRECTIONS

The research we reviewed has a number of limitations that are worthy of note. First, the studies are essentially correlational and cross sectional in nature. Because the research is not longitudinal, it is impossible to tease apart cause and effect relationships: We do not know, for example, whether certain types of daydreaming styles place subjects at risk for depression or whether depression itself engenders specific patterns of cognitive activity characterized by guilt and fear of failure.

Another problem with much of the research reviewed here is its reliance on retrospective reports. Retrospective reports are not without limitations. Persons who are depressed, for example, may bias their reports on daydream measures so as to overestimate the negative qualities or frequency of their ideation. Much can be done to clarify the role of fantasy and daydreams in response to life events and in relation to psychopathology by exploiting alternative measurement strategies that depend less on retrospective report and more on evaluations of contemporary cognitive activity by way of thought sampling in real life situations. There is no reason why a variety of measurement strategies, including structured and open-ended interviews, cannot be applied to the study of fantasy and psychopathology, with the potential benefit of convergent measurement strategies permitting stronger inferences regarding the phenomena in question.

Fantasizers' reports of childhood abuse or maltreatment must be taken with a proverbial grain of salt until prospective research on abused children and children with varying degrees of imaginative propensities is conducted. This research is a high priority because highly fantasy-prone subjects may be prone to confuse fact with fantasy, or to be biased by leading questions or interview procedures, given their relatively high levels of waking suggestibility.

Prospective research is important to support or refute the idea that a causal link exists between childhood abuse and dissociation or fantasy proneness. Although a causal pathway between abuse and dissociation seems intuitive, a case for a causal connection cannot be substantiated on the basis of the correlational data that dominate the literature on this topic (see Tillman, Nash, and Lerner [96]).

Prospective research could examine the way in which individual differences mediate the symptomatic expression of abusive or traumatic life experiences. One possibility is that children who have a predisposition (perhaps biologically based, see Bliss [97]; Braun and Sachs [98]; Kluft [99]) to use fantasy or dissociative strategies before the onset of trauma manifest different symptoms in response to abuse than children who lack such a predisposition. For example, children who lack fantasy or dissociative abilities might be more likely to respond to trauma or abuse with outwardly directed symptomatology (e.g., overt aggression, lying, stealing, truancy), rather than with fantasy or imaginative activity that involves focusing attention inward and regulating affect by way of "escapist" cognitive activity and altering perceptions of the meaning of traumatic events (e.g., denial or minimization). However, there may also be a downside to this latter coping style insofar as exclusive use of denial, for example, may "preempt reflection, reasoning, and planning," and may place such victims at risk for acting impulsively when frustrated, depressed, or anxious [100]. We will consider related issues in some detail below when we examine the relation between fantasy, imagination, and dissociation.

Students of fantasy and psychopathology would do well to venture beyond the college student population. As Lynn, Rhue, and Green have argued, student fantasizers may be particularly well-adapted, insofar as the base-rates of serious psychological disorders is fairly low among students, resulting in an unusually favorable picture of fantasizers' adjustment [101]. Relatively few of the studies reviewed here have examined non-college student populations (e.g., general population) or fantasy and psychopathology in the context of a variety of psychological disorders in which fantasy may play a particularly prominent role.

What would advance the field is a grounding of research in testable hypotheses that link fantasy and psychopathology, and potentially guide treatment efforts. Earlier we noted that cause and effect relationships between and among daydreaming, fantasy, and psychopathology have not been established. One possibility is that daydreaming and psychopathology are related to one another in a recursive fashion. Starker hypothesized that dysphoric daydreaming is integral to a feedback loop in which negative daydreaming is initiated by an internal or external event but then potentiates depression by evoking guilt and diminishing self-esteem which, in turn, facilitate depressed affect in a recursive fashion. Starker observes that this cybernetic model implies that alternative positive fantasies may short-circuit this negative, depressigenic cycle, thereby having a therapeutic effect. This suggests that imagination-based techniques could be productively used in psychotherapy [40].

Starker has also argued that sleep disturbances can be created and perpetuated by a person's daydreaming style [40]. To the extent that a person's daydreams are disturbing and difficult to "turn off," it may be difficult to relax and sleep. By contrast, "the vivid, pleasant fantasies of the positive-vivid daydreamer help him to relax quickly and to drift off easily" [40, p. 30]. As in the case of depression, the use of positive fantasies to compete with dysphoric daydreams, may help the person who suffers from insomnia.

As we have alluded to above, the propensity to daydream and fantasize may place certain persons at risk for psychological disorders. For example, Lynn, Rhue, and Green have reconceptualized certain dissociative phenomena as related to imagination-based activities that play a functional and, at times, defensive role in maintaining a person's psychological equilibrium [101]. Experiences often described as "dissociative" actually appear to be related to the use of imagination to escape the reality of a harsh or frightening situation or environment [102]. Examples of these sorts of experiences include viewing oneself as apart from one's body while one is abused, and retreating to an imaginary "sanctuary" or safe place during abusive treatment by a parent. Notably, out of body experiences and the use of imagination to cope with life stresses are not infrequently reported by fantasizers. One way that dissociation has been described is as a defense mechanism that serves as an "escape from the present" [103]. Dissociation, then, appears to refer to the use of imagination and attention-regulating behaviors to create a credible feeling of distance or separation from aversive events outside the realm of personal control or from feelings that generate guilt, anger, or anxiety.

"Missing time" and non-organic memory problems that interfere with a seamless, integrated experienced of reality have been described as dissociative in nature. If an inordinate amount of time is spent imagining and absorbed in fantasizing, so that the ordinary experiential context in which memories are typically embedded is altered, it is no wonder that persons with dissociative symptoms or disorders often have memory gaps or deficits.

Fine has noted that situations, people, or places associated with childhood abuse can trigger acute emotional reactions [104]. If imaginative activities are used as a coping strategy to regulate anxiety and other emotions, they may be reinforced and likely to occur repeatedly in situations that in some way resemble earlier situations in which imagination was used to cope with anxiety. Lipovsky reports the case of "Debbie," a nine-year-old child subjected to severe sadistic sexual abuse, who presented in therapy as feeling "fine" but had difficulties sleeping, frequent nightmares, and appeared to be distractible in school [105]. During a session in which she suddenly became unresponsive to the therapist for about ten minutes, she initially emerged from her "trance like state" and reported that "nothing had happened" only later to acknowledge that something the therapist had said reminded her of a "scary part of the abuse."

Even anxiety itself, or any sensation associated with trauma, could potentially trigger a pattern of fantasy activity that lacks a sense of being consciously initiated. In short, fantasy-based dissociations become pathological or dysfunctional when they are automatized by way of repetition, not consciously regulated by the person, and triggered by internal cues/sensations or environmental stimuli that resemble or actuate earlier triggers of psychological coping or escape mechanisms.

Imaginative tendencies may place certain persons at risk for experiencing depersonalization and derealization. Virtually any event, if sufficiently traumatic, can evoke symptoms of depersonalization in persons with no history of psychopathology. However, highly fantasy-prone persons, who under ordinary circumstances report that they sometimes have problems differentiating fantasy and reality, might be particularly vulnerable to depersonalization reactions following a traumatic event.

Earlier we noted that the fantasy-prone persons Lynn and Rhue identified who were most psychologically disturbed reported a history of childhood abuse or harsh punishment. Lynn et al. hypothesized that the combination of fantasy proneness and a harsh childhood environment increase the risk that a person will be diagnosed as having a dissociative disorder, specifically multiple personality [101]. A similar line of reasoning was also taken by Bowers, who observed that "fantasized alternatives to reality . . . can become increasingly complex and differentiated with minimal involvement of executive level initiative and control" [106, p. 168]. Bowers further noted that, "when a seriously disturbed individual is also fantasy-prone, 'multiple personality' may well be the result" [106, p. 168]. Putnam [107] has observed that childhood fantasy is an important developmental substrate of multiple personality, whereas Young [108] has maintained that "multiple personality reflects the gradual crystallizing of a fantasy that is amalgamated with dissociative defenses" [108, p. 15]. Fantasizers, with their fluid boundaries between their senses of fantasy and reality, their ability to create diverse "believed in" selves, and their tendency to be suggestible in nonhypnotic as well as hypnotic contexts, may be particularly likely to be diagnosed as multiple personalities when exposed to suggestive procedures in psychotherapy that tend to reinforce or shape behavior consistent with the diagnosis.

Our observations suggest that it should be possible to demonstrate a link between measures of imagination, fantasy, and dissociation. Several lines of research support this hypothetical relationship. First, absorption and imaginative involvement figure prominently as factors or underlying dimensions [109-111] of the most widely used dissociation scale, the Dissociative Experiences Scale (DES; [112]).

Second, moderate to high correlations have been found between measures of dissociation and imaginative involvement in adults and children. Green et al. [113] administered the ICMI to 1,249 college students, along with four measures of dissociation: the DES, the PAS (Perceptual Alteration Scale [114]); the DEQ

(Dissociative Experiences Questionnaire [115]); and the Bliss (Bliss Scale [116]). The measures of fantasy proneness and dissociation correlated in the range of .47 (DES and PAS) to .63 (Bliss). The DEQ correlated at .59 with the ICMI. D. Segal and Lynn found that Bliss and DES measures of dissociation were moderately associated (r = .40-.44) with two dimensions of the SIPI: positive constructive daydreaming and poor attentional control [63]. Finally, Rhue, Lynn, and Sandberg studied children who were seen at a clinic for behavioral problems or problems associated with sexual abuse and physical abuse [94]. A measure of childhood dissociation developed by Shostak and Sanders [117] was found to correlate at .54 with a childhood fantasy inventory and .39 with the ICMI adapted for use with children [118].

Third, Frischolz et al. have recently shown that dissociative disorder patients (MPD and dissociative disorder not otherwise specified) scored higher on measures of hypnotizability than patients with schizophrenia, anxiety disorder, mood disorder, and college student control subjects [119]. Earlier research has also shown that patients with MPD [120] and patients suffering from post-traumatic stress disorder [121-123] are more hypnotizable than control subjects. Because many researchers and theoreticians believe that a link exists between imaginative abilities and hypnosis (see Lynn and Sivec [10]), and that many posttraumatic symptoms are dissociative in nature [124], this research provides indirect evidence for an association between dissociation and imaginative tendencies.

Certain similarities between imaginative activities and dissociation notwithstanding, a person's control over fantasy, imagination, and self-absorbed attention may well be the crucial factor that differentiates what we ordinarily think of as "healthy" imaginative tendencies and more pathological variants such as dissociation. When imagination and drawing attention away from present activities or situations involve gross distortions of reality or lack a willful, purposeful quality or are used as anxiety-based escape or avoidance maneuvers, rather than for energizing present activities or rehearsing future activities, they become a liability rather than an asset.

Indeed, it has been argued that persons with a history of resorting to fantasy, unrealistic thinking, denial, or minimization in the face of threat may be particularly vulnerable to sexual victimization [125-129]. According to Kluft such persons may be "sitting ducks" who have difficulty perceiving and reacting to danger signals in an appropriate and timely manner [127]. For example, one woman described by Kluft, who allowed her victimizer to babysit her own children was engaged in "decatastrophizing" or minimizing the seriousness of the situation which blinded her to potential danger. In summary, if imaginative or fantasy activities preclude accurate perceptions of reality or lead to a reconstruction of threatening events so that normal danger cues are misinterpreted or no longer viewed as threatening, the person may response to potentially dangerous situations in a maladaptive fashion.

Whereas some individuals minimize the threat value of environmental stimuli, other individuals magnify and exaggerate threats by way of the use of imagination. With respect to phobias, Beck and Emery have noted that as a person approaches a phobic stimulus, cognitive distortions, visual imagery, and somatic imagery combine to magnify the real danger, with the belief switching from "it is harmless" to "it is dangerous" [130]. They further argued that many phobic patients have highly specific visual imagery which plays a role in warning a person of the consequences of encountering a particular risky situation. Additionally, the phobic may experience the most feared consequences in fantasy. If the sensory input is of sufficient intensity to activate the internal response set, it triggers anxiety, avoidance, and physiological responses.

Obviously, many phobics are strongly motivated to avoid thinking and imagining the phobic stimulus. However, Wegner has suggested that the suppression of unwanted fearful thoughts typically interferes with the process of habituation [131]. It is possible that the thought suppression of unwanted fearful thoughts not only obstructs habituation but also leads to incubation or sensitization of the fearful stimulus. What may occur in phobics, as well as obsessive compulsive and posttraumatic stress disorder patients, is an unstable mixture of attempts to suppress unwanted cognitive activity, followed by increased sensitization to the stimulus or the distressing thoughts themselves. We believe that, ultimately, an inability to control thoughts and images is close to the root of these disorders.

Our discussion suggests that an inability to engage in adaptive reality testing, and to impose a comfortable degree of control over vivid and intense fantasy and imaginative activities, increases risk for a variety of psychological disorders. If imaginative thoughts are not bounded by normally functioning control mechanisms and have an unbidden quality, become unduly repetitive, seemingly impossible to shut off, or disturbing in content (e.g., obsessive compulsive, phobic, or posttraumatic stress disorders), significant maladjustment or distress may ensue.

Unfortunately, relatively little is known about the psychology or psychophysiology of cognitive control, although recent studies of Wegner et al. have highlighted some of the difficulties in consciously attempting to suppress thoughts, how such attempts can lead to the paradoxical preoccupation with the thought to be suppressed, and how distraction and imagination-based techniques (e.g., imagining other or competing images), rather than active suppression, can be a relatively effective means of controlling negative thoughts [131-133].

IMAGINATION-BASED TREATMENTS

Indeed, techniques that capitalize on a person's imaginative and fantasy abilities have been used to treat a wide variety of psychological and medical disorders. The behavioral techniques of flooding, implosion, and systematic desensitization, used so effectively in the treatment of phobias and obsessive compulsive conditions, rely heavily on imagination-based exposure to anxiety-related stimuli [134]. Hypnosis and guided imagery have been widely used in the treatment of pain, multiple personality disorder, posttraumatic stress disorder, anxiety (see Rhue, Lynn, and Kirsch [135]) and chronic medical conditions [136, 137]. The imagination-based technique of storytelling has been used to treat children in acute pain [138], children who undergo difficult medical procedures [139], and children who were sexually abused [140].

Imagination-based treatments may be useful in problem solving by stimulating and coping with events in fantasy. Although fantasy, by itself, may not guarantee successful coping, it can be an important technique to facilitate that objective. With respect to the use of covert modeling techniques in the treatment of unassertive behavior, Kazdin has noted that it is the imaginative elaboration of scenes, rather than merely vivid imagery ability, that facilitates positive treatment gains [141]. What is needed is controlled research that compares the efficacy of imagination-based approaches with more conventional treatments, as well as research that examines individual differences in daydreaming styles and imaginative abilities as mediators of successful therapy with imagination and conventional techniques.

The picture that emerges from our review is that imagining, daydreaming, and fantasy can be enormously enriching activities that have great adaptive value. However, fantasy, daydreams, and imaginings can have a pathological or maladaptive quality when their content, intensity, and duration are not well controlled, regulated, or subservient to a person's goals and intentions and the requirements of diverse situations. The challenge that faces workers in the field is to understand how fantasy styles and cognitive control mechanisms develop over time, how adaptive control mechanisms fail or become degraded, and how therapeutic technologies can be exploited to instate control over an unsatisfying imaginal life.

REFERENCES

1. T. R. Sarbin, Imagining as Muted Role-taking: A Historical-linguistic Analysis, in *The Function and Nature of Imagery*, P. W. Sheehan (ed.), Academic Press, New York, pp. 333-354, 1972.
2. E. Klinger, *Daydreaming: Using Waking Fantasy and Imagery for Self-Knowledge and Creativity*, St. Martin's Press, New York, 1990.
3. A. Richardson, *Mental Imagery*, Springer, New York, 1963.
4. J. L. Singer, *Daydreaming*, Random House, New York, 1966.
5. S. Starker, *Fantastic Thought: All About Dreams, Daydreams, Hallucinations and Hypnosis*, Prentice-Hall, Englewood Cliffs, New Jersey, 1982.
6. E. Klinger, *Structure and Functions of Fantasy*, John Wiley, New York, 1971.
7. S. Gold and J. P. Reilly, Daydreaming, Current Concerns and Personality, *Imagination, Cognition and Personality, 5,* pp. 117-125, 1985-86.
8. B. Segal, G. J. Huba, and J. L. Singer, *Drugs, Daydreaming, and Personality: A Study of College Youth*, Erlbaum, Hillsdale, New Jersey, 1980.

9. E. Klinger and W. M. Cox, Dimensions of Thought Flow in Everyday Life, *Imagination, Cognition and Personality, 7,* pp. 105-128, 1987-88.
10. S. J. Lynn and H. Sivec, The Hypnotizable Subject as Creative Problem Solving Agent, in *Contemporary Hypnosis Research,* E. Fromm and M. Nash (eds.), Guilford, New York, pp. 292-333, 1992.
11. J. B. Watson, *Behaviorism,* University of Chicago Press, Chicago, 1924.
12. R. R. Holt, The Return of the Ostracized-imagery, *American Psychologist, 19,* pp. 254-264, 1964.
13. S. Freud, The Relation of the Poet to Daydreaming (1908), in *On Creativity and the Unconscious,* B. Nelson (ed.), Harper and Row, New York, pp. 44-54, 1958.
14. J. L. Singer, The Constructive Potential of Imagery and Fantasy Processes, in *Recent Developments in Interpersonal Psychoanalysis,* E. Witenberg (ed.), Gardner Press, New York, 1978.
15. M. Watkins, *Waking Dreams,* Spring, Dallas, 1986.
16. W. Penfield, *The Excitable Cortex in Conscious Man,* Charles C. Thomas, Illinois, 1958
17. W. C. Dement and N. Kleitman, The Relation of Eye Movements during Sleep to Dream Activity: An Objective Method for the Study of Dreaming, *Journal of Experimental Psychology, 53,* pp. 339-346, 1957.
18. E. Kris, *Psychoanalytic Explorations in Art,* International Universities Press, New York, 1952 (original work published 1934).
19. D. Foulkes, P. S. Spear, and J. D. Symonds, Individual Differences in Mental Activity at Sleep Onset, *Journal of Abnormal Psychology, 71,* pp. 280-286, 1966.
20. E. Fromm, The Nature of Hypnosis and Other Altered States of Consciousness: An Ego-psychological Theory, in *Hypnosis: Developments in Research and New Perspectives,* E. Fromm and R. E. Shor (eds.), Aldine, New York, pp. 81-103, 1979.
21. E. Fromm, L. Lombard, S. H. Skinner, and S. Kahn, The Modes of the Ego in Self-hypnosis, *Imagination, Cognition and Personality, 7,* pp. 335-349, 1987-88.
22. E. Kris, *Psychoanalytic Explorations in Art,* International Universities Press, New York, 1952 (original work published 1934).
23. E. Klinger, *Motivation and Emotion in the Flow of Imagery and Cognition,* paper presented to the meeting of the American Association for the Study of Mental Imagery, 1988.
24. J. L. Singer, *The Inner World of Daydreaming,* Harper, New York, 1975.
25. J. L. Singer, Private Personality, *Personality and Social Psychology Bulletin, 10,* pp. 7-31, 1984.
26. J. M. Golding and J. L. Singer, Patterns of Inner Experience: Daydreaming Styles, Depressive Moods, and Sex Roles, *Journal of Personality and Social Psychology, 45,* pp. 663-675, 1983.
27. A. T. Beck, *Depression: Clinical, Experimental, and Theoretical Aspects,* Harper & Row, New York, 1967.
28. J. L. Singer and V. McCraven, Some Characteristics of Adult Daydreaming, *Journal of Psychology, 51,* pp. 151-164, 1961.
29. J. L. Singer and J. S. Antrobus, Daydreaming, Imaginal Processes, and Personality: A Normative Study, in *The Function and Nature of Imagery,* P. W. Sheehan (ed.), Academic Press, New York, pp. 175-202, 1972.
30. J. L. Singer, Daydreaming and the Stream of Thought: An Empirical Research Program, *American Scientist, 2,* pp. 417-424, 1974.
31. A. P. Streissguth, N. N. Wagner, and J. C. Wechsler, Effects of Sex, Illness, and Hospitalization on Daydreaming, *Journal of Consulting and Clinical Psychology, 33,* pp. 218-225, 1969.

32. L. M. Giambra, Sex Differences in Daydreaming and Related Mental Activity from the Late Teens to the Early Nineties, *International Journal of Aging and Human Development, 10*, pp. 1-34, 1979-80.
33. S. J. Blatt, D. M. Quinlan, E. S. Chevron, C. McDonald, and D. Zuroff, Dependency and Self-criticism: Psychological Dimensions of Depression, *Journal of Consulting and Clinical Psychology, 50*, pp. 113-124, 1982.
34. L. M. Giambra, Daydreaming Across the Lifespan: Late Adolescent to Senior Citizen, *International Journal of Aging and Human Development, 5*, pp. 115-140, 1974.
35. L. M. Giambra, Adult Male Daydreaming Across the Life Span: A Replication, Further Analyses, and Tentative Norms Based Upon Retrospective Reports, *International Journal of Aging and Human Development, 8*, pp. 197-228, 1977-78.
36. E. Rosenfield, *The Development of an Imaginal Processes Inventory for Children,* unpublished doctoral dissertation, University of Illinois at Chicago Circle, 1978.
37. G. G. Brannigan, P. A. Hauk, and J. A. Guay, Locus of Control and Daydreaming, *The Journal of Genetic Psychology, 152*, pp. 29-33, 1991.
38. S. R. Gold, J. C. Andrews, and S. W. Minor, Daydreaming, Self Concept and Academic Performance, *Imagination, Cognition and Personality, 5*, pp. 239-247, 1985-86.
39. G. L. Huba, J. L. Singer, C. S. Aneshensel, and J. S. Antrobus, *Short Imaginal Processes Inventory,* Research Psychologists Press, Port Huron, Michigan, 1982.
40. S. Starker, Fantasy in Psychiatric Patients: Exploring a Myth, *Hospital and Community Psychiatry, 30*, pp. 25-30, 1979.
41. G. J. Huba, G. Segal, and J. L. Singer, Consistency of Daydreaming Styles Across Samples of College Males and Females Drug and Alcohol Users, *Journal of Abnormal Psychology, 86*, pp. 99-102, 1977.
42. J. S. Tanaka and G. J. Huba, Longitudinal Stability of Three Second-order Daydreaming Factors, *Imagination, Cognition and Personality, 5*, pp. 231-238, 1985-86.
43. H. J. Eysenck, *Maudsley Personality Inventory,* University of London Press, London, 1959.
44. J. P. Guilford and W. S. Zimmerman, The Guilford-Zimmerman Temperament Survey, *Consulting Psychologists Press,* Beverly Hills, California, 1949.
45. H. Gough, *California Psychological Inventory,* Consulting Psychologists Press, Palo Alto, California, 1964.
46. K. B. Stein and K. H. Craik, Relation between Motoric and Ideational Activity Preference and Time Perspective in Neurotics and Schizophrenics, *Journal of Consulting Psychology, 26*, pp. 460-467, 1965.
47. L. M. Giambra and T. D. Traynor, Depression and Daydreaming: An Analysis Based on Self-ratings, *Journal of Clinical Psychology, 34*, pp. 14-25, 1978.
48. A. T. Beck, C. H. Ward, M. Mendelson, J. Mock, and J. Erbaugh, An Inventory for Measuring Depression, *Archives of General Psychiatry, 4*, pp. 561-571, 1961.
49. W. W. K. Zung, A Self-rating Depression Scale, *Archives of General Psychiatry, 29*, pp. 328-337, 1965.
50. B. Lubin, Adjective Checklist for Measurement of Depression, *Archives of General Psychiatry, 12*, pp. 57-62, 1965.
51. G. Cundiff and S. R. Gold, Daydreaming: A Measurable Concept, *Perceptual and Motor Skills, 49*, pp. 347-353, 1979.
52. S. Starker and J. L. Singer, Daydreaming and Symptom Patterns of Psychiatric Patients: A Factor-analytic Study, *Journal of Abnormal Psychology, 84*, pp. 567-570, 1975.

53. S. Starker and J. L. Singer, Daydream Patterns and Self-awareness in Psychiatric Patients, *Journal of Nervous and Mental Disease, 161,* pp. 313-317, 1975.

54. S. Starker, Dreams and Waking Fantasy, in *The Stream of Consciousness,* K. S. Pope and J. L. Singer (eds.), Plenum, New York, 1978.

55. E. A. Brett and S. Starker, Auditory Imagery and Hallucinations, *Journal of Nervous and Mental Disease, 164,* pp. 394-400, 1977.

56. D. K. Schulz, Imagery and the Control of Depression, in *The Power of Human Imagination,* J. L. Singer and K. Pope (eds.), Plenum Press, New York, 1978.

57. S. Starker, Daydreaming Styles and Nocturnal Dreaming: Further Observations, *Perceptual and Motor Skills, 45,* pp. 411-418, 1977.

58. W. B. Webb, *Sleep, the Gentle Tyrant,* Prentice Hall, Englewood Cliffs, New Jersey, 1975.

59. S. Starker, Daydreaming Styles and Nocturnal Dreaming, *Journal of Abnormal Psychology, 83,* pp. 52-55, 1974.

60. S. Starker, Daydreams, Nightmares, and Insomnia: The Relation of Waking Fantasy to Sleep Disturbances, *Imagination, Cognition and Personality, 4,* pp. 237-248, 1984-85.

61. S. Starker and R. Hasenfeld, Daydream Styles and Sleep Disturbance, *Journal of Nervous and Mental Disease, 163,* pp. 391-400, 1976.

62. B. Segal, Drug Use and Fantasy Processes: Criterion for Prediction of Potential Users, *The International Journal of the Addictions, 9,* pp. 475-480, 1974.

63. D. Segal and S. Lynn, Predicting Dissociative Experiences: Imagination, Hypnotizability, Psychopathology, and Alcohol Use, *Imagination, Cognition and Personality, 12,* pp. 287-300, 1992-93.

64. J. Mayer and W. J. Filstead, The Adolescent Alcohol Involvement Scale: An Instrument for Measuring Adolescent Use and Misuse of Alcohol, *Journal of Studies on Alcohol, 40,* pp. 291-300, 1979.

65. A. Anastasi, *Psychological Testing* (5th Edition), Macmillan, New York, 1982.

66. S. C. Wilson and T. X. Barber, Vivid Fantasy and Hallucinatory Abilities in the Life Histories of Excellent Hypnotic Subjects, in *Imagery:* Vol. 2, *Concepts, Results, and Applications* E. Klinger (ed.), Plenum Press, New York, pp. 133-152, 1981.

67. S. C. Wilson and T. X. Barber, The Fantasy-prone Personality: Implications for Understanding Imagery, Hypnosis, and Parapsychological Phenomena, in *Imagery: Current Theory, Research and Application,* A. A. Sheikh (ed.), John Wiley, New York pp. 340-387, 1983.

68. S. J. Lynn and J. W. Rhue, The Fantasy-prone Person: Hypnosis, Imagination, and Creativity, *Journal of Personality and Social Psychology, 51,* pp. 404-408, 1986.

69. S. A. Myers and H. R. Austrin, Distal Eidetic Technology: Further Characteristics of the Fantasy-prone Personality, *Journal of Mental Imagery, 9,* pp. 57-66, 1985.

70. A. Tellegen, *Brief Manual for the Differential Personality Questionnaire,* unpublished manuscript, University of Minnesota, 1982.

71. A. Tellegen and G. Atkinson, Openness to Absorbing and Self-altering Experiences ("Absorption"): A Trait Related to Hypnotic Susceptibility, *Journal of Abnormal Psychology, 83,* pp. 268-277, 1974.

72. H. J. Irwin, A Study of Paranormal Belief, Psychological Adjustment, and Fantasy Proneness, *The Journal of the American Society for Psychical Research, 85,* pp. 317-331, 1991.

73. J. Council and K. D. Huff, Hypnosis, Fantasy Activity and Reports of Paranormal Experiences in High, Medium, and Low Fantasizers, *British Journal of Experimental and Clinical Hypnosis, 7,* pp. 9-15, 1990.

74. J. W. Rhue and S. J. Lynn, *Fantasy Proneness, ESP, and Magical Thinking*, Meeting of the American Association of Mental Imagery, 1988.
75. J. R. Hilgard, *Personality and Hypnosis: A Study of Imaginative Involvement*, University of Chicago Press, Chicago, 1970.
76. E. R. Hilgard, Toward a Neo-dissociation Theory: Multiple Cognitive Control in Human Functioning, *Perspectives in Biology and Medicine, 17*, pp. 301-316, 1974.
77. J. W. Rhue and S. J. Lynn, Fantasy Proneness: Developmental Antecedents, *Journal of Personality, 55*, pp. 121-137, 1987.
78. J. W. Rhue, S. J. Lynn, P. Boyd, K. Buhk, and J. Henry, Imagination, Hypnosis, and Child Abuse, *Imagination, Cognition and Personality, 10*, pp. 53-63, 1990-91.
79. S. J. Lynn and J. W. Rhue, Fantasy Proneness: Hypnosis, Developmental Antecedents, and Psychopathology, *American Psychologist, 43*, pp. 35-44, 1988.
80. J. W. Rhue and S. J. Lynn, Fantasy Proneness, Absorption, and Hypnosis: A Re-examination, *International Journal of Clinical and Experimental Hypnosis, 37*, pp. 100-106, 1989.
81. J. Siuta, Normative and Psychometric Characteristics of a Polish Version of the Creative Imagination Scale, *International Journal of Clinical and Experimental Hypnosis, 35*, pp. 51-58, 1989.
82. J. Green, S. J. Lynn, J. W. Rhue, C. Mare, and B. Williams, *Fantasy Proneness and Hypnotizability: A Stringent Test*, unpublished manuscript, Ohio University, 1992.
83. S. LeBaron, L. K. Zeltzer, and D. Fanurik, Imaginative Ability and Hypnotizability in Childhood, *International Journal of Clinical and Experimental Hypnosis, 36*, pp. 284-295, 1988.
84. A. B. Plotnick, P. A. Payne, and D. J. O'Grady, Correlates of Hypnotizability in Children: Absorption, Vividness of Imagery, Fantasy Play, and Social Desirability, *American Journal of Clinical Hypnosis, 34*, pp. 51-58, 1991.
85. J. R. Council, D. Chambers, T. A. Jundt, and M. D. Good, Are the Mental Images of Fantasy-prone Persons Really More "Real"?, *Imagination, Cognition and Personality, 10*, pp. 319-327, 1991.
86. L. Johnson, *Magical Ideation, Imagination, and Psychopathology*, unpublished manuscript, Carleton University, 1990.
87. C. S. Newmark, L. Gentry, M. Simpson, and T. Jones, MMPI Criteria for Diagnosing Schizophrenia, *Journal of Personality Assessment, 42*, pp. 366-373, 1978.
88. K. Huff and J. Council, *Fantasy Proneness and Psychological Coping*, paper presented at the meeting of the American Psychological Association, New York, August 1987.
89. K. Kendall-Tackett, L. Williams, and D. Finkelhor, Impact of Sexual Abuse in Children: A Review and Synthesis of Recent Empirical Studies, *Psychological Bulletin, 113*, pp. 164-180, 1993.
90. S. J. Lynn and K. Dudley, *Fantasy Proneness, Magical Thinking, and Perceptual Aberration*, unpublished manuscript, Ohio University, 1987.
91. M. Eckblad and L. J. Chapman, Magical Ideation as an Indicator of Schizotopy, *Journal of Consulting and Clinical Psychology, 51*, pp. 215-225, 1983.
92. L. J. Chapman, J. P. Chapman, and S. Raulin, Scales for Physical and Social Anhedonia, *Journal of Abnormal Psychology, 85*, pp. 374-382, 1976.
93. S. J. Lynn and J. W. Rhue, Fantasy Proneness, Psychopathology, and Multiple Personality, in *Suggestibility in Everyday Life*, J. Schumaker (ed.), Oxford Press, London, 1992.
94. J. W. Rhue, S. J. Lynn, and D. Sandberg, *Fantasy Proneness and Personality Disorders*, unpublished manuscript, Ohio University, 1994.

95. R. L. Spitzer, J. B. Williams, M. Gibbon, and M. B. First, *SCID: User's Guide for the Structured Clinical Interview for DSM-III-R*, American Psychiatric Press, Washington, D.C., 1990.

96. J. G. Tillman, M. R. Nash, and P. M. Lerner, Does Trauma Cause Dissociative Pathology?, in *Dissociation: Clinical, Theoretical and Research Perspectives*, S. J. Lynn (ed.), Washington, D.C., 1994.

97. E. L. Bliss, Multiple Personality, *Archives of General Psychiatry, 37*, pp. 1388-1397, 1980.

98. B. G. Braun and R. G. Sachs, The Development of Multiple Personality Disorder: Predisposing, Precipitating, and Perpetuating Factors, in *Childhood Antecedents of Multiple Personality*, R. P. Kluft (ed.), American Psychiatric Press, Washington, D.C., 1985.

99. R. P. Kluft, Aspects of the Treatment of Multiple Personality Disorder, *Psychiatric Annals, 14*, pp. 51-55, 1984.

100. P. M. Cole and F. W. Putnam, Effect of Incest on Self and Social Functioning: A Developmental Psychopathology Perspective, *Journal of Consulting and Clinical Psychology, 60*, pp. 174-183, 1992.

101. S. J. Lynn, J. W. Rhue, and J. P. Green, Multiple Personality and Fantasy Proneness: Is There an Association of Dissociation?, *British Journal of Experimental and Clinical Hypnosis, 5*:3, pp. 138-142, 1988.

102. D. Spiegel, Dissociating Damage, *American Journal of Clinical Hypnosis, 29*, pp. 123-131, 1986.

103. D. Spiegel, T. Hunt, and H. E. Dondershine, Dissociation and Hypnotizability in Post Traumatic Stress Disorder, *American Journal of Psychiatry, 145*:3, pp. 301-305, 1988.

104. C. G. Fine, The Cognitive Sequelae of Incest, in *Incest-Related Syndromes of Adult Psychopathology*, R. P. Kluft (ed.), American Psychiatric Press, Washington, D.C., pp. 161-182, 1990.

105. J. A. Lipovsky, Assessment and Treatment of Post-Traumatic Stress Disorder in Child Survivors of Sexual Assault, in *Treating PTSD: Cognitive Behavioral Strategies*, D. W. Foy (ed.), Guilford Press, New York, pp. 127-164, 1992.

106. K. S. Bowers, Dissociation in Hypnosis and Multiple Personality, *International Journal of Clinical and Experimental Hypnosis, 39*, pp. 155-176, 1991.

107. F. W. Putnam, *Diagnosis and Treatment of Multiple Personality Disorder*, Guilford Press, New York, 1989.

108. W. C. Young, Observations on Fantasy in the Formation of Multiple Personality, *Dissociation, 1*, pp. 13-20, 1988.

109. M. J. Anguilo and J. F. Kihostrom, *Dissociative Experiences in a College Population*, unpublished manuscript, University of Arizona, 1993.

110. W. J. Ray, M. Faith, and J. Mathieu, *Factor Structure of the Dissociative Experiences Scale: A College Age Population Study*, unpublished manuscript, Pennsylvania, S10, 1994.

111. C. A. Ross, S. Joshi, and G. Anderson, The Dissociative Experiences Scale: A Replication Study, *Dissociation, 1*, pp. 21-22, 1991.

112. E. M. Bernstein and F. W. Putnam, Development, Reliability and Validity of a Dissociation Scale, *Journal of Nervous and Mental Disease, 174*, pp. 727-735, 1986.

113. J. P. Green, S. Kvaal, S. J. Lynn, C. Mare, and D. A. Sandberg, *Hypnosis, Dissociation, Fantasy Proneness and Absorption: The Effects of Context*, paper presented to the annual meeting of the American Psychological Association, San Francisco, California, 1991.

114. S. Sanders, The Perceptual Alteration Scale: A Scale Measuring Dissociation, *American Journal of Clinical Hypnosis, 29*, pp. 95-102, 1986.
115. K. C. Riley, Measurement of Dissociation, *Journal of Nervous and Mental Disease, 176*, pp. 449-450, 1988.
116. M. Wogan, *The Bliss Scale: Development, Reliability, and Validity,* unpublished manuscript, Rutgers University at Camden, 1991.
117. M. Shostak and S. Sanders, *The Childhood Perceptual Alteration Scale (PAS),* unpublished manuscript, 1990.
118. S. A. Myers, The Creative Imagination Scale: Group Norms for Children and Adolescents, *International Journal of Clinical and Experimental Hypnosis, 27*, pp. 265-277, 1986.
119. E. Frischolz, J. Lipman, B. Braun, and R. G. Sachs, *Psychopathology, Hypnotizability, and Dissociation,* unpublished manuscript, University of Illinois, Chicago Circle, 1992.
120. E. L. Bliss, *Multiple Personality, Allied Disorders and Hypnosis,* Oxford University Press, New York, 1986.
121. D. Spiegel, Multiple Personality as a Post-traumatic Stress Disorder, *Psychiatric Clinics of North America, 7,* pp. 101-110, 1984.
122. D. Spiegel, T. Hunt, and H. E. Dondershine, Dissociation and Hypnotizability in Post-traumatic Stress Disorder, *American Journal of Psychiatry, 145,* pp. 301-305, 1988.
123. R. K. Stuntman and E. L. Bliss, Posttraumatic Stress Disorder, Hypnotizability, and Imagery, *American Journal of Psychiatry, 142,* pp. 741-743, 1985.
124. J. Briere and M. Runtz, Multivariate Correlates of Childhood Psychological and Physical Maltreatment among University Women, *Child Abuse and Neglect, 12,* pp. 331-341, 1988.
125. J. A. Chu, The Revictimization of Adult Women with Histories of Child Abuse, *Journal of Psychotherapy Practice and Research, 1,* pp. 259-269, 1992.
126. E. Becker-Lausen, B. Sanders, and J. M. Chinsky, *A Structural Analysis of Child Abuse and Negative Life Experiences,* paper presented at the 100th annual convention of the American Psychological Association, Washington, D.C., 1992.
127. R. P. Kluft, Treating Patients Sexually Exploited by a Previous Therapist, *Psychiatric Clinics of North America, 12,* pp. 483-500, 1989.
128. R. P. Kluft, Dissociation and Subsequent Vulnerability: A Preliminary Study, *Dissociation, 3,* pp. 167-173, 1990.
129. D. Sandberg and S. J. Lynn, *Dissociation and Vulnerability to Subsequent Victimization: A Prospective Analysis,* unpublished manuscript, Ohio University, Athens, Ohio, 1995.
130. A. Beck and G. Emery, *Anxiety Disorders and Phobias,* Basic Books, New York, 1985.
131. D. M. Wegner, *White Bears and Other Unwanted Thoughts: Suppression, Obsession and the Psychology of Mental Control,* Viking, New York, 1985.
132. D. Wegner, D. Schneider, S. R. Carter, and T. White, Paradoxical Effects of Thought Suppression, *Journal of Personality and Social Psychology, 53,* pp. 5-13, 1987.
133. R. Wenzlaff, D. Wegner, and D. Roper, Depression and Mental Control: Resurgence of Unwanted Negative Thoughts, *Journal of Personality and Social Psychology, 55,* pp. 882-892, 1988.
134. D. Rimm and H. M. Cunningham, Behavior Therapies, in *Contemporary Psychotherapies: Models and Methods,* S. J. Lynn and J. P. Garske (eds.), Merrill Press, Columbus, 1985.
135. J. W. Rhue, S. J. Lynn, and I. Kirsch (eds.), *Handbook of Clinical Hypnosis,* American Psychological Association, Washington, D.C., in press.

136. M. R. Johnson, J. K. Whitt, and B. Martin, The Effect of Fantasy Facilitation of Anxiety in Chronically Ill and Healthy Children, *Journal of Pediatric Psychology, 12,* pp. 273-284, 1987.
137. L. K. Zeltzer and S. LeBaron, Fantasy in Children and Adolescents with Chronic Illness, *Developmental and Behavioral Pediatrics, 7,* pp. 195-198, 1986.
138. L. Kuttner, Favorite Stories: A Hypnotic Pain-reduction Technique for Children in Acute Pain, *American Journal of Clinical Hypnosis, 30,* pp. 289-295, 1988.
139. J. R. Hilgard and S. LeBaron, *Hypnotherapy of Pain in Children With Cancer,* William Kaufmann, Los Altos, California, 1984.
140. J. W. Rhue and S. J. Lynn, Storytelling, Hypnosis, and the Treatment of Sexually Abused Children, *International Journal of Clinical and Experimental Hypnosis, 39,* pp. 198-214, 1991.
141. A. E. Kazdin, Imagery, Elaboration and Self-efficacy in the Covert Modeling Treatment of Unassertive Behavior, *Journal of Counseling and Clinical Psychology, 47,* pp. 725-733, 1979.

CHAPTER 5

The Relation of Imagery Vividness, Absorption, Reality Boundaries and Synesthesia to Hypnotic States and Traits

CHARLES M. RADER,
ROBERT G. KUNZENDORF,
AND CARLENE CARRABINO

In this chapter, we present an investigation of four dispositional abilities or traits related to imaginative involvement: vividness of visual images; absorption; thinness of boundaries, particularly the boundary between imaging and perceiving; and synesthesia [1-6]. We explore both their relationships to each other, as they pertain to hypnotic susceptibility, and their possible operation during hypnosis itself, especially concerning the suspension of reality testing. Image vividness and absorption have received considerable attention in the hypnotic literature [3, 6-10]. Boundary thinness and its relations to susceptibility and the hypnotic state have only recently been explored [4-5, 11]. Speculation regarding the relationship of synesthesia to hypnosis has been offered in the past but, heretofore, never systematically explored [12-14].

Our empirical investigation serves to integrate two theoretical perspectives: psychoanalytic theory and source-monitoring theory [11, 15-21]. Both provide a framework for understanding how the above four abilities or traits facilitate the induction of hypnosis and the "primary process" phenomena associated with hypnosis and with regressive or "unmonitored" states like sleep or psychosis. Previous research suggests that hypnosis is a state in which primary process is promoted and imaged sensations are experienced as real [22-26]. Drawing on applications of psychoanalytic theory to hypnosis [27-30], Nash has postulated that hypnosis involves a topographic rather than a temporal regression [31, 32]. Accordingly, he disavows the notion that a temporal return to earlier developmental stages or previous psychic structures is implicated in hypnosis. Rather, hypnosis "involves a shift to more nonlogical, symbolic, imagistic, and primary-process mentation," which implicates a shift in ego functioning or topography [31, p. 180]. In this connection, Fromm's view that hypnotized subjects move from an ego-active to an ego-receptive mode is of particular import, as it not only sheds light on the possible role of absorption but also is consonant with source-monitoring theory. Fromm's work on self-hypnosis suggests that ego activity never stops during hypnosis, but that the focus of self-awareness is narrowed so as to minimize critical judgment, deliberate control of internal experience, and goal-directed thinking. Fromm, in fact, links ego receptivity to the source-monitoring theory of hypnosis:

> When the ego is receptive, defenses are relaxed, allowing into consciousness the emergence of more fluid associations and of images of a fantastic nature. Kunzendorf draws a similar conclusion regarding (hetero-) hypnosis. He suggests it is an "unmonitored" state in which repressed images are allowed to achieve more vivid representation [29, p. 346].

According to Kunzendorf's theory of source monitoring, the illusion of self-consciousness—of a subject "experiencing" imaginal objects and perceptual objects—is the phenomenal quality of a brain mechanism that monitors the central innervation of imaged sensations and the peripheral generation of perceived sensations [17]. Similarly, the illusion of self-control—of an agent "intending" wishful fantasies and willful actions—is the phenomenal quality of a brain mechanism that anticipates the imaginal sensations embodying fantasy and the perceptual sensations paralleling action [21]. During mental states such as hypnosis, sleep, and psychosis, however, the monitoring of actual sensations and anticipated sensations is attenuated, and the boundaries between self and other—self-generated imagery and reality-based perception, intention by a self and possession by an impulse—are diminished. Thus hypnosis, to the extent that it attenuates the source-monitoring process, serves to unleash "unmonitored images" of normally censored material or hallucinations of a primary process nature [11, 15-17, 19]. Furthermore, "hypnosis attenuates: a) the self-consciously monitored boundary between visual sensations and emotional sensations and b) the self-consciously monitored boundary between visual sensations and auditory sensations," which we see later has implications for synesthetic functioning during hypnosis [11, p. 231]. It should be noted that Kunzendorf's equation of reality-testing with self-conscious monitoring processes inherent in the left hemisphere is contrary to the psychoanalytic tendency to equate reality-testing with the development of self-concept or ego [20].

Our integration of psychoanalytic theory and source-monitoring theory has a number of implications regarding absorption, vividness of imagery, thinness of boundaries, and synesthesia, as well as the interactions among such traits during hypnosis. For the purpose of exploring these implications, we shall review theory and research pertaining to each trait individually.

ABSORPTION

Continuing the work of Hilgard's associates and Shor, Orne, and O'Connell [33-36], who developed inventories of hypnotic predispositions and hypnotic-like experiences occurring in daily life, Tellegen and Atkinson constructed their Absorption scale [1]. The original scale primarily contained imaginative involvement items (many taken from Lee-Teng [34]) but also contained items from a previously constructed Trust Rating Scale by Roberts and Tellegen [37]. In the initial study utilizing two samples of female subjects, the Absorption scale correlated significantly with the Harvard Group Scale of Hypnotic Susceptibility [38]—$r = .27$ in the first sample; $r = .43$ in the second sample—and significantly with Field and Palmer's Hypnotic Depth Inventory [39]—$r = .43$ in the first sample, the only one tested for depth. Tellegen and Atkinson defined absorption as an attentional process, "involving a full commitment of available perceptual, motoric, imaginative and ideational resources to a unified representation of the attentional object" [1, p. 274]. In a later paper, Tellegen further defined absorption as an attentional disposition, an inherently interactive functional unit whose expression and utilization will depend upon the circumstances or conditions to which individuals endowed with this ability are exposed [2]. Not surprisingly, later studies investigating the correlation of hypnotizability with absorption, as assessed by the Tellegen scale, have yielded coefficients varying from $r = .13$ to $r = .89$ [3]. Such variability can be attributed to contextual factors [40-42] and to the particular suggestions used to measure hypnotizability [43, 44]. Accordingly, when contexts encourage experiential activity, and when measures focus on internal processing rather than responsiveness, correlations should be higher.

Several facets of Absorption are related to our integrative theory of hypnotic functioning. As Tellegen and Atkinson initially noted, even when the attentional object is constructed by the individual, it is experienced as present and real [1]. Qualifiers such as "this is only my imagination" are not maintained. In essence, reality testing is suspended, ego receptivity predominates, and source monitoring ceases, so that imagination during absorption is indistinguishable from perception. Indeed, Fromm and Kahn have described absorption "as part and parcel of the structure of any hypnotic experience" [45, p. 161], and have explored its role in the fading of the generalized reality orientation in self-hypnosis [46]. And when reality testing fades, primary process functioning should gradually emerge. In the latter regard, Kihlstrom, Register, Hoyt, Albright, Grigorian, Heindel, and Morrison found a .57 correlation between Tellegen's Absorption scale and the Access to the Unconscious scale from their Wisconsin Experience Questionnaire [47]. To the extent that absorption abilities are more likely to be manifested under hypnotic conditions, high absorbers should be more likely than low absorbers to exhibit hypnotic suspension of reality testing (i.e., hypnotic facilitation of hallucinatory imagery) and hypnotic access to "the subconscious."

Given Kunzendorf's evidence that hypnotic hallucinations result merely from the attenuation of source-monitoring, not from the vivification of imaging [15], one would not expect simple interactions between hypnosis, absorption, and image vividness. Roche and McConkey reviewed studies correlating absorption with image vividness and reported coefficients ranging from $r = .26$ to $r = .78$, depending on contextual factors and measuring instruments [3]. In an exemplary study employing Marks' Vividness of Visual Imagery Questionnaire [48], Crawford found a .59 correlation between absorption and image vividness [49]. Likewise, in a noncorrelational study utilizing a phenomenological state instrument, Pekala, Wenger, and Levine found that, relative to low-absorption subjects, higher absorbers report more intense imagery [50]. But in a later study, contrary to what one might expect, Kumar and Pekala found that hypnosis produced no significant imagery differences between high-absorption and low-absorption subjects [51]. The present study was, in part, designed for further assessment of such interactions between absorption, hypnosis, and vividness.

Tellegen and Atkinson, in elaborating the cognitive abilities underlying absorption, included "the ability to operate diverse representation modalities synergistically so that a full but unified experience is realized" [1, p. 275]. Synesthesia, which we will soon discuss in depth, was considered to be a component of the imaginative and integrative aspect of absorption. This led to formal studies of the relationship between absorption and synesthesia 12-14]. Across both sexes in these studies, absorption was moderately correlated with the vividness of synesthetic imagery—as assessed by self-reports of cognitive style ($r = .40$ for females, $r = .46$ for males) and by experimental responses to auditory stimulation ($r = .42$ for females, $r = .39$ for males) [12, 14]. Roche and McConkey observed that such findings "highlight the need for further analysis of the relationship of absorption with cross-modal experiencing of both externally presented and internally generated events" [3, p. 96], a need which we sought to address in the present investigation.

VIVIDNESS OF IMAGERY

Over one hundred years ago, Binet and Féré suggested that vividness of imagery was related to hypnotic responding, particularly hypnotic hallucinating [52]. But as Sutcliff, Perry, and Sheehan point out, image vividness has historically been defined quite narrowly as *percept-like clarity,* rather than more expansively as symbolic and synesthetic *expressivity* or 'fluidity' (the original term for "absorption") [53]. This point is important, because the latter, more expansive definition may better account for the fluctuating relationship between self-reported imagery and hypnotizability in later studies. Furthermore, symbolic and synesthetic expressions of imagination are highly relevant to our integration of psychoanalytic theory and monitoring theory, because such fluid expression entails the ability to suspend ego control and to transcend secondary process thinking.

Empirically, hypnotizability is not fully explained by the ability to generate images of perceptual clarity, as research by Sutcliff, Perry, and Sheehan illustrates [53]. Although these three researchers obtained an overall correlation of .39 between the Betts QMI and the Stanford Hypnotic Susceptibility Scale, Form C [54, 55], the males' correlation of .58 was significant, and the females' correlation of .20 was not. Moreover, the underlying relationship between the two dependent variables departed appreciably from linearity, both for the total sample and for the male sample. That is, nonhypnotic images lacking in perceptual clarity were almost always associated with low hypnotizability, but nonhypnotic images exhibiting perceptual clarity were not necessarily associated with high hypnotizability. Given this finding of nonlinearity, plus the inconsistent findings in subsequent attempts to relate hypnotizability to image clarity [35, 56-59], Heyneman suggests that "the functional properties of the image remain unclear" [60, p. 41]. We suggest, instead, that the functional significance of imagery for highly hypnotizable subjects is related to *imaginative involvement,* as measured by Wilson and Barber's Creative Imagination Scale [61], and to *absorption.* Indeed, recent multivariate hypnosis research is already leading to a better understanding of the hypnotic functioning of imaginative processes, as they interact with traits such as absorption [62, 63]. Up until the present time, however, the imaginative processes measured by such research have not included the process of reality testing. Later in this chapter we will describe Kunzendorf's new paradigm for measuring the latter process [21], and we will show how the state of hypnosis and the trait of absorption interact with reality testing but not with image vividness.

BOUNDARY THINNESS

The concept of boundary thinness had its genesis in Hartmann's investigations of the personality characteristics of frequent nightmare sufferers [64-67]. In these investigations, two separate groups of fifty nightmare sufferers were subjected to psychiatric interviews and psychometric tests. A comparison of mean MMPI profiles indicated that both nightmare groups scored higher than control groups on the "psychotic" side of the profile (Pa, Pt, Sc, Ma) but not on the "neurotic" side (Hs, D, Hy) [68]. On the Rorschach, the nightmare sufferers had more varied protocols than control groups. The nightmare sufferers evidenced a great deal of vivid, emotional, and "primary process" imagery. However, they did not differ significantly from the other groups when protocols were scored according to the Exner Comprehensive System [69]. Interestingly, they did score higher on a scale developed by Sivan to assess "permeable boundaries" [70]. When the TAT was employed in one investigation [71], the nightmare subjects showed no greater interpersonal aggression or hostility in their stories than the control subjects showed. On the basis of psychiatric interviews, only one-third of the nightmare group could be assigned a DSM-III diagnosis: most often an Axis II (personality disorder) diagnosis. However, Hartmann and his fellow interviewers discovered that many nightmare sufferers were strikingly open and trusting, to the point of being undefended, and were extremely sensitive to sensory stimulation from different modalities. Many of them evidenced thin interpersonal boundaries, thin ego boundaries, thin boundaries between masculine and feminine aspects of themselves, as well as thin boundaries upon awakening (and not being able to differentiate whether one is awake or still asleep). Typically, such individuals spent much of their time daydreaming, and described their imagery as so "vivid" that they experienced some difficulty differentiating it from reality. Overall, these characteristics were best captured by the term "thin boundaries."

In an attempt to investigate further the concept of boundaries, Hartmann and his associates developed a questionnaire with 145 items, tapping twelve a priori dimensions of thin versus thick boundaries [5]. Hartmann reported that an exploratory factor analysis of the questionnaire resulted in a best solution of thirteen orthogonal factors, the first four of which exhibited high reliability and accounted for most of the variability [4, 5]. Interestingly, the factor with highest reliability and greatest importance statistically, Factor I, was called *primary process*. The fifty-one items which loaded heavily on this factor describe individuals who have many experiences of merging or switching their identity, who have "vivid" images with little differentiability from perceptual reality, and who have various experiences of synesthesia. Accordingly, Hartmann's Boundary Questionnaire has possible relevance not only for the theoretical integration of psychoanalysis and source monitoring, but also for the empirical integration of hypnotic phenomena, synesthetic experiences, absorption scores, and reality-testing abilities. Indeed, Barrett found that thinness on the Boundary Questionnaire correlated significantly with hypnotic susceptibility as measured by the Harvard Group Scale ($r = .19$), with hypnotic depth as assessed by the Field Inventory ($r = .29$), and with absorption as assessed by Tellegen's scale ($r = .54$) [72]. In contrast, Kunzendorf and Maurer did not find that boundary thinness was significantly correlated with hypnotic susceptibility ($r = .16$) [11]. However, the latter investigators did find that, independently for thin boundaried subjects and for highly susceptible subjects, hypnosis attenuated the boundary between emotional sensations and visual sensations (between imaged feelings of emotion and viewed facial expressions of emotion). Moreover, hypnotic attenuation of this emotional-visual boundary was statistically associated with hypnotic attenuation of the boundary between audible sensations and visual sensations as well. Such confusion of sensory sources—given hypnoidal states and particular traits—has implications for studies of synesthesia, implications which we sought to address within the present study.

SYNESTHESIA

Synesthesia refers to the transposition of sensory "images" from one modality's dimensions to corresponding dimensions in a perceived modality, where the images are "vivid" enough to be perceptual (and correspondent enough not to be hallucinatory). For persons endowed with visual-auditory synesthesia, the most frequently occurring type, hearing a particular sound causes them to "see" something like a corresponding color. For persons endowed with auditory-gustatory synesthesia, tasting a specific flavor causes them to "hear" something like a corresponding melody. For those richly endowed with synesthesia, such intermodal transpositions are automatic and spontaneous.

The intriguing phenomenon of synesthesia was studied in its own right by early psychological scientists such as Galton, Binet, Bleuler, Lehmann, and Werner [73-78]. Unfortunately, like hypnosis, synesthesia was either totally neglected by behavioral scientists or dismissively assimilated into their learning theories. Only relatively recently has real scientific interest in synesthesia been revived, as evidenced by the publication of two books on the subject [79-80]. Still, most of the contemporary research on synesthesia has been limited to psychophysical approaches [81] or to case-history approaches [82]. Psychophysical studies of visual-auditory synesthesia reveal two general principles governing the relation between auditory stimulation and visual imagery: The brightness of the visual image corresponds to the pitch of the auditory stimulus, and the size of the image corresponds to the volume. Studies of individual and group differences in visual-auditory synesthesia reveal considerable variability in the vividness of imagery associated with sound stimuli [79]. The pertinent literature is reviewed in detail [12, 83, 84].

Reapproaching synesthesia from the standpoint of individual differences, Rader and Tellegen factor analyzed visual-auditory phenomena, and studied how the resulting factors relate to individual differences in personality and intellectual functioning [14]. Their factor analyses showed that visual-auditory synesthesia can be partitioned into two dimensions: a *translation factor* (e.g., normal versus deviant *chromotonal correspondence* between particular colors and tones) and an *experiential factor* (e.g., high vs. low vividness of the color images evoked by tonal stimuli). When Rader and Tellegen compared individual differences on their empirically derived norms for chromotonal correspondence and individual differences on similar norms for other correspondences, they obtained a "higher order" general translation factor—a factor indicating that the ability to represent sounds as corresponding colors is a skill manifesting itself across a variety of tasks. When they examined individual differences in the experience of vividness, they obtained evidence for continuously distributed differences (and, thus, no evidence for a typology as proposed by Cytowic [79]). Experienced vividness was statistically independent of chromotonal translation ability, in accord with the results of Marks [81] and Jones [84], but inconsistent with Lehman's report of differences in how "seers" and "nonseers" use color to describe music [85]. Also, vividness of synesthetic imagery was unrelated to MPQ measures of pathology in Rader and Tellegen's study [14], just as it was unrelated to emotional disturbance in Cytowic's [79] and Shindell's studies [86]. Neither vividness nor translation ability was statistically associated with intelligence, as assessed by a modified version of the Mill-Hill [87]. But unlike translation ability, vividness was positively correlated with *absorption*. This latter finding is consistent with Shindell's report [86] that synesthesia correlates positively with both the Creative Personality scale and the A1 scale of the Adjective Check List [88]. Thus confirming the observations of Galton [73] and Cytowic [79], these positive correlations depict "synesthetes" as being creative, as enjoying sensuous experiences, as being skilled in imaginative play.

Integrating hypnosis into this collective depiction of synesthesia and absorption, Rader and Tellegen speculated that "persons endowed with absorption skills may be adept at reinstating the primitive conditions under which synesthetic functioning naturally occurs" [14, p. 987]. In essence, they speculated that high absorbers may be particularly adept in effecting an adaptive regression which, as envisioned by Nash [31, 32] and Shames and the Bowers [89, 90], is topographic and creative. Accordingly, to the extent that hypnosis involves such regression, synesthetic imagery may increase during the hypnotic state. Indeed, in Kunzendorf and Maurer's previously discussed experiments [11], *the hypnotic attenuation of source monitoring* induced both synesthetic imagery and regressive or "primary process" imagery: In the case of synesthetic images (including emotionally symbolic creations), hypnosis attenuated awareness of whether sensations had visual or auditory or emotional origins, and in the case of "primary process" hallucinations, it attenuated awareness of whether sensations had central or peripheral origins. Furthermore, in several experiments [91-93], hypnosis induced eidetic images in accord with Werner's developmental theory, as it pertains to topographic regression during hypnosis [78]. Werner maintained that synesthesia and eidetic imagery were manifestations of an undifferentiated level of functioning, in which a primitive "general sense" operated.

SPECULATIONS BEHIND THE PRESENT INVESTIGATION

Based on the absorption literature reviewed previously, we speculated that hypnotic susceptibility, vividness of visual imagery, boundary thinness, and hours of sleep per night should be positively correlated with absorption. We postulated no relationship between reality discernment prior to hypnosis and absorption, in view of Tellegen's finding that mental health and absorption are unrelated [94]. During hypnosis, however, high absorption should be associated with harder to discern boundaries between sensory reality and sensory imagery, as well as harder to discern boundaries between the sensory modalities. In the latter case, whether or not hypnotic synesthesia improves translation ability is an empirical question of much interest to us.

Based on the hypnosis literature, we surmised that hypnotic susceptibility should be negatively correlated with reality discernment prior to hypnosis [6], with hours of sleep per night [95], and with Marks' Vividness of Visual Imagery Questionnaire (a subjective measure in which vividness is scaled inversely) [48]. But consonant with research reviewed and presented by Kunzendorf [15], we predicted that image vividness should not be enhanced during the hypnotic state, even though image monitoring and reality discernment are diminished during it.

METHOD

Procedure

Two groups of subjects were tested, two to eight subjects at a time, in a laboratory with nine IBM PS2s. On these computers, both groups were administered first a warm-up exercise (described below), then a succession of questionnaires—Hartmann's Boundary Questionnaire [5], Marks's Vividness of Visual Imagery Questionnaire [48], and the Absorption Scale of Tellegen's Multidimensional Personality Questionnaire [96, 97]. Upon completion of these questionnaires, one group was administered Kunzendorf and Carrabino's test for *reality discernment* [21], and the other group was administered three tests for synesthesia (all described below). Thereafter in both groups, hypnosis was induced and tested with the Stanford Group Hypnotic Susceptibility Scale [98], Form C (behavioral scoring only). Prior to the ninth suggestion on Form C (anosmia), the three tests for synesthesia were administered to the group that had not received them before hypnosis, and the test for *reality discernment* was administered to the other group of subjects. After the twelfth suggestion, terminating hypnosis, subjects confirmed the number of hours that they reportedly sleep in a typical twenty-four-hour school day.

Warm-up Exercise. This exercise was designed to provide prehypnotic familiarization with procedures employed in the second test for synesthesia—a test which some subjects received under hypnosis, and others prior to hypnosis. Throughout the warm-up, synesthetic correspondences between color and emotion were assessed with queries like this first one involving anger:

Which of the following colors do you most strongly associate with feeling *angry?* Suppose you have FIVE POINTS to distribute to the colors most strongly associated with this feeling, and suppose you can assign more than one point to a color if you want to.
For each point, press first letter of the color to which you assign the point.

R = red	B = blue	W = white
O = orange	V = violent	G = gray
Y = yellow	D = dark brown	I = ink black
L = leaf green	P = pink	

The experimenter explained that subjects should press "O" five times if anger is associated only with orange, for example, whereas they should press "O" three times, and "G" two times if anger is associated mostly with orange but also with gray. Following anger, ten more emotions were assessed, so that subjects became completely familiar with the 5-point procedure.

Three Tests for Synesthesia. The first test—a new *objective* measure of synesthetic *correspondences* between color and sound—was inspired by Marcia Johnson's paradigm for measuring confusions between imagination and perception [99]. At the outset of this new test for synesthesia, the subjects turned their attention to one centrally situated computer, and the experimenter read aloud the following instruction:

> Pay close attention, while the speaker in this computer generates pure tones, then the middle of the screen changes colors, then the speaker generates tones again, and so on. When you are done paying attention to the colors and the tones, your own computer will ask you some questions about them.

The central computer then presented 5 blocks of pure tones and rectangular colors (10-row by 40-column rectangles of color, surrounded by low-intensity white). The first block contained 9 half-sec tones—3 low tones (200 Hz, 120 Hz, 242 Hz), 3 medium tones (1000 Hz, 1100 Hz, 1210 Hz), and 3 high tones (4000 Hz, 4400 Hz, 4840 Hz)—followed by 9 half-sec colors—3 dark colors (black, gray, brown), 3 medium colors (blue, green, red), and 3 light colors (pink, yellow, white). Across all 5 blocks, 1 of the 3 tones in each category (low, medium, high) was presented 5 times; the other 2 low tones were presented 8 times; the other 2 medium tones were presented 2 and 8 times apiece; and the other 2 high tones were presented twice. Additionally across all blocks, 1 of the 3 colors in each category (dark, medium, light) was presented 8 times, 1 of the 2 remaining colors in each category was presented 5 times, and the last color in each category was presented twice. At the conclusion of this first test for synesthesia, the 9 colors were individually presented on each subject's computer screen, and the subject estimated how many times he or she had just seen each color. It was expected that subjects with synesthesia would experience low tones as dark colors and (because low tones are presented more often than other tones) would overestimate the frequency of dark colors.

The second and third tests for synesthesia were based on procedures developed by Rader and Tellegen [13, 14]. For each of 9 tones, the second test—a *subjective* measure of synesthetic *correspondences* between color and sound—displayed the following query:

> Which of the following colors do you most strongly associate with the [half-sec] tone that is being presented?
> (Wait for the experimenter to play the tone.)
> Suppose you have FIVE POINTS to distribute to the colors most strongly associated with this tone, and suppose you can assign more than one point to a color if you want to.

For each point, press first letter of the color to which you assign the point.

R = red	B = blue	W = white
O = orange	V = violet	G = gray
Y = yellow	D = dark brown	I = ink black
L = leaf green	P = pink	

After the second test and before the next tone, the third test—a *subjective* measure of synesthetic *experiences*—was manifested as a succession of five yes-no inquiries:

> Did you feel that your experiences of color while listening to this tone could best be described as "very vivid," as though watching colored movies or patterns inside your head?
> The tone "sounded like" colors, but you didn't actually see them.
> The tone made you feel like certain colors make you feel.
> Are you unsure whether your color experiences fit any of the categories above?
> You had no color experiences at all.

The 9 tones for the second and third tests of synesthesia were half-sec tones at 200 Hz, 4840 Hz, 1100 Hz, 220 Hz, 4400 Hz, 242 Hz, 4000 Hz, 1000 Hz, and 1210 Hz—in that order.

Test for Reality Discernment. Throughout this two-phase test [21], all light sources in the laboratory were turned off, except for the computer screens. In the first phase, each subject adjusted the vividness of colored circles on the screen, until they matched the vividness of a circle imaged by the subject. In the second phase, the subject attempted to discern between a circular percept, the vividness of which was controlled in this manner, and a circular image.

At the beginning of the first phase, the bottom of the computer screen displayed three filled circles—a red circle on the left, a green circle in the center, plus a yellow circle on the right—and the top of the computer screen displayed the following instruction:

> Take a good look at the red, green, and yellow circles. When you have taken a good look, press G and the green circle will go away. With the green circle gone, try visually to imagine that there is still a green circle between the red and yellow circles. Image the green circle to be as VIVID as the two circles still on the screen. If your imaginary circle is less vivid than the other two, then turn down the CONTRAST KNOB (the closer knob) on the left side of the monitor, until the image is as vivid as the other two circles. When your image seems equally vivid, KEEP THAT CONTRAST until told otherwise and call the experimenter to CONTINUE.

The three circles—each 20 points in diameter—were horizontally separated by 5 points, and from left to right, were filled by Colors 2, 1, and 3 of BASICA Palette 0. The medium-resolution background was Color 13 (light magenta), which made Color 3 appear yellow rather than brown. At the outset of the experiment, the screen was set at maximum contrast, minimum brightness, and the illuminance of the yellow circle was maximized at 20 ft-candles. After the subject lowered the contrast to match his or her imagery, the yellow circle was covered with the probe of a Gossen Panlux 2 light meter, and the circle's illuminance was entered into the computer as an image-vividness score. Thus concluded the first phase.

Immediately thereafter, as the second phase commenced, the green circle reappeared between the red and yellow circles, and the following instruction appeared:

> Take another good look at the red, green, and yellow circles. In a moment you will be instructed to close your eyes and vividly image the three circles. While imaging the three circles with your eyes closed, you will hear a BEEP. As soon as you hear the beep, open your eyes while continuing to image the three circles, AND MERGE YOUR IMAGINARY CIRCLES WITH THE REAL CIRCLES. Keep imaging until the screen turns black. Reread these instructions if necessary. Immediately before you close your eyes and image the three circles, press C.

Three seconds after the subject pressed the letter "C," the red circle disappeared from the screen, and the computer beeped the subject to open both eyes and to merge the three imaginary circles with the real circles—only two of which remained on the light magenta background. Then, three seconds after the beep, the green and yellow circles also disappeared from the screen, and on a black background, the following succession of questions appeared one after another:

> NOW TURN THE CONTRAST ALL THE WAY UP
> After you opened your eyes, how many circles did you see? (Type 0-5)
> . . . .
> After you opened your eyes, was the red or green or yellow circle less vivid than the other circles? (Answer Y or N)
> If Y, which circle was less vivid? (Type R for the red circle, G for the green circle or Y for the yellow one)

The former of these questions served to differentiate "discerners of reality" who reportedly saw two circles, the number of real circles, from "nondiscerners of reality" who reportedly saw three circles, the number of imaginary circles. It also served to screen out subjects who reportedly saw zero circles, presumably because they failed to open their eyes before the background turned black. The latter question served to screen out subjects whose red imagery was not as vivid as the green and yellow screen, either because they failed to turn down the screen's contrast sufficiently or because they failed to image.

Subjects

From introductory psychology classes at the University of Massachusetts-Lowell, 136 subjects were sampled. All 136 subjects were included in data analyses of the synesthesia tests. However, forty-four subjects who failed to meet one of the two screening criteria above (usually the latter criterion) were excluded from statistical analyses of the reality-discernment test.

RESULTS

Hypnotic Susceptibility and Absorption

As Table 1 reveals, subjective ratings of higher absorption were not significantly correlated with behavioral indications of higher hypnotic susceptibility, but were strongly correlated with subjective ratings of more vivid imagery (lower ViVilm scores) and of thinner boundaries. Higher hypnotic susceptibility was associated with thinner boundaries and with fewer hours of sleep.

For purposes of computing noncorrelational analyses (ANOVAs), both the hypnotic susceptibility of each subject and the absorption of each subject were classified into a high, medium or low grouping. A subject scoring between 12 and 9 on Form C was classified in the high susceptibility group, between 8 and 6 in the medium susceptibility group, and between 5 and 0 in the low susceptibility group. Independently, a subject scoring between 34 and 25 on Tellegen's scale was classified in the high absorption group, between 24 and 17 in the medium absorption group, and between 16 and 0 in the low absorption group.

Image-Vividness and Reality-Discernment

Table 2 shows that vividness of imagery, as objectively measured in image-matching foot-candles, is enhanced neither by the trait of hypnotic susceptibility nor by the state of hypnosis. Accordingly, with foot-candles as the dependent variable, an analysis of variance reveals no main effect of the trait of susceptibility, $F(2,86) = 0.33$, no main effect of the state of arousal, $F(1,86) = 0.62$, and no two-way interaction, $F(2,86) = 1.08$.

Table 2 also shows that reality-discernment—discernment of two real circles while imaging a third of equal vividness—is diminished by being in the high susceptibility group and, independently, by being in the hypnotic state. With the

Table 1. Correlations Between the Stanford Group Hypnotic Susceptibility Scale (Form C), Tellegen's Absorption Scale (Absorp), Hartmann's Boundaries Questionnaire (Bounds), Marks' Vividness of Visual Imagery Questionnaire (ViVilm), and Hours of Sleep (HrsSlp)

	Form C	Absorp	Bounds	ViVilm	HrsSlp
Form C		.12	.20*	−.04	−.18*
Absorp			.67*	−.23*	−.13
Bounds				−.13	−.15
ViVilm					.13
HrsSlp					

*$df = 134$, two-tailed $p < .05$.

Table 2. Hypnotic States and Traits, Related Not to Greater
Imagery-vividness but to Poorer Reality-discernment

State of Arousal Trait of Susceptibility	Objective Measure of Imagery-vividness (of foot-candles corresponding to the imaged circle)	Probability of *Poor* Reality-discernment (of "seeing" 3 circles when 2 are presented and 1 is imaged)
Pre-hypnotic arousal		
Low suscept. ($n = 14$)	5.7 (*SD* = 5.8)	.07
Med. suscept. ($n = 14$)	8.6 (*SD* = 7.3)	.14
High suscept. ($n = 17$)	6.4 (*SD* = 5.8)	.53
Hypnotic trance		
Low suscept. ($n = 18$)	7.4 (*SD* = 7.0)	.17
Med. suscept. ($n = 18$)	7.1 (*SD* = 6.7)	.39
High suscept. ($n = 11$)	9.8 (*SD* = 6.7)	.73

probability of "seeing" three circles as the dependent variable, an analysis of variance confirms both a main effect of the trait of susceptibility, $F(2,86) = 10.79$, $p < .001$, and a main effect of the state of arousal, $F(1,86) = 3.89$, $p = .05$, but no two-way interaction, $F(2,86) = 0.25$.

Poor discerners of *pre*-hypnotic reality tend to be more susceptible in a subsequent hypnotic state (as Table 2 indicates), and more susceptible subjects tend to sleep less (as Table 1 indicates). Accordingly, Table 3 confirms that poor discerners of *pre*-hypnotic reality tend to sleep fewer hours. An analysis of variance for sleep verifies the significance of this interaction between poor versus good reality-discernment and the *pre*-hypnotic versus hypnotic state, $F(1,88) = 11.06$, $p = .001$.

In contrast with Table 2, Table 4 shows that reality-discernment is diminished neither by the *trait of absorption* nor by the state of hypnosis. Rather, reality-discernment is enhanced through the interaction of the high absorption group with the *pre*-hypnotic state, and reality-discernment is diminished through the interaction of the high absorption group with the hypnotic state. Thus, controlling for hypnotic susceptibility, an analysis of covariance with reality-discernment as the dependent variable reveals no main effect of the trait of absorption, $F(2,85) = 0.26$, and no main effect of the state of arousal, $F(1,85) = 2.77$, but a significant interaction between absorption and arousal, $F(2,85) = 3.06$, $p = .05$. For Table 4 as for Table 2, an analysis with imagery-vividness as the dependent variable reveals no main effect of trait, $F(2,85) = 0.50$, no main effect of state, $F(1,85) = 0.69$, and no two-way interaction, $F(2,85) = 1.29$.

Table 3. Poorer Pre-hypnotic Reality-discernment, Related to Fewer
Hours of Sleep in a Typical Twenty-four-hour Period

	Hours of Sleep
Poor discerners of pre-hypnotic reality (12 Ss who "saw" 3 circles incl. 1 image)	5.2 (SD = 1.7)
Good discerners of pre-hypnotic reality (33 Ss who saw only 2 real circles)	6.9 (SD = 1.5)
Poor discerners of hypnotic reality (18 Ss who "saw" 3 circles incl. 1 image)	6.9 (SD = 0.7)
Good discerners of hypnotic reality (29 Ss who saw only 2 real circles when 2 were presented and 1 was imaged)	6.8 (SD = 0.9)

Table 4. Absorption, Related to Better Reality-discernment before
Hypnosis and Poorer Reality-discernment during Hypnosis

State of Arousal Level of Absorption	Objective Measure of Imagery-vividness (of foot-candles corresponding to the imaged circle)	Probability of *Poor* Reality-discernment (of "seeing" 3 circles when 2 are presented and 1 is imaged)
Pre-hypnotic arousal		
Low absorption (n = 15)	7.1 (SD = 7.0)	.33
Med. absorption (n = 18)	7.0 (SD = 6.4)	.28
High absorption (n = 12)	6.5 (SD = 5.7)	.17
Hypnotic trance		
Low absorption (n = 17)	6.1 (SD = 6.0)	.29
Med. absorption (n = 19)	7.7 (SD = 7.5)	.37
High absorption (n = 11)	10.7 (SD = 6.3)	.55

Synesthesia

Subjective Experience. Table 5 indicates that subjective reports of
"seeing color" during tones were more frequent in the high absorption group and,
independently, in the hypnotic state. However, subjective reports of "thinking
about color" during tones were more frequent only across higher levels of absorption, not across states of arousal. Analyses of covariance controlling for hypnotic

susceptibility confirmed both of these indications. An analysis for "seeing color" revealed a main effect of absorption levels, $F(2,129) = 8.20$, $p < .001$, a main effect of arousal states, $F(1,129) = 4.74$, $p < .05$, and no interaction, $F(2,129) = 0.51$. An analysis for "thinking about color" revealed a main effect of absorption, $F(2,129) = 3.03$, $p = .05$, *no* main effect of arousal, $F(1,129) = 0.06$, and no interaction, $F(2,129) = 0.21$.

Subjective Chromatonal Correspondence. In Table 6, the subjective matching of low tones with dark colors, medium tones with medium colors, and high tones with light colors is lowest in highly absorbed subjects in the *pre*-hypnotic state, but highest in highly absorbed subjects in the hypnotic state. *It is noteworthy that this facilitative effect of hypnosis on highly absorbed subjects' chromotonal matches is paralleled, in Table 4, by the attenuating effect of hypnosis on highly absorbed subjects' reality-discernment. Furthermore, this hypnotically facilitated rise in highly absorbed subjects' chromotonal matches—from 49 percent to 67 percent—is paralleled, in Table 5, by the hypnotically facilitated rise in "seeing color" during tones—from 40 percent to 65 percent. (The lack of change in less absorbed subjects' chromotonal matches—from 60 and 60% to 59 and 61%—is paralleled, in Table 5, by the lack of change in their "thinking about color"—from 60 and 66% to 57 and 73%.)* Controlling susceptibility, an analysis of covariance for chromotonal matching confirms a significant interaction between levels of absorption and states of arousal, $F(2,129) = 3.60, p < .05$, as well as no main effect of absorption, $F(2,129) = 0.24$, and no main effect of arousal, $F(1,129) = 2.14$.

Objective Chromotonal Correspondence. For the test of frequency memory for colors (and frequency confusion with corresponding tones), the slope

Table 5. Absorption, Related to Tendency to See Colorful Tones—
Especially in Hypnosis—and to Think of Colorful Tones

State of Arousal Level of Absorption	Proportion of Tones Wherein Colors were Reportedly "Seen"	Proportion of Tones Wherein Colors were Reportedly "Thought Of "
Pre-hypnotic arousal		
Low absorption (*n* = 20)	.17 (*SD* = .23)	.60 (*SD* = .37)
Med. absorption (*n* = 33)	.34 (*SD* = .32)	.66 (*SD* = .37)
High absorption (*n* = 13)	.40 (*SD* = .34)	.80 (*SD* = .29)
Hypnotic trance		
Low absorption (*n* = 24)	.26 (*SD* = .31)	,57 (*SD* = .35)
Med. absorption (*n* = 28)	.42 (*SD* = .35)	.73 (*SD* = .33)
High absorption (*n* = 18)	.65 (*SD* = .35)	.80 (*SD* = .28)

Table 6. Absorption, Related to Chromotonal Independence
before Hypnosis and Chromotonal Correspondence
during Hypnosis

State of Arousal Level of Absorption	Proportion of Low, Medium, and High Tones Matched with Dark, Medium, and Light Colors, Respectively
Pre-hypnotic arousal	
Low absorption (n = 20)	.60 (SD = .19)
Med. absorption (n = 33)	.60 (SD = .18)
High absorption (n = 13)	.49 (SD = .13)
Hypnotic trance	
Low absorption (n = 24)	.59 (SD = .18)
Med. absorption (n = 28)	.61 (SD = .17)
High absorption (n = 18)	.67 (SD = .20)

of each subject's estimated color frequencies, over actual frequencies (2, 5, or 8 depending on the color), was computed by the method of least squares regression. For subjects tested in the pre-hypnotic state, the average slope of estimated frequencies over actual frequencies was .17 (SD = .24), and for subjects tested in the hypnotic state, the average slope was .10 (SD = .27). In addition, each subject's slope was computed for estimated color frequencies over corresponding tone frequencies. Because the 3 low tones corresponding to the 3 dark colors in this experiment were presented more frequently, it was expected that the latter slope would be closer to unity, especially during hypnosis. However, for pre-hypnotic subjects, the average slope of estimated color frequencies over corresponding-tone frequencies was .15 (SD = .41), and for hypnotized subjects, the average slope was .03 (SD = .43). If the primary effect of hypnosis on our "objective" measure of chromotonal correspondence is to promote amnesia for all frequencies, rather than confusion between color frequencies and tone frequencies, then our "objective" measure has little value in the context of hypnosis.

CONCLUSIONS

In this study of hypnosis, we have examined two cognitive boundaries that are supposedly obscured during regressive or "primary process" mentation: the boundary between visual and auditory *modalities* of sensation, and the boundary between imaginal and perceptual *sources* of sensation. We have found that auditory tones in the hypnotic state are more likely to be experienced as colorful, in accordance with recently proposed laws of chromotonal correspondence [13, 14, 80, 81, 83]. In addition, we have confirmed that hallucinatory images are not more vivid than normal [15, 17, 100]; such images, during hypnosis or following very little sleep, are simply less differentiable from percepts of equivalent vividness. As Hilgard notes, a faint hallucination like "an apparition, ghost or wraith need not be fully lifelike to be seen 'out there' " rather than in one's imagination [101, p. 14].

Finally, we have discovered that cognitively differentiable boundaries are not only thinnest in highly absorbed subjects under hypnosis, but also thickest in highly absorbed subjects outside hypnosis. This discovery proved true both for *modality* differentiation as measured by chromotonal independence and for *source* differentiation as measured by reality discernment. Accordingly, the psychological regression underlying hypnotic synesthesia and hypnotic hallucination reflects neither a psychological state nor a personality trait. Rather, the hypnotic attenuation of both modality monitoring and source monitoring reflects an interaction between the state of hypnosis and the trait of absorption—an interaction best described as "adaptive regression" in the service of high absorbers, who normally are the very best discerners of reality [30, p. 139].

REFERENCES

1. A. Tellegen and G. Atkinson, Openness to Absorbing and Self-altering Experiences ("Absorption"), a Trait Related to Hypnotic Susceptibility, *Journal of Abnormal Psychology, 83,* pp. 268-277, 1974.
2. A. Tellegen, Practicing the Two Disciplines for Relaxation and Enlightenment: Comment on "Role of the Feedback Signal in Electromyograph Biofeedback: The Relevance of Attention: by Qualls and Sheehan, *Journal of Experimental Psychology: General, 110,* pp. 217-226, 1981.
3. S. M. Roche and K. M. McConkey, Absorption: Nature, Assessment, and Correlates, *Journal of Personality and Social Psychology, 59,* pp. 91-101, 1990.
4. E. Hartmann, Thin and Thick Boundaries: Personality, Dreams, and Imagination, in *Mental Imagery,* R. G. Kunzendorf (ed.), Plenum, New York, pp. 71-78, 1990.
5. E. Hartmann, *Boundaries in the Mind: A New Psychology of Personality,* Basic, New York, 1991.
6. S. C. Wilson and T. X. Barber, The Fantasy-prone Personality: Implications for Understanding Imagery, Hypnosis, and Parapsychological Phenomena, in *Imagery: Current Theory, Research, and Application,* A. A. Sheikh (ed.), Wiley, New York, pp. 340-387, 1983.
7. R. Nadon, J.-R. Laurence, and C. Perry, The Two Disciplines of Scientific Hypnosis: A Synergistic Model, in *Theories of Hypnosis: Current Models and Perspectives,* S. J. Lynn and J. W. Rhue (eds.), Guilford, New York, pp. 485-519, 1991.
8. M. de Groh, Correlates of Hypnotic Susceptibility, in *Hypnosis: The Cognitive-Behavioral Perspective,* N. P. Spanos and J. F. Chaves (eds.), Prometheus Books, Buffalo, New York, pp. 32-63, 1989.
9. J. F. Kihlstrom, Hypnosis, *Annual Review of Psychology, 36,* pp. 385-418, 1985.
10. P. W. Sheehan, Hypnosis and the Process of Imagination, in *Hypnosis: Developments in Research and New Perspectives* (2nd Edition), E. Fromm and R. Shor (eds.), Aldine, New York, pp. 381-411, 1979.

11. R. G Kunzendorf and J. Maurer, Hypnotic Attenuation of the 'Boundaries' between Emotional, Visual, and Auditory Sensations, *Imagination, Cognition and Personality, 8,* pp. 225-234, 1988-89.
12. C. M. Rader, *Explorations in Synesthesia,* unpublished doctoral dissertation, University of Minnesota, 1979.
13. C. M. Rader and A. Tellegen, A Comparison of Synesthetes and Nonsynesthetes, in *Imagery: Vol. 2, Concepts, Results, and Applications,* E. Klinger (ed.), Plenum, New York, pp. 153-163, 1981.
14. C. M. Rader and A. Tellegen, An Investigation of Synesthesia, *Journal of Personality and Social Psychology, 52* pp. 981-987, 1987.
15. R. G. Kunzendorf, Hypnotic Hallucinations as 'Unmonitored' Images: An Empirical Study, *Imagination, Cognition and Personality, 5,* pp. 255-270, 1985-86.
16. R. G. Kunzendorf, Repression as the Monitoring and Censoring of Images: An Empirical Study, *Imagination, Cognition and Personality, 5,* pp. 31-39, 1985-86.
17. R. G. Kunzendorf, Self-consciousness as the Monitoring of Cognitive States, *Imagination, Cognition and Personality, 7,* pp. 3-22, 1987-88.
18. R. G. Kunzendorf, Posthypnotic Amnesia: Dissociation of Self-concept or Self-consciousness?, *Imagination, Cognition and Personality, 9,* pp. 321-334, 1989-90.
19. R. G. Kunzendorf and A. A. Sheikh, Imaging, Image-monitoring, and Health, in *The Psychophysiology of Mental Imagery: Theory, Research, and Application,* R. G. Kunzendorf and A. A. Sheikh (eds.), Baywood, Amityville, New York, pp. 185-202, 1990.
20. R. G. Kunzendorf, S. M. Beltz, and G. Tymowicz, Self-awareness in Autistic Subjects and Deeply Hypnotized Subjects: Dissociation of Self-concept versus Self-consciousness, *Imagination, Cognition and Personality, 11,* pp. 129-141, 1991.
21. R. G. Kunzendorf, C. Carrabino, and D. Capone, 'Safe' Fantasy: The Self-consciousness Boundary between Wishing and Willing, *Imagination, Cognition and Personality, 12,* pp. 177-188, 1992.
22. A. Tellegen, On Measures and Conceptions of Hypnosis, *American Journal of Clinical Hypnosis, 21,* pp. 219-237, 1979.
23. R. J. Wiseman and J. Reyher, Hypnotically Induced Dreams Using the Rorschach Inkblots as Stimuli: A Test of Freud's Theory of Dreams, *Journal of Personality and Social Psychology, 27,* pp. 329-336, 1973.
24. A. G. Hammer, W. Walker, and A. D. Diment, A Nonsuggested Effect of Trance Induction, in *Hypnosis at its Bicentennial: Selected Papers,* F. H. Frankel and H. S. Zamansky (eds.), Plenum, New York, pp. 91-100, 1978.
25. D. Gruenewald, E. Fromm, and M. I. Oberlander, Hypnosis and Adaptive Regression: An Ego-psychological Inquiry, in *Hypnosis: Research Developments and Perspectives,* E. Fromm and R. E. Shor (eds.), Aldine, Chicago, pp. 495-509, 1972.
26. D. Barrett, The Hypnotic Dream: Its Relation to Nocturnal Dreams and Waking Fantasies, *Journal of Abnormal Psychology, 88,* pp. 584-591, 1979.
27. M. M. Gill and M. Brenman, *Hypnosis and Related States: Psychoanalytic Studies in Regression,* International Universities Press, New York, 1959.
28. E. Fromm, The Nature of Hypnosis and Other Altered States of Consciousness: An Ego-psychological Theory, in *Hypnosis: Developments in Research and New Perspectives* (2nd Edition), E. Fromm and R. Shor (eds.), Aldine, New York, pp. 81-103, 1979.
29. E. Fromm, L. Lombard, S. H. Skinner, and S. Kahn, The Modes of the Ego in Self-hypnosis, *Imagination, Cognition and Personality, 7,* pp. 335-349, 1987-88.
30. E. Fromm, An Ego-psychological Theory of Hypnosis, in *Contemporary Hypnosis Research,* E. Fromm and M. R. Nash (eds.), Guilford, New York, pp. 131-148, 1992.

31. M. R. Nash, Hypnosis as a Special Case of Psychological Regression, in *Theories of Hypnosis: Current Models and Perspectives,* S. J. Lynn and J. W. Rhue (eds.), Guilford, New York, pp. 171-194, 1991.
32. M. R. Nash, Hypnosis, Psychopathology, and Psychological Regression, in *Contemporary Hypnosis Research,* E. Fromm and M. R. Nash (eds.), Guilford, New York, pp. 149-169, 1992.
33. A. Ås, J. W. O'Hara, and M. P. Munger, The Measurement of Subjective Experiences Presumably Related to Hypnotic Susceptibility, *Scandinavian Journal of Psychology, 3,* pp. 47-64, 1962.
34. E. Lee-Teng, Trance-susceptibility, Induction-susceptibility, and Acquiescence as Factors in Hypnotic Performance, *Journal of Abnormal Psychology, 70,* pp. 383-389, 1965.
35. J. R. Hilgard, *Personality and Hypnosis: A Study of Imaginative Involvement,* University of Chicago Press, Chicago, 1970.
36. R. E. Shor, M. T. Orne, and D. N. O'Connell, Validation and Cross-validation of a Scale of Self-reported Personal Experiences which Predicts Hypnotizability, *Journal of Psychology, 53,* pp. 55-75, 1962.
37. A. H. Roberts and A. Tellegen, Ratings of Trust and Hypnotic Susceptibility, *International Journal of Clinical and Experimental Hypnosis, 21,* pp. 289-297, 1973.
38. R. E. Shor and E. C. Orne, *Harvard Group Scale of Hypnotic Susceptibility,* Consulting Psychologists Press, Palo Alto, California, 1962.
39. P. B. Field and R. Palmer, Factor Analysis: Hypnosis Inventory, *International Journal of Clinical and Experimental Hypnosis, 17,* pp. 50-61, 1969.
40. H. P. de Groot, M. I. Gwynn, and N. P. Spanos, The Effects of Contextual Information and Gender on the Prediction of Hypnotic Susceptibility, *Journal of Personality and Social Psychology, 54,* pp. 1049-1053, 1988.
41. R. Nadon, I. P. Hoyt, P. A. Register, and J. F. Kihlstrom, Absorption and Hypnotizability: Context Effects Reexamined, *Journal of Personality and Social Psychology, 60,* pp. 144-153, 1991.
42. I. Kirsch and J. R. Council, Situational and Personality Correlates of Hypnotic Responsiveness, in *Contemporary Hypnosis Research,* E. Fromm and M. R. Nash (eds.), Guilford, New York, pp. 267-291, 1992.
43. K. M. McConkey, P. W. Sheehan, and H. G. Law, Structural Analysis of the Harvard Group Scale of Hypnotic Susceptibility, Form A, *International Journal of Clinical and Experimental Hypnosis, 28,* pp. 164-175, 1980.
44. C. G. Balthazard and E. Z. Woody, The Spectral Analysis of Hypnotic Performance with Respect to "Absorption," *International Journal of Clinical and Experimental Hypnosis, 40,* pp. 21-43, 1992.
45. E. Fromm and S. Kahn, *Self-Hypnosis: The Chicago Paradigm,* Guilford, New York, 1990.
46. R. E. Shor, Hypnosis and the Concept of the Generalized Reality-orientation, *American Journal of Psychotherapy, 13,* pp. 582-602, 1959.
47. J. F. Kihlstrom, P. A. Register, I. P. Hoyt, J. S. Albright, E. M. Grigorian, W. C. Heindel, and C. R. Morrison, Dispositional Correlates of Hypnosis: A Phenomenological Approach, *International Journal of Clinical and Experimental Hypnosis, 37,* pp. 249-263, 1989.
48. D. Marks, Visual Imagery Differences in the Recall of Pictures, *British Journal of Psychology, 64,* pp. 17-24, 1973.
49. H. J. Crawford, Hypnotizability, Daydreaming Styles, Imagery Vividness, and Absorption: A Multidimensional Study, *Journal of Personality and Social Psychology, 42,* pp. 915-926, 1982.

50. R. J. Pekala, C. F. Wenger, and R. L. Levine, Individual Differences in Phenomenological Experience: States of Consciousness as a Function of Absorption, *Journal of Personality and Social Psychology, 48,* pp. 125-132, 1985.
51. V. K. Kumar and R. J. Pekala, Hypnotizability, Absorption, and Individual Differences in Phenomenological Experience, *International Journal of Clinical and Experimental Hypnosis, 36,* pp. 80-88, 1988.
52. A. Binet and C. Féré, *Animal Magnetism,* Kegan, Paul, and French, London, 1887.
53. A. Ås, J. P. Sutcliff, C. W. Perry, and P. W. Sheehan, Relation of Some Aspects of Imagery and Fantasy to Hypnotic Susceptibility, *Journal of Abnormal Psychology, 76,* pp. 279-287, 1970.
54. G. H. Betts, The Distribution and Functions of Mental Imagery, *Teachers College Contributions to Education, whole no. 26,* 1909.
55. A. M. Weitzenhoffer and E. R. Hilgard, *Stanford Hypnotic Susceptibility Scale, Form C,* Consulting Psychologists Press, Palo Alto, California, 1962.
56. M. J. Diamond and R. Taft, The Role Played by Ego Permissiveness and Imagery in Hypnotic Responsivity, *International Journal of Clinical and Experimental Hypnosis, 23,* pp. 130-138, 1975.
57. C. Perry, Imagery, Fantasy and Hypnotic Susceptibility, *Journal of Personality and Social Psychology, 26,* pp. 217-221, 1973.
58. A. H. Morgan and D. Lam, The Relationship of the Betts Vividness of Imagery Questionnaire and Hypnotic Susceptibility: Failure to Replicate, *Research Memorandum No. 103,* Hawthorne House, Stanford, California, 1969.
59. N. P. Spanos, Imagery, Hypnosis and Hypnotizability, in *Mental Imagery,* R. G. Kunzendorf (ed.), Plenum, New York, pp. 79-88, 1991.
60. N. E. Hayneman, The Role of Imagery in Hypnosis: An Information Processing Approach, *International Journal of Clinical and Experimental Hypnosis, 38,* pp. 39-59, 1990.
61. S. C. Wilson and T. X. Barber, The Creative Imagination Scale as a Measure of Hypnotic Responsiveness: Applications to Experimental and Clinical Hypnosis, *American Journal of Clinical Hypnosis, 20,* pp. 235-240, 1978.
62. R. Nadon, J.-R. Laurence, and C. Perry, Multiple Predictors of Hypnotic Susceptibility, *Journal of Personality and Social Psychology, 53,* pp. 948-960, 1987.
63. N. P. Spanos, J. L. D'Eau, A. E. Pawlak, C. D. Mah, and G. Ritchie, A Multivariate Study of Hypnotic Susceptibility, *Imagination, Cognition and Personality, 9,* pp. 33-48, 1989-90.
64. E. Hartmann, Boundaries of Dreams, Boundaries of Dreamers: Thin and Thick Boundaries as a New Personality Measure, *Psychiatric Journal of the University of Ottawa, 14,* pp. 557-560, 1989.
65. E. Hartmann, D. Russ, B. van der Kolk, R. Falke, and M. Oldfield, A Preliminary Study of the Personality of the Nightmare Sufferer: Relationship to Schizophrenia and Creativity?, *American Journal of Psychiatry, 138,* pp. 794-797, 1981.
66. E. Hartmann, R. Harrison, J. Bevis, I. Hurwitz, A. Holevas, and H. Dawani, The Boundary Questionnaire: A Measure of Thin and Thick Boundaries Derived from Work with Nightmare Sufferers, *Sleep Research, 16,* p. 274, 1987.
67. E. Hartmann, D. Russ, M. Oldfield, I. Sivan, and S. Cooper, Who Has Nightmares? The Personality of the Lifelong Nightmare Sufferer, *Archives of General Psychiatry, 44,* pp. 49-56, 1987.
68. S. R. Hathaway and J. C. McKinley, *The Minnesota Multiphasic Personality Inventory Manual,* Psychological Corporation, New York, 1951, 1967.
69. J. E. Exner, *The Rorschach: A Comprehensive System, Vol. 1: Basic Foundations,* Wiley, New York, 1986.

70. I. Sivan, *Anxiety and Ego Functions of Nightmare Dreamers,* unpublished Master's thesis, Haifa University, Israel, 1983.
71. H. A. Murray, *Thematic Apperception Test Manual,* Harvard University Press, Cambridge, Massachusetts, 1943.
72. D. Barrett, *The Relationship of Thin versus Thick Boundaries to Hypnotic Susceptibility,* paper presented to the Eastern Psychological Association, Boston, 1989.
73. E. Galton, *Inquiries into Human Faculty and Its Development,* Macmillan, London, 1883.
74. A. Binet, Le Problème de L'Audition Colorée, *Revue des Deux-Mondes, 113,* pp. 586-614, 1892.
75. A. Binet, L'Application de la Psychométrie à l'Etude de L'Audition Colorée, *Revue Philosophique, 36,* pp. 334-336, 1893.
76. E. Bleuler and K. Lehmann, *Zwangsmassige Lichtempfindungen durch Schall und verdwandte Erscheinungen,* Fues' Verlag, Leipzig, 1881.
77. H. Werner, L'Unite de Sens, *Journal de Psychologie Normale et Pathologique, 31,* pp. 190-205, 1934.
78. H. Werner, *Comparative Psychology of Mental Development,* International Universities Press, New York, 1948.
79. R. E. Cytowic, *Synesthesia: A Union of the Senses,* Springer Verlag, New York, 1989.
80. L. E. Marks, *The Unity of the Senses: Interrelations among the Modalities,* Academic, New York, 1978.
81. L. E. Marks, On Associations of Light and Sound: the Mediation of Brightness, Pitch, and Loudness, *American Journal of Psychology, 87,* pp. 173-188, 1974.
82. L. A. Riggs and T. Karwoski, Synaesthesia, *British Journal of Psychology, 25,* pp. 29-41, 1934.
83. L. E. Marks, On Colored-hearing Synesthesia: Cross-modal Translations of Sensory Dimensions, *Psychological Bulletin, 82,* pp. 303-331, 1975.
84. H. Jones, *Synesthesia and Its Role in Memory,* unpublished doctoral dissertation, University of Texas, 1976.
85. R. E. Lehman, *Imagery, Imagination, and Hypnosis,* unpublished doctoral dissertation, University of Oregon, 1972.
86. S. M. Shindell, *Personality Characteristics Associated with Reported Synesthesia,* unpublished manuscript, 1986.
87. J. Raven, *Mill Hill Vocabulary Scale,* H. K. Lewis, London, 1943.
88. H. G. Gough, The Adjective Check List as a Personality Assessment Research Technique, *Psychological Reports, 6,* pp. 107-122, 1960.
89. K. S. Bowers and P. G. Bowers, Hypnosis and Creativity: A Theoretical and Empirical Rapproachement, in *Hypnosis: Developments in Research and New Perspectives* (2nd Edition), E. Fromm and R. Shor (eds.), Aldine, New York, pp. 371-379, 1979.
90. V. A. Shames and P. G. Bowers, Hypnosis and Creativity, in *Contemporary Hypnosis Research,* E. Fromm and M. R. Nash (eds.), Guilford, New York, pp. 334-363, 1992.
91. N. S. Walker, J. B. Garrett, and B. Wallace, Restoration of Eidetic Imagery via Hypnotic Age Regression: A Preliminary Report, *Journal of Abnormal Psychology, 85,* pp. 335-337, 1976.
92. B. Wallace, Restoration of Eidetic Imagery via Hypnotic Age Regression: More Evidence, *Journal of Abnormal Psychology, 87,* pp. 673-675, 1978.
93. H. Crawford, B. Wallace, K. Nomura, and H. Slater, Eidetic-like Imagery in Hypnosis: Rare but There, *American Journal of Psychology, 99,* pp. 527-546, 1986.
94. A. Tellegen, *Personal Communication,* September 30, 1992.

95. R. G. Kunzendorf, C. Brown, and D. McGee, Hypnotizability: Correlations with Daydreaming and Sleeping, *Psychological Reports, 53,* p. 406, 1983.
96. A. Tellegen, *Multidimensional Personality Questionnaire,* 1982. (Available from Dr. Auke Tellegen, Department of Psychology, University of Minnesota, Minneapolis, MN 55455.)
97. A. Tellegen, *Brief Manual for the Differential Personality Questionnaire* [renamed Multidimensional Personality Questionnaire], 1982. (Available from Dr. Auke Tellegen, Department of Psychology, University of Minnesota, Minneapolis, MN 55455.)
98. H. J. Crawford and S. N. Allen, *Stanford Group Hypnotic Susceptibility Scale, Form C,* 1982. (Available from Dr. Helen Crawford, Department of Psychology, Virginia Polytechnic and State University, Blacksburg, Virginia 24061.)
99. M. K. Johnson, C. L. Raye, A. Y. Wang, and T. H. Taylor, Fact and Fantasy: The Roles of Accuracy and Variability in Confusing Imaginations with Perceptual Experience, *Journal of Experimental Psychology: Human Learning and Memory, 5,* pp. 229-240, 1979.
100. N. P. Spanos and H. L. Radtke, Hypnotic Visual Hallucinations as Imaginings: A Cognitive-social Psychological Perspective, *Imagination, Cognition and Personality, 2,* pp. 195-210, 1982-83.
101. E. R. Hilgard, Imagery and Imagination in American Psychology, *Journal of Mental Imagery, 5,* pp. 5-66, 1981.

CHAPTER 6

Fantasizers and Dissociaters: Two Types of High Hypnotizables, Two Different Imagery Styles

DEIRDRE BARRETT

Wilson and Barber studied a group of high hypnotic susceptibles and reported that all but one of them were what they termed "fantasizers": people with an extreme degree of involvement in imaginative activity [1, 2]. Their fantasizers had a hallucinatory degree of vividness to their imagery, they spent 50 percent or more of their time fantasizing often while carrying out everyday tasks, and they experienced dramatic physiologic reactions to their imagery. Subsequent studies have confirmed a relationship of hypnotizability and fantasy proneness but found it to account for a minority of their variance [3-5].

In addition to standard criteria for high hypnotizability, Wilson and Barber included the ability to reenter hypnosis rapidly without a formal induction as one of their inclusion factors. This was their most unusual requirement; standard measures of hypnotic susceptibility such as the Harvard Group Scale of Hypnotic Susceptibility [6] and the Stanford Scale of Hypnotic Susceptibility, Form C [7] give subjects about fifteen minutes of hypnotic induction before beginning the specific suggestions to be scored for hypnotizability. It seemed likely that this criteria might distinguish the fantasizers from other high hypnotizables.

The present study set out to examine the replicability of Wilson and Barber's findings about fantasy activity among high hypnotizables and to explore what traits might characterize high hypnotizables who were not extreme fantasizers. Thirty-four subjects, twenty-two women and twelve men, who scored 11 or 12 on both the HGSHS and the SSHS-C were selected from a pool of approximately 1200 undergraduate college students. Thus, they represented about the 3 percent most hypnotizable, approximately the same level as in Wilson and Barber's study. Subjects completed an absorption scale [8] and an inventory of hypnotic experience [9]. They were tested for both suggested and spontaneous amnesia for hypnosis. Their response to a rapid re-hypnosis suggestion similar to Wilson and Barber's was tested.

These thirty-four subjects were initially interviewed for two-and-one-half to four hours about their hypnotic and waking experiences including asking them whether their waking imagery was entirely realistic, whether they experienced amnesia for daydreaming, what was the age of their earliest recollection, and about whether hypnosis was very different from their other experiences. Details of the procedure have been described elsewhere in more detail [10, 11].

In a later follow-up with the twenty-four subjects who were still geographically available (15 women, 9 men) they were hypnotized again, given suggestions for hypnotic deafness before the first four lines of a recorded nursery rhyme were played at a clear volume, and then tested for the Hilgard's hidden observer phenomena [12]. These twenty-four were then interviewed with detailed queries about childhood trauma, dream content, and diagnostic questions for dissociative disorders. This follow-up study's method has been described in detail elsewhere [13].

Statistical analyses were performed contrasting subjects who responded positively to the instant re-hypnosis suggestion with those who did not for all other variables. Chi-square analyses were employed where expected cell size allowed; for smaller subsamples, significance was computed by Fisher's Exact Probability Test.

WAKING IMAGERY, FANTASY, AND MEMORIES

The first subgroup of deep trance subjects was selected by their ability to enter a deep trance rapidly and to pass SHSS-C items without the scale's formal induction. These nineteen people, twelve women, seven men, also differed significantly from subjects who did not achieve their deep trances immediately on the other variables in the study. These characteristics on which they scored higher clustered around vividness of fantasy processes, so they are referred to for the rest of this discussion by Wilson and Barber's term "fantasizers."

Waking imagery was very realistic for the fantasizers. Sixteen of them said their imagery was entirely realistic. When asked about amnesia for daydreams— whether they "startled" out of daydreams which they could not recall, four said they experienced this occasionally although usually then had a "tip of the tongue" feeling about the fantasy and its memory would "come back" to them shortly.

Their vivid fantasies began in childhood. They had at least one, most many, imaginary companions. These included a real playmate who had moved out of state, a princess, an entire herd of wild horses, and space aliens among others. The fantasizers greatly enjoyed stories, movies, and drama; they tended to prolong their experience of these by incorporating them into their fantasy lives, providing another source of imaginary companions. For example one subject described that after seeing the movie Camelot, he had spent two years engaging daily in an elaborate scenario in which he was the son of Arthur and Guinivere and commanded the King's court. Periodically he would appoint new knights of his own invention to the roundtable. His real-life brother was cast in the role of Mordred, but all the other characters were either from the film, or completely from his own imagination. The fantasizers described these imaginary companions as every bit as vivid as real persons.

Their adult fantasy continued to occupy the majority of their waking hours. They all fantasized throughout the performance of routine tasks and during any unoccupied time. Six of them said they did not "fantasize" or "daydream" when dealing with the most demanding tasks, but still continued to have vivid images in response to any sensory words or geometric tasks that occurred. The other thirteen said they continued to have elaborate ongoing fantasy scenarios. Some experienced these superimposed and intertwined with the ongoing tasks: "I'm listening to my boss's directions carefully, but I'm seeing the "Saturday Night Live" character "Mockman" next to him mocking all his gestures." Others experienced the fantasies as simultaneous or separate, happening "on a side stage," as one subject described it: "somehow I'm seeing the real world and experiencing my fantasy one at the same time."

All of these subjects described some of the dreamlike, surreal content, sudden transitions, and surprise that two earlier studies have reported for deep trance subjects' daydreams [1, 2, 14]. Seven of them reported that they occasionally had "daymares"—frightening fantasies that seemed not to be under their control.

All of the fantasizers described sometimes experiencing physical sensations to visual stimuli such as feeling hot, dry, and impulsively getting something to drink in response to looking at desert photos, getting motion sickness at a film set on a tossing submarine, or feeling pain when seeing someone injured on TV. Fourteen of the fantasizers could experience orgasm through fantasy in the absence of any physical stimulation, and all of them reported frequent, vivid and varied sexual fantasies.

Fantasizers all had some experiences which they considered "psychic." This is in keeping with Wilson and Barber's reports and similar to another study in which the present author found high hypnotizability to correlate with "psychic" dreams and out-of-body experiences [15].

The earliest memories of the fantasizers were all subjectively identified as being before the age of three, and before the age of two for eleven subjects. For randomly selected college students, the average age of subjectively recalled first memory is about three-and-a-half and two to six is the usual range [16, 17].

Fantasizers all scored high on the Absorption Scale: with a range of 32-37 of 37 items and a mean of 34 (see Table 1).

The other subgroup of fifteen subjects was selected for scoring as very highly hypnotizable but not meeting Wilson and Barber's additional criterion of being able to enter a trance rapidly. They did not display many of Wilson

Table 1. Waking Imagery Characteristics of Fantasizers
Compared with Dissociaters

Characteristic	Fantasizers (12 Women, 7 Men)		Dissociaters (10 Women, 5 Men)		Chi Square $df = 1$
	Yes	No	Yes	No	$\chi =$
Waking image less than real	3	16	15	0	20.05**
Daydream amnesia	3	16	14	1	15.22**
Earliest memory > 3	0	19	11	4	14.44**
Absorption score low	0	19	7	8	6.19*

*$p < .02$
**$p < .001$

and Barber's fantasizers' characteristics. The distinguishing traits of this group cluster around amnestic and dissociative phenomena and they are referred to as "dissociaters."

None of the dissociaters initially described their waking imagery as entirely realistic. Five of them said they rarely or never were able to produce imagery in any sensory modality. When asked about daydream amnesia, fourteen of them said their fantasizing was often characterized by inability to remember some or all of the content. The fantasies which the dissociaters did recall from both childhood and currently were usually much more mundane than the other subgroup's. They tended to be pleasant, realistic scenarios about events they would like to happen in their near future.

When reinterviewed four years after the first study, two dissociaters described that their imagery had gotten much more vivid since the first interview. They both described that the study's questions had gotten them to thinking about whether they could image things entirely realistically and they could. These still remained static images or very short fantasies. The content had not changed as the vividness did. The eight other dissociaters who returned for the follow-up study reported that their imagery had stayed the same between interviews. Most did not appear interested in questions about imagery and fantasy.

Dissociaters were somewhat more like the fantasizers in how they reacted to external drama. They described that as both children and adults, they could become so absorbed in books, films, plays, and stories being told to them that they could lose track of time, surroundings, or their usual sense of identity. However, unlike fantasizers, dissociaters described how this absorption in external stimuli was often intertwined with amnestic phenomena; several subjects commented that they thought they got very caught up in horror movies, but then could not remember their content shortly afterwards.

Dissociaters experienced dramatic psychophysiological reactions even more extreme than those of fantasizers. Five of the ten women had experienced symptoms of false pregnancy. They reported getting cold watching arctic scenes and becoming nauseated after eating supposedly spoiled food that they later learned was fine. One developed a rash after being told by a prankster friend that a harmless vine she had handled was poison ivy. Three of them also reported feeling pain when witnessing others' traumas. This might have been true of more of them, as six remarked that they often could not remember moments around witnessing injuries.

None of this group said they achieved orgasms solely from fantasy. Six subjects remarked that they knew that they had sexual fantasies but usually couldn't remember them afterward. The fantasies which they did report were mundane compared with those of the fantasizers, and dissociaters were much more likely to report guilt about them.

Fewer subjects in this subgroup believed they had psychic experiences, and for nine of the eleven who did so, these experiences were confined solely to altered states of consciousness: dreams most commonly for seven of them, automatic writing for two, and trance-like seance phenomena for two.

The earliest memories of the dissociaters were later than average and all over the age of three (mean = 5 and for 6 subjects between ages 6 and 8). This was opposite the trend for the fantasizers. Seven dissociaters scored below the norm on the Absorption Scale; eight scored at or above the norm (range 16-33, mean = 26).

RESPONSE TO HYPNOSIS

Fantasizers experienced hypnotic amnesia only when it was specifically suggested—and not always absolutely then. Six of the eight fantasizers scoring 11 rather than 12 on the HGSHS-A had the amnesia suggestion as their only failed item. Some had partial recall although they had formally passed it. Others described that it seemed not as completely real an effect as the other hypnotic phenomena, citing working to keep items out of consciousness or being very aware they could counter the suggestion if they chose. On the Field inventory, eleven of them scored higher than the norm, eight scored equal to or lower than the norm, and the group mean was 18. They scored extremely low on the six Field items which reported unusualness of hypnotic phenomena, mean = .9 (see Table 2).

They also verbally stated that hypnosis was similar to what they did when fantasizing, although most could describe some differences. These differences included hypnotic imagery being more consistently hallucinatory for six subjects, and two saying they felt much more subjective time had gone by in hypnosis than

Table 2. Hypnotic Experience of Fantasizers
versus Dissociaters

Characteristic	Fantasizers (12 Women, 7 Men)		Dissociaters (10 Women, 5 Men)		Chi Square $df = 1$
	Yes	No	Yes	No	$\chi =$
Need time to reach deep trance	0	19	15	0	30.06**
Spontaneous amnesia for trance details	0	19	9	6	11.61**
Suggested Amnesia Total	5	14	15	0	15.06**
Hypnosis very different from other experiences	2	17	15	0	22.99**
Field score high	11	8	15	0	6.08*

*$p < .02$
**$p < .001$

it would if they were fantasizing for a similar amount of real time. One drama major said:

> Hypnosis is a lot like what I do with method acting only you can get more into it. When I'm doing an acting exercise, I can only get so far into the experience because some part of me has to keep watching that I don't become the character so much that I'd just walk out of the class if he was mad, but with the hypnosis you don't have to watch that sort of thing at all. During the age regression I could leave my adult self behind completely.

Fantasizers were all quite aware that hypnosis was a phenomenon which they produced themselves. None of them conceptualized it at all in terms of something the hypnotist was doing to them. They were likely to know hypnotic hallucinations were not real without needing to be told this. When asked how they were sure they knew there had not been a real candle lit in the room for instance, fourteen of them cited some cognitive strategy which they had long practiced for differentiating the hallucinations of their waking fantasies from reality. Nine of them also usually retained memory of suggestions to hallucinate—which made the deduction simple.

All fantasizers awoke from the trance immediately alert. Some began talking about their trance experience before the experimenter asked any questions. The most common response upon awakening from hypnosis for the fantasizers was a big smile.

Dissociaters experience of hypnosis was characterized by much amnesia. Amnesia was consistent and total for them whenever it was suggested, and it sometimes persisted even once removal cues had been given. Half of them experienced some degree of spontaneous amnesia for trance events when it had not been suggested.

Dissociaters scored very high on the Field questionnaire, mean = 33, usually answering "true" to all six items which express unusualness of hypnotic phenomena. During the interviews many of them described hypnotic hallucinations as a very surprising response while amnesia was much less remarked on as unusual. Dissociaters were likelier than fantasizers to believe their hypnotic hallucinations were real until told otherwise. The few who realized they were not real, distinguished them on the basis of their implausibility rather than by any other method for telling hallucinations from reality. They almost never remembered the verbal suggestions for the hallucinations, and when they did, still ignored the association with their perceptions. One subject remained convinced that, coincidentally at the moment that I suggested the HGSHS-A fly hallucination to a roomful of subjects, a real fly happened to begin to buzz around him.

They were much likelier to conceptualize hypnotic phenomena as due to some amazing talent of the hypnotist rather than as produced by themselves. They were resistant to hearing that it was something within their control, and in some sense this may really be less true for this group: for them it is less consciously controlled.

When dissociaters were asked to awaken, they would usually open their eyes, but most blinked and looked confused at first. Four asked disoriented questions such as "what happened"? or "Where was I?" Some struggled for a moment to talk, and were slow to begin to answer questions. All of these behaviors were transient and all subjects were fully alert within a couple minutes. Several dissociaters described some hypnotic phenomena as mildly unpleasant and/or asked questions seeking reassurance that responses such as hallucinations were normal in the hypnotic situation.

HIDDEN OBSERVER

The hidden observer phenomena was slightly more common in dissociaters. Seven of nine dissociaters manifested a hidden observer, while seven of fifteen fantasizers did (see Table 3). What was much more clearly pronounced was the difference in content of hidden observers for dissociaters versus fantasizers. All dissociaters who manifested a hidden observer gave accurate descriptions of the stimulus. Four recited it flawlessly, two first named it or said "nursery rhyme" and when asked for the complete rhyme recited it with only minor mistakes. Three dissociaters gave hidden observer responses in a flat monotone similar to all other

Table 3. Hidden Observer Phenomenon of
Fantasizers versus Dissociaters

Characteristic	Fantasizers N = 15 (9 Women, 6 Men)		Dissociaters N = 9 (6 Women, 3 Men)		Fischer Exact Probability Test
	Yes	No	Yes	No	p <
Some hidden observer response	7	8	7	2	.1
Hidden observer with detailed accuracy	7	8	4	5	.85
Recurring nightmares	0	15	6	3	.005
Trauma known	2	13	5	4	.05
Trauma known or suggested	2	13	9	0	.005

requested vocalizations they had ever made in trance. Two spoke in a more childlike voice than usually characterized their waking or trance vocalizations.

The final dissociater with a hidden observer responded quite dramatically to the suggestion: opening her eyes (not suggested), saying, "Hi I think I'm who you want to talk to" in a much more aggressive demeanor than the subject's usual waking or hypnotized style, reciting the rhyme in a sarcastic tone, glaring for about fifteen seconds, and then closing her eyes again. This response will be discussed later in the section on dissociative diagnoses.

None of the six dissociaters remembered the rhyme or their hidden observer responses upon awakening, nor did the three who failed to exhibit a hidden observer recall the rhyme upon awakening.

The four fantasizers who gave fairly realistic accounts also described an intentional strategy of "not listening." A typical response was, "It was the rhyme 'Twinkle, Twinkle, Little Star.' The voice was there but I kept telling myself I didn't hear it."

Three fantasizers said something additional in response to hidden observer suggestions that did not contain the majority of the poem. All of these contained some confabulated, visual or dream-like content either related and unrelated to the poem. One contained a star in the night sky, one heard a "nursery rhyme" which they could not name or recite while experiencing apparently unrelated rich visual imagery, the third heard ". . . something about diamonds; I know I could have heard more but I tried not to listen."

After awakening from hypnosis, all seven of the fantasizers had some memory of the rhyme and their hidden observer responses. They appeared integrated with the hidden observer identity although they could also still recall the point in time at which they had been unable to recall the stimulus. For them the hidden observer seemed to have much the same effect as a simple amnesia removal cue.

DREAMS

When asked to recount the most recent dream that they could recall clearly, eleven of the fifteen fantasizers gave a dream from the previous night. All others were from the past four days. They were typically lengthy, fantastic accounts.

There was one out-of-body account, one lucid dream, and a false awakening. All of these are very rare categories, albeit ones that have been found to correlate with hypnotizability in another study on a different sample by the present author [15]. Three of the dreams were sexual, another rare category [18], most were pleasant, and none were nightmares. When asked if they had nightmares, four fantasizers reported that they had at least one a month. None of them reported any recurring nightmares.

In contrast, when dissociaters were asked to recount the most recent dream they could recall, many had trouble thinking of one. Although two recalled dreams from the previous night, several dated the last dream they could recall as years before. One gave a recurring nightmare which had happened only a few times as the only dream she believes she has ever recalled in her lifetime. Two more dissociaters gave a recurring nightmare as their most recent well-recalled dream and three others reported they experienced recurring nightmares at least once a month. All of these subjects also experienced some nonrecurring nightmares and one additional dissociater reported nonrecurring nightmares only. Three reported sexual content in their most recent dreams, but these were all within the context of nightmares or other unpleasant dreams. Their nightmares had even more obviously disturbing content than those of the fantasizers including things such as suffocating, the dreamer's body coming apart, and horribly injured babies and children.

TRAUMA HISTORIES

When asked about how their parents had disciplined them and about any possible abuse, eleven of the fantasizers said that their parents had disciplined them solely by some combination of two strategies: 1) rewards or withholding of rewards, and 2) reasoning with them, often emphasizing empathy:

One time I'd gotten in a fight at nursery school with another little girl because there was this doll there that was her favorite or regular toy to play with. I'd gotten it first that day; she tried to take it away from me and I pushed her down. The teacher called my mother and told her about it. Mother told me I should think about what she had felt like when she fell down, and it became like I really was her hitting the floor, scraping one knee, and crying. I could also feel her desperation and thinking it really was her doll (even though it was the school's); she had named it and everything. After that I wouldn't have done that again.

Eight of this group reported discipline that they experienced as harsh including frequent spankings, being locked in their rooms for extended periods, and verbal belittling. They typically used fantasy and imaginary companions to restore self esteem after these incidents. Most of these fantasies were of retaliation against parents, albeit tempered by leniency on the part of the offended child. Usually powerful beings acted against the parent, sometimes for the parents mistreatment of the child, sometimes for unrelated reasons. Parents were kidnapped by aliens, chained in King Arthur's dungeon, arrested by the police, or sent back to grade school. In most cases however, the next step was that the child intervened on the parents' behalf and the parents were released feeling repentant and/or indebted.

None of the nineteen fantasizers reported any severe beatings or sexual abuse by immediate family or caretakers. Two female subjects in this group did report abusive sexual behavior on the part of other adults, in one case a social acquaintance of the family, in the other a stranger. Fantasizers in this study actually reported less physical and sexual abuse than the 20 to 25 percent rate reported by general college populations [19]. Their higher than average recollection for early childhood events would make it unlikely they are underreporting, although this finding is inconsistent with Lynn and Rhue's finding that a history of abuse correlates with their fantasy-proneness questionnaire [4].

When asked about parental discipline and possible abuse, four of the fifteen dissociaters initially remembered abusive behavior. For three of them this involved physical violence and for two of them it involved sexual abuse. In addition to these four with direct memories, two subjects said they did not remember but had been told that they had been battered as children (in one case an older sibling remembered witnessing this, in another case a social worker had monitored the parents following a teacher's report of abuse). One additional subject in this group described a severe history of early childhood multiple fractures and burns for which his parents presented improbable explanations. Another subject experienced nausea and vomiting whenever anyone touched a certain portion of her thigh. Six of the remaining seven subjects reported some signs such as the recurring nightmares outlined in the previous section and the lack of recollections before the ages of seven or eight described earlier. These signs have been associated with an increased likelihood of childhood abuse [19, 20]. Two of the dissociaters reported regaining abuse memories in the four years between the initial and follow-up interviews, which further suggests the rate for this group may approach 100 percent.

In addition to this suggestion that between six and fourteen of the dissociaters had been abused by parents, three of them reported other major traumas in childhood, in one case a very painful and extended medical condition, and for two the deaths of a parent when they were under ten.

DISSOCIATIVE DIAGNOSES AND POST-TRAUMATIC STRESS DISORDER

No fantasizer came close to meeting DSM3-R [21] Dissociative Disorder or Post-Traumatic Stress Disorder, although 100 percent of the fantasizers fit what would constitute Dissociative Disorder Not Otherwise Specified: "trance states, i.e., altered states of consciousness with markedly diminished or selectively focused responsiveness to environmental stimuli" [21, p. 277]. However, DSM defines mental disorders to be diagnosed as "a psychological syndrome with present distress or disability . . . or increased risk of suffering" [21, p. xxii]. The fantasizers do not appear to be distressed by their ability for selectively focused responsiveness.

Although the interview did not include all diagnostic questions for every other possible disorder less obviously related to content of the study, fantasizers did not obviously meet any other diagnoses. Two fantasizers did demonstrate some bipolar tendencies, and one some schizotypal ones; however in no case did they exhibit enough of the criteria and/or the severity of distress or impairment necessary for the formal diagnosis. Overall, the fantasizers appeared to be a mentally healthy group of people.

Four dissociaters met Dissociative Disorder NOS criteria, one with features of multiple personality—the person whose hidden observer exhibited such autonomy and distinctness had other brief amnestic episodes of speaking as a very different persona. A fifth dissociater met formal criteria for Psychogenic Amnesia. Again most of the remaining dissociaters could be seen as meeting the symptom criteria for this disorder by their daydream amnesia alone except that they did not appear to experience distress or impairment from their amnestic tendencies.

Even the five dissociaters with enough distress to qualify for dissociative diagnoses were toward the mild level of impairment from these disorders. Only one of them had sought long-term psychotherapy or therapy directed at trauma and dissociative symptoms. One of the other four with diagnoses and two other dissociaters had been in brief counseling around other issues. None of the subjects in this study have married abusive spouses, been unable to hold a job, made serious suicide attempts, or been hospitalized in psychiatric settings. However, all these events are common for other people with a serious trauma history and/or dissociative disorders.

SUMMARY AND CONCLUSIONS

In summary, this study found two distinct subgroups of people who were highly hypnotizable. Wilson and Barber's concept of many highly hypnotizable people having vivid fantasy and imagery ability is confirmed. However, it appears there is another, perhaps smaller, group characterized by amnesia and dissociative phenomena who do not achieve trance as rapidly, but are nevertheless capable of eventually reaching as deep a trance as fantasizers. This distinction does not seem to be synonymous with previously recognized ones such as high susceptibles who manifest Hilgard's hidden observer versus those who do not.

Although the two dissociaters who developed some fantasizer-type imagery suggest these people may have some of the same fantasy ability masked by amnesia, for the most part the people in this study constitute two remarkably distinct groups. The present author and other clinicians have certainly seen patients who seem like hybrids of the two types—with dissociative disorders, but also with voluntary vivid imagery [22, 23]—however this seems to be rare. On the basis of this research, it seems most accurate to think of high hypnotizables as composed of two groups whose life histories have specialized them primarily toward one of the major hypnotic phenomena: hallucinatory imagery or dissociative abilities.

REFERENCES

1. S. C. Wilson and T. X. Barber, Vivid Fantasy and Hallucinatory Abilities in the Life Histories of Excellent Hypnotic Subjects ("Somnambules"): A Preliminary Report, in *Imagery: Volume 2: Concepts, Results, and Applications,* E. Klinger (ed.), Plenum Press, New York, 1981.
2. S. C. Wilson and T. X. Barber, The Fantasy-prone Personality; Implications for Understanding Imagery, Hypnosis, and Parapsychological Phenomena, in *Imagery: Current Theory, Research, and Application,* A. A. Sheikh (ed.), Wiley, New York, pp. 340-390, 1983.
3. S. J. Lynn and J. W. Rhue, The Fantasy Prone Person: Hypnosis, Imagination, and Creativity, *Journal of Personality and Social Psychology, 51,* pp. 404-408, 1986.
4. S. J. Lynn and J. W. Rhue, Fantasy Proneness: Hypnosis, Developmental Antecedents, and Psychopathology, *American Psychologist, 43,* pp. 35-44, 1988.
5. N. P. Spanos, *Imagery and Hypnosis: Some Recent Developments,* paper presented at the Third World Conference on Imagery, Washington, D.C., June 1989.
6. R. E. Shor and E. C. Orne, *The Harvard Group Scale of Hypnotic Susceptibility, Form A,* Consulting Psychologists Press, Palo Alto, California, 1962.
7. A. Weitzenhoffer and E. Hilgard, *Stanford Scale of Hypnotic Susceptibility, Form C,* Consulting Psychologists Press, Palo Alto, California, 1962.
8. A. Tellegen and G. Atkinson, Openness to Absorbing and Self-altering Experiences ("Absorption"), a Trait Related to Hypnotic Susceptibility, *Journal of Abnormal Psychology, 83,* pp. 268-277, 1974.
9. P. Field, An Inventory Scale of Hypnotic Death, *International Journal of Clinical and Experimental Hypnosis, 13,* pp. 238-249, 1965.

10. D. L. Barrett, Deep Trance Subjects: A Schema of Two Distinct Subgroups, in *Mental Imagery*, Plenum, New York, pp. 101-111, 1991.
11. D. L. Barrett, Fantasizers and Dissociaters: An Empirically Based Schema of Two Types of Deep Trance Subjects, *Psychological Reports, 71*, pp. 1011-1014, 1992.
12. E. R. Hilgard, Divided Consciousness in Hypnosis: The Implications of the Hidden Observer, in *Hypnosis: Developments in Research and New Perspectives* (2nd Edition), E. Fromm and R. E. Shor (eds.), Hawthorne, Aldine, New York, 1979.
13. D. Barrett, Fantasizers and Dissociaters: Two Types of High Hypnotizables and Their Differences in Hidden Observers, Trauma Histories, and Diagnostic Indicators, in *Contemporary Hypnosis,* in press.
14. D. L. Barrett, The Hypnotic Dream: Its Content in Comparison to Nocturnal Dreams and Waking Fantasy, *Journal of Abnormal Psychology, 88*, pp. 584-591, 1979.
15. N. Zamore and D. L. Barrett, Hypnotic Susceptibility and Dream Characteristics, *Psychiatric Journal of the University of Ottawa, 14*, pp. 572-574, 1989.
16. D. L. Barrett, The First Memory as a Predictor of Personality Traits, *Journal of Individual Psychology, 36*, pp. 136-149, 1980.
17. D. L. Barrett, Early Recollections as Predictors of Self-disclosure and Interpersonal Style, *Journal of Individual Psychology, 39*, pp. 92-98, 1983.
18. C. Hall and R. Van de Castle, *The Content Analysis of Dreams,* Appleton-Century-Crofts, New York, 1966.
19. K. Belicki, *Nightmares of Abused vs. Non-abused Women,* invited address at the ninth international conference of the Association for the Study of Dreams, Santa Cruz, California, June 1992.
20. D. L. Barrett and H. J. Fine, A Child was Being Beaten: The Therapy of Battered Children as Adults, *Psychotherapy: Theory, Practice, and Research, 17*, pp. 285-293, 1980.
21. *Diagnostic and Statistical Manual of Mental Disorders* (3rd Edition-Revised), American Psychiatric Association, Washington, D.C., 1987.
22. M. Schatzman, *The Story of Ruth,* Putnam, New York, 1980.
23. D. L. Barrett, Dreams in Multiple Personality and Other Dissociative Disorders, in *Trauma and Dreams,* D. Barrett (ed.), Harvard University Press, Cambridge, Massachusetts, 1996.

CHAPTER 7

Breaching Posthypnotic Amnesia: A Review

WILLIAM C. COE

Posthypnotic amnesia is a failure to recall what has taken place during hypnosis. Amnesia is usually suggested by the hypnotist while the subject is hypnotized, although it may occur spontaneously without the suggestion. The suggestion for amnesia may be that the subject will not remember *anything* that happened during hypnosis or that the subject will forget specific events that occurred during hypnosis [1].

In the usual experimental setting, subjects are told that they will not remember anything that has happened while they were hypnotized until they are later told that they can remember. After awakening, they are asked to tell everything that happened since they entered hypnosis. The events that they recall are recorded. After they recall no more, they are told: "Now you can remember everything." Anything else that they recall is then recorded.

The usual way to judge whether or not subjects "passed" posthypnotic amnesia is to employ an objective criterion: for example, if subjects recall fewer than four out of twelve items on the Stanford Hypnotic Susceptibility Scale, Forms A and B [2], they are scored as passing posthypnotic amnesia. Such a measure is called "recall" amnesia. The additional number of items recalled after they are told that they can remember may also be used as a criterion for amnesia. This is called a measure of "reversibility." The combination of low recall and high reversibility is a more valid measure than either one by itself; that is, it assures the investigator that subjects have not simply forgotten.

In experimental settings, amnesia may also be suggested for specific isolated events during hypnosis [3, 4]. However, suggestions for selective amnesia are probably more common in clinical practice. Therapists may have special reasons for not wanting their clients to remember some specific material. For example, a therapist may think it unwise at an early point in therapy for the client to remember a traumatic event that came up during hypnotic age regression.

The amnesia suggestion may be given in a very specific and emphatic way, which is often the case in experiments, or it may be permissive and open-ended, which is often the case in clinical settings [5]. An experimenter may say, "You will not remember *anything* until I tell you that you can remember," while a hypnotherapist may say, "You will remember only what you are ready to remember."

Spontaneous posthypnotic amnesia seems to occur more often in clinical settings, where clients fail to recall certain aspects of a session, than it does in experimental settings. Complete spontaneous amnesia is quite rare. In any event, it is difficult to determine whether amnesia is ever really "spontaneous," since the hypnotherapist might give subtle indications which act as suggestions for amnesia, or subjects may give themselves suggestions with the same effect. However, when spontaneous amnesia does seem to occur, the content of the forgotten material may help the clinician to understand the psychodynamics of the client.

Laboratory research has led to the development of standardized, reliable measurements of suggested posthypnotic amnesia. These measures may be separated into two groups: 1) those that subjects can easily modify, and 2) those that they cannot.

Most standard scales of hypnotic susceptibility use measures that depend solely on the subjects' reports and are, therefore, easily modified. Subjects are asked to recall everything that happened during hypnosis; the number of items recalled is used to judge the degree of amnesia (recall amnesia). After the amnesia suggestion is lifted, subjects are asked to recall anything else they remember (reversibility of amnesia). Only recall amnesia is used on most scales, reversibility being used more often in research studies. Other methods of recall have also been employed, for example, the "forgotten" items may be presented to subjects for recognition memory. The degree of recognition recall in posthypnotic amnesia is usually higher than free recall, as it also is in studies of normal memory. The way in which subjects recall, judged by their nonverbal behavior (Do they appear puzzled? Are they trying?), may also be employed as a subjective estimate of the process of recall.

All the above measures could be easily simulated should subjects be so inclined; therefore, their validity as indicators of actual experience during recall is unknown. Because of this difficulty, measures that are not easily modified have been used in attempts to determine whether the temporarily forgotten material still affects subjects, even though they claim not to remember it.

Difficult-to-modify measures generally fall into two categories: 1) physiological responses, and 2) subtle measures of recall. Physiological measures, like those used in lie detection, can be taken in order to determine whether the material which subjects claim not to remember is nevertheless affecting their physiological responses (responses which subjects presumably cannot control voluntarily). For example, galvanic skin response (GSR) may be monitored during recall. Subjects are given suggestions to forget certain "key" words while they are hypnotized. During recall, the key words are interspersed with neutral

BREACHING POSTHYPNOTIC AMNESIA / 139

words, and subjects are asked which words they recognize. If subjects claim nonrecognition yet show different GSRs to the neutral and key words, the words probably are available at some level. The subtle ways of testing recall also are not easy to modify (see [1, 6] for more details). An example is the effect of retroactive inhibition. If subjects learn two lists of similar words, the efficiency of recalling the first list is decreased by their learning the second list. Subjects learn one list before they are hypnotized and one list while they are hypnotized. Posthypnotic amnesia is suggested for the second list. They are then asked to recall both lists. If subjects do not recall the second list (amnesia), that should not interfere with their recalling the first list (by comparison to subjects who are not amnesic). However, when amnesic subjects recall the first list no better than nonamnesic subjects do, the forgotten material apparently still actively affects recall on some level.

Research with difficult-to-modify measures has generally supported the notion that the amnesic material is still active. That is, subjects judged amnesic by easily modified measures do not appear amnesic on difficult-to-modify measures. Since the unreported and presumably forgotten material is clearly available at some level, rather than being temporarily ablated from memory, the question of accounting for these observations is raised [7].

THEORIES

The major theoretical differences surrounding posthypnotic amnesia revolve around the issue of whether posthypnotic amnesia should be viewed as a "happening" or a "doing." Special-process theorists prefer "happenings." In opposition, social psychological theorists prefer "doings."

Special-process theorists postulate that subjects *cannot* remember. Posthypnotic amnesia is viewed like other everyday disruptions of memory, for example, forgetting where one left one's car keys, or blocking out someone's name at a cocktail party [8]. Cooper, for example, states that "amnesia . . . has been traditionally viewed as being outside of the subject's volitional control and carried out automatically" [9, p. 248].

Social psychological theories, on the other hand, postulate that subjects are best viewed as "doing" something not to recall, even to the extent that their failure to recall may be interpreted by them as out of their control, for example, involuntary. Variables in the setting are believed to interact with subject variables in important ways, interactions are therefore emphasized [6, 10].

Kihlstrom, a special process theorist, stated that

> we have analyzed the wider social context and determined the relative importance of contextual variables in amnesia. . . . Thus, we are led to shift our emphasis from the social context "in which" amnesia occurs to the cognitive processes "by which" it occurs [8, p. 252].

Unusual, special processes, like dissociations of materials and amnesic barriers, are postulated as accounting for subjects' inability to recall. It is postulated that memories are dissociated from conscious control so that they cannot be accessed voluntarily [8, 11-16]. Special process theorists also imply that hypnosis is best viewed as a special state of consciousness [8, 13]. However, they are also careful to spell out that "special state" or "hypnosis" represents a "category of phenomena, not a causal agent" [8, p. 250].

The paradox of subjects seeming to know, but at the same time not to know, is explained by special process proponents by comparing it to other memory findings. Posthypnotic amnesia should not be considered unusual, because other findings in memory research have shown that material can be available in memory storage but cannot be retrieved for recall. "A failure to remember simply means that the person cannot 'now' gain access to the target memory" [17] or that he or she cannot construct a complete account based on what he has accessed [8, p. 251; 18]. The posthypnotic cue lifting amnesia presumably operates like other cues that help increase recall, e.g., recognition cues.

The social psychological view argues that the hypnosis setting and subject characteristics interact in important ways to determine both self-reports *and* personal experiences [6, 10, 19-23]. Rather than trying to hold the setting constant in order to obtain one sort of self-report, interactions among setting and subject variables may be studied systematically. Predictions may be made as to what and how subjects report; post-hoc explanations are not necessary. Subject variables are clearly recognized as important, but the emphasis is on their interactions with setting variables. However, the subject variables of interest are not those of memory, they are concepts like "expectations," "response-expectations," or "cognitive skills." Thus, subjects who respond to the suggestion for posthypnotic amnesia are viewed as actively employing their skills or abilities to fulfill their expectations for the role of "good" subject. Subjects of interest are those who objectively demonstrate posthypnotic amnesia by 1) reporting very little or none of the critical material, 2) reporting the experience as involuntary, and 3) recovering the materials on cue.

BREACHING POSTHYPNOTIC AMNESIA

One experimental paradigm has been used in an attempt to resolve the theoretical issue of "happenings" versus "doings." It is the breaching study. Breaching amnesia addresses the question whether subjects who initially respond to posthypnotic amnesia will report more *before* the reversal cue, when external pressures to recall are placed on them. If amnesia cannot be breached, subjects presumably have no control over remembering, which would support the view of posthypnotic amnesia as a "happening" (or a special process).

In 1978 [6], I evaluated two studies that had claimed to demonstrate that posthypnotic amnesia cannot be breached [15, 24]. They will be reviewed briefly along with my earlier conclusions.

Bowers designed a rather elaborate study to deceive subjects into believing that the experiment had ended before amnesia was removed [24]. All subjects were high susceptibles. Half were hypnotized when given the posthypnotic amnesia suggestion. Half were read the same suggestion while awake, then asked to pretend that they had been hypnotized when they heard it. All showed high responsiveness to the suggestion with a second experimenter. Bowers then asked them to see a third person who needed subjects for pilot data, but he did not give the cue removing amnesia. He said, "And listen, since we're all finished here, *I want you to be completely honest with him, regardless of what I've said before*" [24, p. 45, italics his]. The responses to the third experimenter's questions showed that all of the simulators and 43 percent of the reals were aware of the amnesia suggestion. Also, all simulators, but only 14 percent of the reals, rated amnesia as voluntary.

Bowers interpreted the results as support for posthypnotic amnesia as a happening, for example, a demand for honesty did not breach amnesia. I qualified his interpretation by pointing out that almost half of the real subjects reported being aware of their "amnesic" response (even though only a small percentage claimed that it was voluntary). I further criticized his procedures on the ground that the demands on simulators to "confess" were much stronger than the demands on the reals.

My evaluation of the Kihlstrom et al. study [15] raised the issue of the differential strengths that various situational circumstances hold for breaching amnesia. Their design tested four groups. Following the administration of the Harvard Group Scale of Hypnotic Susceptibility (HGS) [25], all subjects were tested for posthypnotic amnesia (3 minutes to write down everything that they remembered), then different instructions were given to each group: 1) *retest*, asked to recall again, 2) *cue*, list the items in chronological order, 3) *challenge*, overcome amnesia by exerting more effort to recall, and 4) *honestly* cautioned not to fail to report voluntarily what they actually remembered. Amnesia was tested a second time, was then lifted on cue, and then followed by a final recall.

The initially amnesic subjects in all four samples did not differ from each other on recalls 2 or 3. Because the three "breaching" groups did not recall more than the "retest" group at recall 2, the results were interpreted as evidence that posthypnotic amnesia was not breached. However, my examination of the data made it clear that about 50 percent of the subjects in *all four* samples breached. That is, each of the instructions led about half of the initially amnesic subjects to recall significantly more. Thus, the results could have as easily been interpreted as showing that *all four* instructions had a considerable effect on breaching amnesia. Kihlstrom did not agree [8]. He offered the alternative hypothesis that posthypnotic amnesia, "at least in inexperienced subjects, remits with time regardless of demands" [8, p. 258]. His hypothesis is evaluated later.

I concluded that the potency of the situational demands for breaching was an important variable. Kihlstrom agreed, but also argued that until someone obtained positive evidence with stronger demands, posthypnotic amnesia remained robust in the face of demands for extra effort to recall and for honesty in reporting [8]. Since my review, a number of studies have addressed the question of breaching.

We have evaluated the effects of stronger breaching demands and also the interaction of breaching with subjects' ratings of their control over remembering [26-29]. In the first four studies, we introduced "honesty demands" and "lie detector demands" after the initial testing for amnesia. In the "honesty" condition subjects were told that they should be completely honest and report *everything* that they could remember. In the "lie detector" condition they were told that the physiological apparatus to which they were attached acted like a lie detector; in some cases they were told nothing more, and in some cases they were told that it indicated they were *not* telling all they knew. Controls who were only asked to recall again were also included. In general, each breaching condition, compared to the control condition, created significantly more breaching. No one breaching manipulation was especially more effective than the others. However, breaching was not complete in the breaching samples, and it interacted with subjects' ratings of their control over remembering. That is, those who rated themselves as being in control of remembering (voluntaries) were more likely to breach, even in the control condition, than were those who rated themselves as not in control of remembering (involuntaries). Compared to the Kihlstrom et al. [15] results, our breaching subjects recalled more at the second recall than our controls. Thus, we supported the hypothesis that stronger demands created more breaching, but there was still a considerable number of the initially amnesic subjects who did not breach—about 50 percent, mostly "involuntaries."

Our most recent study considerably increased the demands for breaching [30]. As in the earlier studies, we preselected only highly susceptible subjects who had demonstrated amnesia on the HGS [25]. Approximately half were categorized as "voluntaries" and half as "involuntaries" on the basis of their control ratings from the HGS amnesia response. They were then administered the individual Stanford Hypnotic Susceptibility Scale, Form C (SHSS:C) [31] with the usual posthypnotic amnesia item. After testing amnesia and obtaining another control rating, subjects were assigned to a breaching condition or a control condition (half voluntaries and half involuntaries, based on their HGS ratings). Breaching consisted of three manipulations over approximately fifty minutes. First, "honesty" instructions were administered, followed by a second recall and control rating. Next, subjects were told that the physiological equipment indicated they were not telling all they knew ("lie"), followed by a third recall and control rating. (Subjects simply sat in their chairs in between breaching manipulations.) They were next shown a videotape replay of their hypnosis session, then asked if they could really recall anything else [32]. A fourth recall and control rating followed. Finally, the reversal cue for amnesia was given followed by a fifth recall.

The control sample sat quietly for the same amount of time. At the times matching the breaching subjects' critical recalls, the controls were only asked if they recalled anything else, followed by the recall and control ratings. Amnesia was lifted in the same way as for the breaching sample.

All but one of nineteen breaching subjects breached *completely* before amnesia was lifted. About 50 percent, nearly all voluntaries on the HGS, breached completely in the control condition. The involuntaries in the control condition recalled significantly more items at reversibility than they did over the three preceding recalls. Thus, for subjects who had initially claimed control over remembering (voluntaries), amnesia appeared to dissipate over time, whether or not they were under pressure to breach. However, involuntaries not under pressure to breach remained amnesic, while their counterparts who were under pressure breached.

Coe and Tucibat [33] recently selected twenty-one subjects (half voluntaries, half involuntaries) who had scored 9 or higher and passed posthypnotic amnesia on the HGS and tested them following the individual SHSS:C under the first two breaching conditions of the Coe and Sluis study ("honesty" and "lie") [30]. Sixteen of the twenty-one breached almost completely. Three of the five remaining subjects were "pseudoamnesics," recalling only one or two items over all four recalls. Only two subjects remained amnesic until the reversal cue. The HGS voluntary/involuntary designation was not related to breaching. In fact, all but three subjects rated their first recall on the SHSS:C as *involuntary*. As they recalled more items at breaching trials, their ratings changed in the voluntary direction.

CONCLUSION

Our results in general support the hypothesis that most amnesic subjects will breach under adequate pressure. They *do not* appear to be passive persons who experience some sort of special process that interferes with their memory abilities. As pressure is added for them to remember more, they do so, to the extent that they have nothing left to remember when amnesia is lifted. Our results represent the "positive evidence" Kihlstrom [8] requested that demonstrates that posthypnotic amnesia *does not* remain robust in the face of strong demands.

Our series of studies on breaching may also shed some light on the issue of spontaneous memory recovery in posthypnotic amnesia over time. In the first four studies, only one breaching recall was given after the challenge recall. Controls who were only asked to recall again (no breaching pressure) did not uniformly show increased recall at recall two. Generally, across the studies, subjects who had rated their first recall attempt as "mostly not in their control" (involuntaries) were not likely to recall more at the second recall. But, subjects who had rated their recall as "mostly in their control" (voluntaries) were likely to recall more at recall two. In the Coe and Sluis study, control subjects were given three recalls after the challenge trial and before amnesia was removed [30]. The voluntary controls (no breaching pressures) recalled more items at each recall, and at a level equal to the voluntary or involuntary subjects in the breaching conditions. However, the involuntary controls did not increase their recall significantly until amnesia was lifted, even over about forty-five minutes and three recall requests.

Thus, it may be accurate to say that without added pressures to breach, the amnesia of about half of the subjects who are initially amnesic dissipates over *recalls*. It remains to be tested, however, whether time alone is also an important factor. If time is important, then subjects given three post-challenge recalls over forty-five minutes, would not show greater recall than subjects given only one post-challenge recall at the end of forty-five minutes.

Taken together, our studies have suggested that, even with additional post-challenge recall requests, amnesia may be maintained for at least forty-five minutes in subjects who view their amnesia as mostly out of their control. However, the fact that their involuntary counterparts who were under strong breaching pressures did not maintain amnesia qualifies the observation. They should not be viewed as having no control over remembering because of inner cognitive workings like amnesic barriers or dissociated subsystems. When pressures to recall are added, they will be able to recall. Nevertheless, a subject's report of control-over-remembering may be an important variable to consider in future research on the spontaneous recovery of amnesia.

All in all, as more research becomes available, posthypnotic amnesia appears to be most parsimoniously understood in the framework of social-psychological views. Responsive hypnotic subjects can be viewed as engaged in strategic enactment to fulfill the role of good hypnotic subject as they perceived it.

REFERENCES

1. W. C. Coe, Posthypnotic Amnesia: Theory and Research, in *Hypnosis: The Cognitive Behavioral Perspective,* N. P. Spanos and J. F. Chaves (eds.), Prometheus, Buffalo, New York, 1989.
2. A. M. Weitzenhoffer and E. R. Hilgard, *Stanford Hypnotic Susceptibility Scale, Forms A and B,* Consulting Psychologists Press, Palo Alto, California, 1959.
3. N. P. Spanos and H. L. Bodorick, Suggested Amnesia and Disorganized Recall in Hypnotic and Task-motivated Subjects, *Journal of Abnormal Psychology, 86,* pp. 295-305, 1977.
4. N. P. Spanos and M. L. Ham, Cognitive Activity in Response to Hypnotic Suggestion: Goal-directed Fantasy and Selective Amnesia, *American Journal of Clinical Hypnosis, 15,* pp. 191-198, 1973.
5. M. V. Kline, Hypnotic Amnesia in Psychotherapy, *International Journal of Clinical and Experimental Hypnosis, 14,* pp. 112-120, 1966.
6. W. C. Coe, The Credibility of Posthypnotic Amnesia: A Contextualist's View, *International Journal of Clinical and Experimental Hypnosis, 26,* pp. 218-245, 1978.

7. W. C. Coe, B. Basden, D. Basden, and C. Graham, Posthypnotic Amnesia: Suggestions of An Active Process in Dissociative Phenomena, *Journal of Abnormal Psychology, 85,* pp. 455-458, 1976.
8. J. F. Kihlstrom, Context and Cognition in Post Hypnotic Amnesia, *International Journal of Clinical and Experimental Hypnosis, 26,* pp. 246-267, 1978.
9. L. M. Cooper, Hypnotic Amnesia, in *Hypnosis: Research, Developments, and Perspectives,* E. Fromm and R. Shor (eds.), Aldine, Chicago, Illinois, 1972.
10. N. P. Spanos, Hypnotic Behavior: A Social Psychological Interpretation of Amnesia, Analgesia and "Trance Logic," *Behavioral and Brain Sciences, 9,* pp. 449-567, 1986.
11. E. R. Hilgard, Toward a Neodissociation Theory: Multiple Cognitive Controls in Human Functioning, *Perspectives in Biology and Medicine, 17,* pp. 301-316, 1974.
12. E. R. Hilgard, The Problem of Divided Consciousness: A Neodissociation Interpretation, *Annals of the New York Academy of Sciences, 296,* pp. 48-59, 1977.
13. E. R. Hilgard, *Divided Consciousness: Multiple Controls in Human Thought and Action,* Wiley, New York, 1977.
14. J. F. Kihlstrom, Instructed Forgetting: Hypnotic and Nonhypnotic, *Journal of Experimental Psychology: General, 112*(a), pp. 73-79, 1983.
15. J. F. Kihlstrom, F. J. Evans, E. C. Orne, and M. T. Orne, Attempting to Breach Posthypnotic Amnesia, *Journal of Abnormal Psychology, 89,* pp. 603-626, 1980.
16. J. F. Kihlstrom and R. E. Shor, Recall and Recognition during Posthypnotic Amnesia, *International Journal of Clinical and Experimental Hypnosis, 26,* pp. 330-349, 1979.
17. E. Tulving and Z. Perlstone, Availability vs. Accessibility of Information in Memory for Words, *Journal of Verbal Learning and Verbal Behavior, 5,* pp. 381-391, 1966.
18. R. Brown and D. McNeill, The "Tip of the Tongue" Phenomenon, *Journal of Verbal Learning and Verbal Behavior, 5,* pp. 325-337, 1966.
19. W. C. Coe and T. R. Sarbin, Hypnosis from the Standpoint of a Contextualist, *Annals of the New York Academy of Sciences, 296,* pp. 2-13, 1977.
20. T. R. Sarbin and W. C. Coe, *Hypnosis: A Social Psychological Analysis of Influence Communication,* Holt, Rinehart and Winston, New York, 1972.
21. T. R. Sarbin and W. C. Coe, Hypnosis and Psychopathology: Replacing Old Myths with Fresh Metaphors, *Journal of Abnormal Psychology, 88,* pp. 506-526, 1979.
22. N. P. Spanos, Hypnotic Responding: Automatic Dissociation or Situation-relevant Cognizing?, in *Imagery: Concepts, Results and Applications,* E. Klinger (ed.), Plenum, New York, 1981.
23. N. P. Spanos, A Social Psychological Approach to Hypnotic Behavior, in *Integrations of Clinical and Social Psychology,* G. Weary and H. Mirels (eds.), Oxford University Press, New York, pp. 231-271, 1982.
24. K. S. Bowers, Hypnotic Behavior: The Differentiation of Trance and Demand Characteristics Variables, *Journal of Abnormal Psychology, 71,* pp. 42-51, 1966.
25. R. E. Shor and E. C. Orne, *Harvard Group Scale of Hypnotic Susceptibility,* Consulting Psychologists Press, Palo Alto, California, 1962.
26. W. C. Coe and E. Yashinski, Breaching Posthypnotic Amnesia: Volitional Experiences and Their Correlates, *Journal of Personality and Social Psychology, 48,* pp. 716-722, 1985.
27. M. L. Howard and W. C. Coe, The Effects of Context and Subjects' Perceived Control in Breaching Posthypnotic Amnesia, *Journal of Personality, 48,* pp. 342-359, 1980.
28. B. A. Schuyler and W. C. Coe, A Physiological Investigation of Volitional and Nonvolitional Experience during Posthypnotic Amnesia, *Journal of Personality and Social Psychology, 40,* pp. 1160-1169, 1981.

29. B. A. Schuyler and W. C. Coe, More on Volitional Experiences and Breaching Posthypnotic Amnesia, *International Journal of Clinical and Experimental Hypnosis, 37,* pp. 320-331, 1989.
30. W. C. Coe and A. S. E. Sluis, Increasing Contextual Pressures to Breach Posthypnotic Amnesia, *Journal of Personality and Social Psychology, 57,* pp. 885-894, 1989.
31. A. M. Weitzenhoffer and E. R. Hilgard, *Stanford Hypnotic Susceptibility Scale, Form C,* Consulting Psychologists Press, Palo Alto, California, 1962.
32. K. M. McConkey and P. W. Sheehan, The Impact of Videotape Playback of Hypnotic Events on Posthypnotic Amnesia, *Journal of Abnormal Psychology, 90,* pp. 46-54, 1981.
33. W. C. Coe and M. Tucibat, The Relationship between Volition and Breaching Posthypnotic Amnesia, *British Journal of Clinical and Experimental Hypnosis,* in press.

[Portions of this chapter summarize material in Coe [3] and Coe [5].]

CHAPTER 8

Hypnotic Responsiveness, Nonhypnotic Suggestibility, and Responsiveness to Social Influence

MAXWELL I. GWYNN
AND NICHOLAS P. SPANOS

The concept of suggestibility has played an important role in the history of social psychological theory. Allport stated that suggestion and its related concepts, sympathy and imitation, "compose the principal triumvirate of theories in social psychology" [1, p. 23]. Definitions of suggestion and suggestibility vary. MacDougall provided an early definition of suggestion as "a process of communication resulting in the acceptance with conviction of the communicated proposition in the absence of logically adequate grounds for its acceptance" [2, p. 100]. MacDougall postulated that the essence of suggestion involves an instinct of submission that was aroused by any person exhibiting prestige [2]. More recently, Eysenck, Arnold, and Meili included the central elements of both Allport's and MacDougall's interpretations in their definition of suggestion as "a process of communication during which one or more persons cause one or more individuals to change (without critical response) their judgments, opinions, and attitudes" [3, p. 1077]. Some definitions of suggestibility are worded in general terms with little reference to context. Schumaker defines suggestibility as a term "used to indicate a person's propensity to respond to suggested communications" [4, p. 3]. Eysenck, Arnold, and Meili, on the other hand, specifically include the concept of hypnosis when defining suggestibility as "the individual degree of susceptibility to influence by suggestion and hypnosis" [3, p. 1076]. Hypnosis had been viewed by many early theorists (e.g., Bernheim [5], Braid [6], Forel [7], Hull [8], and Sidis [9]) as an extreme instance of the suggestive process, and its precursor (i.e., "animal magnetism") involved an early naturalistic explanation of phenomena that are today described as resulting from suggestion [1].

As indicated by this brief overview, the varied definitions given to the term suggestion all include the idea of communication from an authoritative source that asserts (implicitly or explicitly) some proposition without requisite supportive evidence. Relatedly, suggestibility is taken to refer to individual differences in the extent to which the proposition is accepted by people as factual in the absence of critical examination and/or supportive evidence. In laboratory experiments the authoritative communication frequently defines some aspect of the subjects' situation as counterfactual (e.g., your arm is getting lighter and lighter and rising in the air). In many other situations, however, the communication may include propositions that are intuitively more believable and that, in fact, may be accurate (e.g., This car runs like a dream).

A moment's reflection makes it clear that the terms suggestion and suggestibility, as commonly defined, encompass a very large range of social behavior. Almost everything that we do, from stopping at a stop light, to getting at the end of the line at the supermarket, to kissing your wife or husband goodbye in the morning, to following instructions or directions, to holding religious beliefs of almost any kind, to chatting with an acquaintance, can be defined as fitting the above definitions of responses to suggestion. All of these situations involve tacit or explicit communications from others. In each case a shared set of tacit assumptions about the structure of the social world is also involved. Moreover, because these assumptions are taken for granted, people guide their behavior in terms of them without critical reflection or supportive evidence. For instance, when your wife meets you at the door as you return from work, closes her eyes, lifts her head toward yours, and puckers her lips, she is tacitly communicating a proposition (e.g., I feel affectionately toward you) which you understand intuitively and without critical reflection, and to which you respond more or less unthinkingly by kissing her.

Despite the fact that formal definitions of terms like suggestions and suggestibility encompass almost all human behavior, investigators who conduct studies on suggestibility often limit their analyses to behaviors that, from the taken-for-granted perspective of the experimenters, are not intuitively understandable [10]. Experimenters, of course, are members of particular cultures at particular points in historical time, and their intuitive beliefs about what is reasonable or easily understandable reflect their cultural backgrounds. In our culture reaching out one's hand to collect change from the store clerk makes intuitive sense and is unlikely to be studied as an example of suggestibility. Lifting one's hand when told it is being pulled upwards by a nonexistent balloon makes less intuitive sense in our culture and therefore, is likely to be "explained" in terms of suggestibility. In many contexts the term suggestibility has slightly pejorative connotations (e.g., non-rational, gullible) and often reserved for behaviors that appear to be inconsistent with implicitly held social values (e.g., independence is valued therefore conformity in response to social pressure is labeled negatively as "suggestibility" as opposed to, for example, cooperativeness). Because notions of suggestibility are employed to account for a very wide range of behavior, and because the concept is often invoked only when the behaviors in question appear to involve violations of implicit cultural understandings or cultural values, we should be prepared to find that the behaviors labeled as examples of suggestibility often share few intrinsic communalities.

While the term "suggestion" is defined in terms of certain kinds of communications, responsiveness to suggestions (i.e., suggestibility) is frequently conceptualized as a stable characteristic that differs in degree from one person to the next. The assumption that suggestibility is a stable trait is pervasive, and consequently much of the literature on this topic has been devoted to developing measures of this supposedly stable trait, and to assessing its correlates. Frequently, studies conducted from a trait perspective tend to de-emphasize the importance of contextual variables in shaping subjects' interpretations of and responses to different "suggestive" situations. As will be seen, however, contextual factors and tacit interpretations are often of great importance for understanding both why subjects respond as they do to persuasive communications and why different measures of suggestibility sometimes correlate substantially with one another and sometimes do not.

HISTORICAL BACKGROUND:
SUGGESTION AND HYPNOSIS

The phenomena that eventually were designated as hypnosis and suggestion first began to be systematically investigated as a result of interest in behaviors brought about by "animal magnetism" in the late eighteenth century. A French Royal Commission, headed by Benjamin Franklin, was called to investigate claims that diseases could be healed by the powers of animal magnetism [11]. Animal magnetism was also known as "mesmerism," so-named after the founder of the procedure, Franz Anton Mesmer. Mesmer claimed that his "cures" involved the transmission of subtle fluids between the magnetizer and patient [12]. However, the commission concluded that any healing powers in the animal magnetism procedure could be attributed to the effects of imagination, and expectant desire; in short to what later would be called the "power" of suggestion [13].

The findings of the Royal Commission did not lead to the demise of magnetism. Nevertheless, by the middle of the nineteenth century scientific and medical thinking were increasingly influenced by the popularity and rise in status of neurology. As a result "fluidist" accounts of magnetic phenomena increasingly gave way to accounts based on contemporary notions of neurological functioning [14].

The best known neurological alternative to fluidist accounts was developed by James Braid [6]. Braid was initially misled by the lethargic appearance of his patients into concluding that their behavior occurred automatically as a result of spreading neural inhibition. Supposedly, sustained visual attention (from staring at a shiny object) produced eye muscle fatigue. The resultant neural inhibition was thought to spread backwards from the optic nerves to the brain to produce a state resembling sleep in which the phenomena of magnetism (now relabeled with the Greek word for sleep, "hypnosis") occurred.

Braid soon became dissatisfied with these early speculations and, as an alternative, developed the notion of monoideism [6]. Monoideism was based on the concept of ideo-motor action. According to this hypothesis ideas that remain uncontradicted by other ideas lead automatically to the corresponding action. For example, if a subject who believes that her arm is becoming light and rising in the air remains oblivious to such competing thoughts as "I know I'm only imagining this," her arm will supposedly rise. Moreover, because the arm rising flows directly from the corresponding idea, and is not generated by volitional action, it is experienced as "going up by itself."

The concept of monoideism strongly influenced the work of Liebault, Bernheim, and other members of the so-called "Nancy school," who made it the central tenet in their theory of suggestion. Bernheim's notion of suggestion as ideo-motor action became the cornerstone of much of the theorizing about hypnosis that developed in the early twentieth century [5]. Bernheim argued that suggestion was both a cause and an explanation for hypnotic phenomena, and viewed hypnosis as simply a state of hypersuggestibility [5].

Charcot was the premier neurologist in nineteenth-century France, and his interest in hypnosis lent credibility to a topic that had been officially shunned in that country since its dismissal by the Royal commission. Charcot rejected Bernheim's notion of suggestion as an adequate account of hypnotic phenomena and hypothesized instead that hypnosis was a neuropathological state that possessed certain invariant behavioral characteristics, and that could be produced only in hysterics [14].

Although many of Charcot's ideas about hypnosis were dismissed by most of the scientific community before the end of the nineteenth century, he greatly influenced Janet, who developed the concept of dissociation [15]. According to the dissociation hypothesis the neural substrates of ideas or behavioral patterns that normally occur together or in sequence could be separated or dissociated from one another. Supposedly, dissociations occurred when people who were predisposed with a constitutionally weak nervous system were exposed to trauma or stress. In such people, dissociations could also be produced by the suggestions of the hypnotist. Dissociation theory was used to explain complex behaviors like multiple personality as well as such relatively simple "automatisms" as limb catalepsy. Dissociation theory gained numerous adherents in both Europe and America around the turn of the century. Nevertheless, by the end of the first quarter of the twentieth century, it had been largely displaced in theories of hypnosis by variants of Bernheim's theory of suggestibility [14]. One reason for the decline of interest in dissociation was described by White and Shevach:

. . . the pattern of dissociative barriers is in a great many cases directly dependent on what is suggested, following in minute detail even the most bizarre conceits of the operator. . . . In short, the operator can impose a dissociative barrier almost wherever he chooses. This fact tends to shift our interest from dissociation to suggestion . . . [16, p. 327].

Around the turn of the twentieth century, researchers such as Seashore, Sidis, Binet, and Bernheim began to investigate the phenomenon of suggestibility outside of the context of hypnosis. Binet indicated that to fully understand suggestibility in its broad sense, one must take into account the individuals' attitudes, expectations, and imagination [17]. Relatedly, Seashore recognized the importance of wording and contextual cues when assessing suggestibility. With regard to the influence of sensory processes, Seashore wrote: "A seemingly insignificant word, thing or circumstance may determine what the observer shall see or not" [18, p. 63]. Sidis believed that he had discovered the main laws of suggestible behavior, leading him to argue for the elitist proposition that, "not sociability, nor rationality, but suggestibility is what characterizes the average specimen of humanity, man is a suggestible animal" [9, p. 17]. Less pejoratively, Bernheim also argued that suggestibility comes into play in the waking state as well as during hypnosis [5]. He believed that outside of hypnotic behavior, suggestibility manifested itself in the daily influence of one individual upon another resulting in a change in beliefs and attitudes; indeed, such was the "stuff" of formal education.

Implicit in all of the above formulations was a mechanistic view of human functioning in which suggested behaviors were conceptualized as automatically caused by discrete stimuli. During the first quarter of the twentieth century, however, social philosophers like Cooley [19] and Mead [20] began laying the ground work for what would eventually become symbolic interactionist views of human functioning. According to these views, people are active, cognizing beings whose social reality is structured through interaction with others. Language is the symbol system through which people come to conceptualize themselves and others and is the major vehicle through which they construct shared and mutually understandable social realities. Implicit in these ideas is the notion that all communications including "suggestions" involve the tacit, contextually shaped understandings of the participants. Behavior flows from these understandings in terms of the role requirements associated with the statuses of the individuals involved in the interactions.

These ideas influenced White who became the first modern investigator to critically challenge the notion that behavior was elicited automatically from the suggestions of the hypnotist [21]. White held instead that hypnotic responding involved goal-directed behavior. Hypnotic behavior was but a form of social behavior determined by subjects' implicit expectations, guided by their attempts to portray themselves in terms of what they believed the hypnotist expected of them.

Contemporary research in hypnosis has tended to follow one of two paths. The "social psychological" approach [22-25] stems from White's [21] conceptualizations of hypnotic behavior as goal-directed enactment. Investigators who adopt this perspective emphasize the role enactment and situational aspects involved in the subject-hypnotist relationship. According to this perspective, subjects who enact the "hypnotized" role base their responses on preconceptions and expectations concerning hypnosis, and use cues in the hypnotic context and from the hypnotist to guide them in carrying out what they interpret to be appropriate behavior.

On the other hand, investigators espousing "special process" or "state" conceptualizations [26-29] tend to view hypnotic responses as occurring automatically, and as explicable in terms of traditional notions like ideo-motor and dissociative responding. Typically these investigators downplay the goal-directed nature of hypnotic responding and the importance of interpretations, expectations, and contextual influences in guiding hypnotic enactments.

Many special process theorists tend to view hypnotizability as a trait-like capacity that remains relatively stable over time [26, 28]. On the other hand, social psychological theorists, while acknowledging the stability of hypnotic responsiveness across repeated testing, usually emphasize that this stability reflects subjects' stable attitudes, expectations, and interpretations concerning hypnotic responding [30, 31]. As has now been demonstrated, altering subjects' interpretations and expectations can produce substantial changes in their responsiveness to suggestion (see Spanos [32] for a review).

TESTS OF WAKING SUGGESTIBILITY

Interest in individual differences among experimental psychologists at the turn of the century led to the development of many tests of suggestibility outside of the hypnotic context. The majority of these early suggestibility tests dealt with the effects of suggestion on the sensory system. On many of these tasks, subjects were tested indirectly, without knowing that attempts were being made to influence their perceptions or judgments, or to induce them to report the presence of a stimulus (tactile, visual, or olfactory) when in fact no stimulus was present. Binet's progressive weights and lines tests are examples of this type of indirect suggestion [17]. The progressive weights test involves having subjects lift, one at a time, each of a series of boxes. The first few boxes are each slightly heavier than the one before it, but subsequent boxes are of equal weight. The extent to which subjects report differences between the weights when none exist is taken as a measure of suggestibility. The progressive lines test operates in the same manner, involving the discrimination of line lengths rather than weights.

Hull later labeled tasks of this type as tests of "impersonal suggestion" [8]. Tests of "personal suggestion," on the other hand, involved explicit statements by an operator that a particular behavioral effect (the suggested effect) was occurring.

Examples are Hull's "postural sway" test in which the subjects, standing with eyes closed, are told repeatedly that they are falling forward, and the hand rigidity test of Aveling and Hargreaves which informed subjects that their hand was becoming stiff and tight and unable to bend [33]. Bird later emphasized a similar distinction between suggestibility tests, but preferred to use the labels direct versus indirect suggestibility [34]. Historically, these distinctions have been confounded with particular suggestibility-testing procedures [35], particularly following the influential empirical work of Eysenck and Furneaux [36]. Tests involving *motor* aspects of suggestibility, such as the body sway test and Chevreul pendulum task, have a direct character. That is, they explicitly tell the subject to do or try to experience the suggested effect (e.g., "Feel yourself leaning forward, falling forward . . ." or "Notice the pendulum starting to swing, swinging more and more . . ."). *Sensory* tests, such as the Binet progressive weights test, on the other hand, are typically worded *indirectly*. As explained by Sidis "instead of openly telling the subject what he should do, [with indirect suggestion] the experimenter produces some object or makes a movement, a gesture which in silent fashion tells the subject what to do" [9, p. 19]. Subsequent research, however, has established that both motor and sensory processes can each be influenced by direct or indirect processes [37, 38] indicating that the historical confound can be avoided.

From its conception, the generality of waking suggestibility as a stable, unitary, cross-test "trait" has evoked controversy. Sidis [9] and Otis [39] argued, on the basis of experimental findings, that there exists a general trait of suggestibility. Brown [40] and Estabrooks [41], on the other hand, found little empirical evidence of a such generality. Allport believed that suggestibility is a trait which may characterize only a few individuals consistently; on the whole, he concluded, suggestibility was not a unitary trait [1].

Eysenck and Furneaux [36] made distinctions similar to earlier conceptions by Hull [8] between types of suggestibility tests. Using a factor-analytic approach, these researchers distinguished between "primary" and "secondary" suggestibility. Primary suggestibility involved subjects' responding to direct verbal suggestions, supposedly without their volitional participation. Examples of such measures include Hull's body sway and Chevreul pendulum tests [8]. For the latter test, the subject is asked to hold a pendulum above a ruler, and is told that the pendulum will start to swing. These tests were found to correlate with hypnotizability, and were associated by early researchers with the ideo-motor theory of action [8, 36].

Secondary suggestibility was said to be measured by indirect sensory test procedures such as the progressive lines and weights tests of Binet [17]. These tests tended to correlate negatively with intelligence, and not at all with hypnotic responsiveness. Eysenck and Furneaux stated that "possibly a better name for this secondary kind of suggestibility might be 'gullibility' " [36, p. 494]. Eysenck and Furneaux also reported the emergence of a third factor which they related to prestige suggestibility. This factor involved attitude change resulting from persuasive communication from an authority figure.

Subsequent empirical attempts to corroborate the findings of Eysenck and Furneaux [36] with different samples have produced equivocal results. Grimes administered various tests of suggestibility to 233 orphan boys ranging in age from eight to fifteen years [42]. Some evidence of a primary suggestibility factor emerged, but even so, inter-test correlations were small, and the three remaining emergent factors obtained by these investigators did not lead to ready explanation.

Benton and Bandura, using a smaller ($n = 50$) sample of undergraduate students, found mostly nonsignificant intercorrelations between tests of suggestibility [43]. Yates [44] criticized Benton and Bandura's use of a sample that was homogeneous with respect to intelligence, because, according to Eysenck [45], intelligence is strongly related to suggestibility. Benton and Bandura's sample was found to be relatively nonsuggestible according to the body sway test. However, Evans [27] found that a similar sample of undergraduate students displayed a level of body sway resembling that of Eysenck and Furneaux's original sample of neurotic army personnel. Subsequent factor-analytic studies [27, 38, 46, 47] found general support for a factor of primary suggestibility, but little or no evidence for a secondary factor of suggestibility as described originally by Eysenck and Furneaux [36].

Duke administered a series of tests to ninety-one domiciled veterans between the ages of thirty-four and seventy-two [46]. Four tests similar to measures of primary suggestibility exhibited moderately high intercorrelations (average r value of .36). On the other hand, five tests that supposedly tapped secondary suggestibility produced lower intercorrelations (average r value = .14). Duke arbitrarily divided tests into four categories: tests of "task set" (progressive weights and lines), "sensory suggestibility" (heat and odor illusions, in which subjects' reports of warmth or odors when none existed was taken as a measure of suggestibility), "conformity" (picture report tests involving leading questioning), and standard geometric illusions. The correlations of tests placed both within each category and between categories were generally low or zero, indicating a lack of empirical support for either the factorial uniqueness of his arbitrary categories or for a unitary concept of secondary suggestibility.

Evans [27], after reviewing the empirical research concerning nonhypnotic suggestibility, concluded that Eysenck and Furneaux's [36] original classification of primary and secondary suggestibility was not justified. Evans' reanalysis of the Eysenck and Furneaux data led him to identify three independent factors: "primary" (passive and/or motor) suggestibility as described originally by Eysenck and Furneaux (i.e., the body sway and pendulum tests, along with tests of hypnotic and posthypnotic responding); "challenge" suggestibility as measured by tests worded in the imperative mood (e.g., the arm rigidity suggestion, where the operator suggests to the subject that they cannot bend their arm, then challenges them to overcome the induced rigidity); and "imagery" suggestibility, which purportedly involve uncritical acceptance of an implied situation, such as the heat and odor illusions and picture report tests.

Stukat's research with a sample of Swedish adults and children indicated a secondary suggestibility factor, which he claimed involved the effect of subjective factors (such as need for conformity and expectation) on cognitive functions (such as perception and memory) [47]. This interpretation reflected that of Binet who had earlier conceptualized several tests of suggestibility (e.g., prestige and interrogatory suggestibility, progressive weights and lines) as involving four precursors: obedience to mental influence from another person; tendency to imitate; influence of a preconceived idea that paralyzed the individual's critical sense; and expectative attention [17]. Binet's obedience and imitative characteristics corresponded to Stukat's need for conformity, while Binet's latter two characteristics (loss of critical sense and expectative attention) correspond closely to Stukat's expectation factor.

In summary, the available findings concerning the construct of waking (nonhypnotic) suggestibility are mixed and inconclusive. It is not at all clear what factors, or how many, make up this construct. There is general evidence, however, that suggestibility is not a unitary dimension. The majority of studies have employed tests of primary (motor) suggestibility. This may be due to the availability and popularity of oft-used tests of motor suggestibility (even though there were no generally accepted and established rules concerning how to carry out these primary suggestibility tests [48]). Fewer studies have examined relationships between sensory suggestibility, social influence, and hypnotic responsiveness. Discussion of the phenomena now turns to a review of the research in the areas of social influence and hypnotic susceptibility.

STUDIES OF SOCIAL INFLUENCE

As indicated earlier, the concept of suggestibility includes the idea of communication from an authoritative source that is aimed at influencing the thought processes and behavior of recipients. Implied in this definition is the notion of social influence; a topic that has been of central importance in social psychology since the early years of the discipline. Most of the research on this topic has concentrated on the effects of groups or implied norms on individual behavior. However, investigators have followed increasingly divergent research paths. Thus, topics investigated under the general rubric of social influence include: personality correlates and the generality of suggestibility, (i.e., whether or not suggestibility is a consistent trait: [49-53]); age and sex differences in suggestibility and influencibility [40, 42, 54]; attitudinal and situational factors in suggestibility [55-57]; as well as interactions between the above factors [58-60].

Maass and Clark pointed out that the field of social influence has been dominated by research into conformity [61]. In fact, until the late 1960s, the term "social influence" and "conformity" were nearly interchangeable [62]. More recently, interest in social influence has expanded to include topics such as consumer susceptibility to interpersonal influence [63], concern for social appropriateness [64], the role of self-focused attention on susceptibility to suggestion [65], normative versus informational mechanisms of conformity [66], and suggestibility within the context of a police interrogation [67]. Generally speaking, however, studies of social influence have tended to follow one of two separate paths: research into suggestibility, in the older ideo-motor sense, and persuasibility, in the form of opinion change and influential communication [68]. In only a few studies have attempts been made to integrate the constructs of suggestibility and persuasibility/influencibility.

Using a sample of eighty adults, Stukat found a significant correlation ($r = 0.35$) between the pendulum test (a classic test of primary suggestibility) and a test of responsiveness to leading questions (a test of persuasibility) [47]. Stukat also reported a second-order suggestibility factor, which correlated significantly both with primary suggestibility and the tendency to conform to majority opinion.

Abraham tested 101 undergraduate students in an attempt to determine the relationship between sensory and verbal susceptibility to suggestion [49]. Correlations of moderate magnitude ($r_{pb's}$ of .30 to .48) were found among the heat test, odor test, and a persuasibility test devised by Hovland and Janis [69]. Abraham concluded that

> there are measurable personality needs (autonomy and deference) which predispose individuals towards high or low suggestibility, irrespective of the sources of the suggestion . . . individuals who are susceptible to suggestion in sensory tests tend also to be susceptible to persuasion in opinion change tests" [49, p. 183].

Moore [70] obtained measures of susceptibility to social influence from eighty male undergraduates; these measures included Hovland and Janis's [69] persuasibility test of written communications of opinion from authoritative sources, Schachter's [71] influencibility test with false peer group norm feedback data, and Sherif's [72] autokinetic test of perceptual judgment in the presence of a confederate's influence. Although Moore hypothesized significant positive relationships among these three measures, the results of her study indicated only small nonsignificant correlations among the tests (r's ranging from .08 to .13) [70]. Further, only the influencibility test was found to be significantly correlated ($r_{pb} = .64$) with a measure of suggestibility (the postural sway test). In short, Abraham's [49] findings of consistent, moderately sized correlations between various measures of suggestibility and persuasibility were not replicated by Moore [70].

EFFECTS OF SEX ON SOCIAL INFLUENCIBILITY

Gender has often been identified as important in studies of social influence, conformity, and compliance. Most of the early research that compared the responses of males and females to influence-communications found that males resisted group pressures toward conformity to a greater extent than females in a wide variety of testing situations. For example, greater resistance to the persuasive attempts of the experimenter by males than females was found in studies that used: a synonym matching task with high school students [73]; the judgment of geometric areas and line lengths [74]; the autokinetic effect [75]; and size estimation of different objects by children [76].

Females were more swayed than males by reciprocity appeals [77, 78], and more likely than males to describe conformity as a positive virtue [79]. In a review of the literature on conformity, Nord concluded that "it has also been well established, at least in our culture, that females supply greater amounts of conformity under almost all conditions than males" [80, p. 198]. Most investigators account for gender differences in influencibility in terms of cultural role prescriptions, females having been raised to "go along" and behave as expected, while males are more often rewarded for independence and innovation. For example, a series of studies by Janis and Field that assessed susceptibility to influence by persuasive communications, found that males were significantly less persuasible than females [58]. Janis and Field interpret these findings as due to "different sex roles in our society, particularly with respect to intellectual independence and docility in many aspects of everyday life" [58, p. 59]. They cautioned that it is "necessary to consider separately the male and female subsamples when studying the correlations between personality factors and persuasability" [58, p. 59].

Sistrunk and McDavid cited fourteen studies published between 1955 and 1963 (the "heyday" of conformity research) with results supporting the proposition that women yield more to social pressures than men [81]. However, these investigators also described several studies in which significant sex differences failed to emerge. Sistrunk and McDavid concluded that situational, personality, and motivational factors, as well as the sex of the influencer, all play critical roles in the conformity process, and that studies finding significant sex differences may have failed to adequately account for these mediating factors [81]. Sistrunk and McDavid concluded that:

> it appears clear that the simple and sovereign explanation of sex differences in conforming behavior as a function of cultural prescriptions for the female role is grossly inadequate, and that a disregard for particular characteristics of the behaving male or female together with the particular nature of the judgmental tasks which have been employed in experimental studies of conformity may have contributed to artificially inflated observations of sex-determined differences [81, p. 64].

The results of a meta-analysis by Eagly and Carli supported the contention that women conform more in group situations than men [77]. However, they noted that almost 80 percent of the influencibility studies they reviewed were carried out by males, and that these male researchers tended to obtain larger sex differences (in the direction of greater female conformity) than did female researchers. In general, experiments authored by women showed no sex difference. These findings suggest that the sex differences in conformity research may be due in part to an artifact of the experimental methodology [77]. Another reason may be the stimuli involved in conformity studies. Sistrunk and McDavid varied the nature of the items used to elicit group pressure [81]. Females were found to conform most on items that were familiar to men, while males conformed most on items more familiar to females. On items that were equally familiar to males and females, no sex differences in conformity were found. In light of these findings it is apparent that differences between male and female influencibility are unlikely to be explained by positing a general trait of conformity.

HYPNOTIZABILITY AND RESPONSIVENESS TO SOCIAL INFLUENCE

Hull found a positive correlation between responses to direct, verbal (nonhypnotic) suggestions and hypnotizability, but no relationship when the suggestions were worded in an indirect manner [8]. Relatedly, two studies found that hypnotizability tended to correlate with primary suggestibility (which involves direct tests) but not secondary suggestibility (which involves more indirect tests) [27, 36].

Moore [70] examined relationships between persuasibility, influencibility, the autokinetic effect, and responsiveness to suggestion following a hypnotic induction, as measured by the Stanford Hypnotic Susceptibility Scale (SHSS; [82]). Moore hypothesized that hypnotizability and social suggestibility were essentially independent, on the premise that the former taps "primary" suggestibility, while the latter appears to be more related to conceptions of "secondary" suggestibility. The correlations between hypnotizability and two of the measures approached significance, however that with persuasibility was negative ($r = -.17$, $p < .10$), while the correlation with influencibility was positive ($r = .21$, $p < .05$). The moderate correlation of influencibility with the SHSS may be partially accounted for by the inclusion of the waking postural sway suggestion in the total SHSS score. The autokinetic test was found to be uncorrelated with the SHSS ($r = -.08$, n.s.). Moore concluded that hypnotizability and social suggestibility were independent of one another because the measures of suggestibility were related to hypnotizability only marginally and in different directions [70].

Shames, on the other hand, found strong correlations between hypnotizability and a measure of conformity to majority group opinion in an Asch-type experiment involving judgments of line lengths [83]. Based on these results, Shames concluded that "hypnotic susceptibility is a reasonable predictor of conformity, and both appear to be tied to the construct of suggestibility" [83, p. 563]. However, the "hypnotizability" test used in Shames' study, the Eye-roll Levitation method [84], correlates only very poorly with conventional suggestion-based tests of hypnotic responsiveness [85, 86].

Miller [87] found that subjects high and medium in hypnotizability were more likely than lows to incorrectly report "seeing" suggested tachistoscopically-presented syllables when in fact none were presented, and Farthing, Brown, and Venturino [88] reported that high hypnotizables made more false alarms (i.e., adopted a more lax criterion for evidence constituting a signal) than lows in a visual signal detection task. Farthing et al. interpreted false alarms as representing a nonhypnotic measure of suggestibility [88]. On the other hand, both Graham and Schwartz [89] and Jones and Spanos [90] found no differences between high and low hypnotizables in baseline criterion placement in an auditory detection task.

Wallace, Garrett, and Andstadt [91] found a significant correlation between hypnotic responsiveness and (suggested) perceived changes in autokinetic movement, while Hajek and Spacek [92] reported a small but significant correlation between hypnotic responsiveness and the tendency to report that a light (of constant intensity) had, in the subject's opinion, increased in brightness after such an effect was suggested.

Council and Loge found that high hypnotizables reported significantly larger increases in heaviness (on the incremental weights task) and odors (on an odors test) than low hypnotizables [93]. As well, highs were significantly more confident in their reports than lows. No significant hypnotizability by context interactions were found, indicating that the greater responsiveness of high hypnotizables was evident both with and without the prior administration of an hypnotic induction procedure. The authors concluded that these results provided evidence of a general factor underlying suggestibility in hypnotic and nonhypnotic contexts.

Graham and Greene found that individuals who previously scored high in hypnotic responsiveness were more likely than those scoring low to contribute to the college alumni fund [94]. They interpreted these findings as an indication that "hypnotic susceptibility should be related to a person's response to persuasive communications that are emotional and imaginative" [94, p. 353]. These authors did not claim that alumni giving was the result of waking suggestibility, but the possibility of a relationship between response to persuasive communication (requests for charitable donations) and hypnotic responsiveness presents itself.

Support for this position also comes from a study by Malott, Bourg, and Crawford designed to assess the impact of a hypnotic induction and hypnotizability level on response to a persuasive communication (advocating mandatory pregraduation comprehensive examinations) [95]. High hypnotizables agreed more often than lows with the communication and produced significantly more favorable thoughts in line with the arguments presented in the communication, in both the hypnotic and nonhypnotic contexts. The authors concluded that both context and "trait" (hypnotizability level) play a significant role in responsiveness to persuasive communication.

In summary, the findings with respect to the relationship between hypnotic responsiveness and social influencibility are inconsistent. It appears that higher levels of hypnotizability may be associated with greater responsiveness to

persuasive communication when these communications (like hypnotic suggestions) are presented in a direct, authoritarian manner [8, 95], but when the attempts
at influence are less direct, the relationship becomes more tenuous [8, 70, 92].

Attempts to find stable correlates between hypnotizability and measures of
waking suggestibility are premised on the notion that hypnotizability is a stable
trait as opposed to a dimension on which subjects vary as a function of context-
specific attitudes, expectations and interpretations. Numerous studies indicate
high test-retest correlations for hypnotizability and, in addition, different tests of
hypnotizability usually correlate to a substantial degree (see Bertrand [96] for a
review). As pointed out by several investigators [30, 97], however, all of the
standardized hypnotizability tests are similar in structure and all define the situation to subjects (explicitly or implicitly) as hypnosis. Moreover, subjects are
unlikely to encounter information that will change their attitudes, expectations, or
interpretations of hypnosis and hypnotic responding from one test session to the
next. In short, the high test-retest and cross-test correlations found for hypnotizability scales may largely reflect the fact that the hypnotizability testing
situation remains stable across both time and tests.

Spanos, Gabora, Jarrett, and Gwynn examined these ideas by testing subjects'
responsiveness to suggestions in two sessions [98]. In session 1 the suggestibility
test was explicitly defined as a test of hypnotizability for all subjects. In session 2
all subjects were tested with a different suggestibility scale. For half of these
subjects this was defined as a test of hypnotizability, while for the other half it was
defined as a test of creative imagination. When both tests were defined as hypnosis the correlation between them was significantly and substantially higher than
when one test was defined as hypnosis and the other as measuring creative
imagination.

In a second experiment subjects who were either high or low in hypnotizability
were administered a test of waking suggestibility [98]. Half of the highs were led
to expect that they would perform in the same way on the waking test as they had
on the hypnotizability test while the remaining half were informed that they were
likely to score poorly on the waking test because it lacked a necessary hypnotic
induction procedure. Relatedly, half the lows were informed that waking and
hypnotic suggestibility involved similar psychological processes and therefore
that they were likely to respond poorly to the waking test. The remaining lows
were informed that they had the creative ability to respond to the waking suggestions, and that hypnosis had previously inhibited their native talents. Now, without
hypnosis to interfere, they should perform well on the waking test.

Lows given positive expectation attained much higher waking suggestibility
scores than lows given the negative expectations. Relatedly, highs given positive
expectations scored higher on waking suggestibility than highs given negative
expectations. Importantly, when initial hypnotizability scores were correlated
with waking suggestibility scores for subjects who had been given information
implying consistent performance in the two test situations (i.e., highs-positive

expectations, lows-negative expectations), the correlation was very high and significant. However, for subjects who had been led to expect performance differences across the sessions (i.e., highs-negative expectations, lows-positive expectations) the correlation between session 1 hypnotizability and session 2 suggestibility was very low and nonsignificant. The findings of these two experiments indicate that the stability usually found in hypnotizability scores is much more strongly related to situation specific expectations and interpretations than is commonly acknowledged. They further suggest that correlations between hypnotizability and other variables are likely to vary in magnitude as a function of the expectations and beliefs held by subjects about the variables on which they are assessed, and about how they believe those variables are interrelated.

SUGGESTIBILITY, HYPNOTIZABILITY, AND FALSE MEMORY REPORTS

Numerous studies have investigated the roles of hypnosis and hypnotizability on reports of false memory. Typically, subjects are presented with a stimulus event, such as hypnotic instructions to "relive" a previous night [99-102], a series of slides [103], or a videotape depicting a simulated crime [100 (study 2), 104-106]. After a hypnotic induction, subjects are given false information in the form of a suggestion or misleading questions. Subjects who "accept" the suggested information and report it posthypnotically as an actual memory of the original event are defined as exhibiting a hypnotically-induced pseudomemory.

In several studies highly hypnotizable subjects reported more pseudomemories than low hypnotizables regardless of whether they were first administered an hypnotic induction procedure [103-106]. In some studies highs also made more errors in response to misleading questions than did lows, regardless of whether they were administered an hypnotic induction [104, 107 (Experiment 6), 108-110]. However, in a number of these studies, hypnotizability was confounded with experimental condition (hypnotic induction for the highs vs. task-motivation or simulation of hypnosis for the lows), rendering impossible an examination of the effects of hypnotizability level alone on errors in response.

In a recent study, Barnier and McConkey presented subjects with a series of slides of a purse snatching, and then asked them to recall the events of the crime in hypnotic or waking conditions [103]. After suggestions (in the form of misleading questions implying that the offender wore a scarf and helped the victim pick up a bunch of flowers), more high- than low-hypnotizables reported this false information.

Spanos et al. [106] found that hypnotic responsiveness and reaction to social influence tactics were interrelated. In that study subjects viewed a videotape of a simulated crime (a convenience store robbery and shooting). Approximately one week later, they viewed a short videotape which they were told to treat as if it was a news clip from the evening news. This video portrayed the arrest of a suspect in the convenience store shooting. This suspect was *not* the offender from the original video, although he was similar to the offender in age and clothing. In a subsequent session, subjects were interrogated about the offender. During the interrogation subjects were asked a series of leading questions which falsely implied that the offender in the first video possessed a number of characteristics that were only true for the suspect in the second video (e.g., "Did you see the tattoo on the offender's left arm?"). Regardless of whether or not the interrogation involved hypnotic procedures, high hypnotizables reported the offender as possessing more of the suggested false characteristics than did lows. Highs also incorrectly selected a mug shot as portraying the offender more frequently than lows. In addition, when cross-examined in a further session, highs changed their testimony in the direction espoused by the cross-examiner more often than did lows. The social demands of the experimental situation called for subjects to 1) misattribute characteristics when questioned about the offender, 2) misidentify the offender by choosing a mug shot, and 3) admit that their earlier testimony might have been mistaken when questioned by the cross-examiner. Highs responded to each of these demands to a greater extent than did lows.

The greater tendency of highs to be led during interrogation and then to disavow their testimony under cross-examination may reflect a tendency of highs to comply more than lows to social influence regardless of their private beliefs. Alternatively, the highs may have created more vivid but accurate images than the lows in response to the leading questions. Because their images were vivid, the interrogation may have swayed the highs to report their image of the offender as being an actual memory. During cross-examination, "the vivid and highly salient images that initially led highs to misattribute characteristics may have also made plausible to them during cross-examination that their images were interrogator-induced suggestions" [106, p. 282]. Although these two interpretations suggest differing reasons for high-low differences, both suggest that highs are more likely than lows to give in to the interpersonal pressure exerted by different experimenters (the interrogator and the cross-examiner) during two separate questioning sessions.

A possible confound exists in several of the studies that found a relationship between hypnotic responsiveness and false memory reporting. In these studies, subjects were tested for hypnotic responsiveness and nonhypnotic suggestibility in the same testing session or at least in the same experimental laboratory as part of the same study, i.e., within the same context [106-110]. This raises the possibility that cross-over effects occurred in these studies. Subjects in these studies knew their pretested hypnotizability levels. Consequently, they may have responded to subsequent suggestibility testing based on their conceptions of how a "highly hypnotizable" or "nonhypnotizable" subject should respond. The findings of four recent studies, provide evidence that expectancies generated by the context of testing influence whether or not questionnaires that assess such attributes as absorption in imaginings and dissociation correlate significantly with hypnotizability [111-114]. Relatedly, Spanos, Quigley, Gwynn, Glatt, and Perlini provided evidence for context effects in a study that assessed the confidence displayed by hypnotic and nonhypnotic witnesses in their incorrect mug shot identifications [115].

In the Spanos, Quigley et al. study, high and low hypnotizables witnessed a videotaped mock murder and then attempted to choose the offender from a mug shot lineup [115]. One to two weeks later subjects returned to the laboratory and again made a mug shot selection. Before their second selection attempt, however, half of the highs and half of the lows were administered an hypnotic procedure and half were not. In fact, for the nonhypnotic subjects care was taken to not inform them that they had been selected for the present study on the basis of their earlier hypnotizability scores. Neither hypnotizability nor the administration of the hypnotic induction influenced the accuracy of mug shot identifications. On the other hand, hypnotizability correlated significantly with the amount of confidence displayed by hypnotic subjects in their incorrect identifications. Hypnotizability failed to correlate significantly with confidence in nonhypnotic subjects. These findings support the hypothesis that relationships between hypnotizability and other indexes of persuasability or suggestibility are strongly influenced by a carry-over of expectation effects that are generated by the context of testing.

INTERROGATIVE SUGGESTIBILITY

Individual differences in responsiveness to social influence and the reporting of false memories have been investigated in a productive line of research carried out by Gudjonsson and his colleagues [67, 116-119]. These studies, similar to the Spanos, Gwynn et al. [106] and Sheehan [107, 109, 110] studies, involved investigating the effects of leading questioning on recall. In particular, Gudjonsson has assessed the effects on individual responding of the interpersonal pressure exerted during police questioning. This form of social responsiveness has been labeled "interrogative suggestibility."

Binet first introduced the concept of "interrogatory" suggestibility at the turn of the century [17]. To measure this form of suggestibility Binet used the picture report test, which involved asking subjects a series of leading questions concerning a picture they had been shown. The degree to which they were led by the suggestive questions provided an index of interrogatory suggestibility. Similar procedures were used by subsequent researchers such as Stern [120] and Burtt [121] in applied settings, and more recently by Loftus [122] in a forensic setting. Binet's conceptions of the suggestive effect of leading questioning on memory were largely ignored, and studies that did attempt to investigate interrogative suggestibility involved complicated laboratory settings that are not easily replicated [123-125]. The major reason for the lack of research into Binet's interrogatory suggestibility is probably the fact that his groundbreaking work has never been completely translated into English. As well, a suitable objective psychometric instrument for measuring this type of suggestibility was not available until recently [126].

THE GUDJONSSON SUGGESTIBILITY SCALE

Gudjonsson developed a scale of interrogative suggestibility to measure individual differences in response to leading questioning [117, 119, 127-129]. The Gudjonsson Suggestibility Scale (GSS) is considered an indirect test of suggestibility because subjects are not aware of the real reason that they are being tested. Instead, they are told that the scale involves a test of memory. Interrogative suggestibility is defined as "the extent to which, within a closed social interaction, people come to accept messages communicated during formal questioning, as a result of which their subsequent behavioral response is affected" [119, p. 84].

In short, the procedure of the GSS is as follows: subjects are read a short narrative story about a robbery, given an opportunity to verbally recall the story, and then asked a series of twenty questions related to the story. Many of the questions contain false premises, questioning subjects on details not actually presented in the story. After responding to these "suggestive" questions, subjects are told that many of their answers were incorrect, and therefore the questioning must be repeated. Subjects are told at this point to try to be more accurate in their answering. The scale allows for a measure of the tendency of the subjects to *yield* to leading questions, and to *shift* their answers from previous responses following the interpersonal pressure of criticism and negative feedback. Yield scores are calculated as the number of suggestive questions on which the subject simply acquiesces or provides one of the false alternatives after initial questioning. Shift scores represent the number of questions to which the subject provides differing responses on the two recall trials.

The narrative passage is similar to that in the Wechsler Memory Scale, but considerably longer so that subjects are unable to remember all of the details. As in the Wechsler scale, the passage can be parsed into individual facts, and the number of these facts recollected (out of a possible 40) provides a continuous measure of memory recall.

PROPERTIES OF THE GSS

The GSS possesses adequate levels of internal consistency [117, 130] and high test-retest reliability [129]. The construct validity of the GSS as a measure of suggestibility has been demonstrated in several studies [116, 117, 127, 128, 131-134]. For example, Gudjonsson compared the GSS scores of two groups of criminal suspects: alleged "false confessors" (individuals who had retracted earlier confession statements) and "deniers" (those who had made no admissions despite forensic evidence against them) [127]. False confessors scored significantly higher on interrogative suggestibility than deniers. Further, it was found in another study that the GSS scores of grade-school students correlated significantly with teachers' ratings of suggestibility [135].

Interrogative suggestibility has been found to relate to a number of external variables. *Positive* correlations have been found with measures of compliance [136, 137], social desirability [116, 138], neuroticism [116], the EPI Lie scale [117], perceptual defensiveness and belief in witchcraft and precognition [134], acquiescence [128], fear of negative evaluation, evaluative and state anxiety [139], external locus of control, and perceived distance between the self and the experimenter in terms of competence, power, and control [132]. GSS scores have been found to correlate *negatively* with intelligence and memory recall [116, 137], self-esteem and internal locus of control [132, 140], assertiveness [131], and suspiciousness and anger [141].

The one study of interrogative suggestibility that included gender as an independent factor [132] found no significant mean differences between males and females on suggestibility. There was, however, a tendency for the sexes to show different correlational patterns. The correlations between suggestibility and locus of control, competence, and potency were higher for males than females.

Manipulated factors found to influence interrogative suggestibility include the form of questioning (i.e., misleading vs. objective) [142], negative feedback [138], and manipulated expectations and anxiety level [143].

Other factors have been hypothesized to influence interrogative suggestibility, but were found in one or more studies to be nonsignificant predictors. Such factors include age [117], hypnotizability level (when the GSS is administered after a hypnotic induction) [142], manipulated stress levels [138], instructions to the subject to "fake a bad performance on the test" [144], perceptions of the experimenter [140], psychoticism and extraversion (as measured by the EPI) [116, 134], traditional religious beliefs, superstition, and beliefs in psi phenomena and extraordinary life forms [134].

INTERROGATIVE SUGGESTIBILITY AND HYPNOTIC RESPONSIVENESS

The relationship between interrogative suggestibility and hypnotizability has yet to be adequately investigated. The results of one study [145, cited in 119] suggest a nonsignificant relationship between interrogative suggestibility and hypnotizability as measured by the Harvard Group Scale of Hypnotic Susceptibility. The methodology and bases for interpretation of this study are not available for critique, however, since the research was conducted as an undergraduate thesis in Reykjavik, Iceland, and has never been published.

The only published study to involve both Gudjonsson's scale and a measure of hypnotic responsiveness was conducted by Register and Kihlstrom [142]. These researchers attempted to induce memory errors through the use of the GSS following a hypnotic induction. Although this study included subjects pretested for hypnotizability (also on the Harvard Scale), several procedural modifications render assessment of the impact of hypnotizability level on interrogative suggestibility unclear. One half of the subjects received a version of the GSS which included "objective" rather than misleading questioning, a major procedural digression from the original GSS. Only low (0-4 HGSHS scores) and high (8-12) hypnotizables were utilized, so correlational assessments were not available. All subjects were tested for yielding on the second questioning trial only *following* a hypnotic induction; there was no nonhypnotic control group employed. Thus, it was not possible to compare nonhypnotic high- versus low-susceptibles in a repeated measures format similar to the original procedures of the GSS. Further, Gudjonsson's measure of total suggestibility was not reported by the researchers, and shifts were scored in a manner differing from usual procedures. Given the results of the false memory studies described earlier [103-106], it might be hypothesized that high hypnotizables would be more likely than lows to be influenced by the misleading questioning, and to subsequently report some of the misleading information in later recall trials. An effect of this kind would be evidenced in the Register and Kihlstrom study by a significant three-way interaction of hypnotizability, condition, and trials [142]. Although errors of fact were tabulated in the study, and a three-way interaction between these variables was reported to have reached significance, the authors stated that the interaction was uninterpretable. The only data from this study which can be used to assess the effect of hypnotizability level on an interrogative suggestibility measure prior to the hypnotic induction involves the number of Yields during the first interrogation. An inspection of the relevant means indeed indicates a tendency for high hypnotizables ($M = 12.50$, $s = 3.89$) to yield slightly more to misleading questioning than lows ($M = 11.20$, $s = 4.49$). Unfortunately, although confidence was assessed for each response, reported confidence scores were transformed into pre-post confidence change scores, and raw confidence scores for Trial 1 were not presented. Thus, the procedures and reported results of the Register and Kihlstrom study do not allow for any firm conclusions concerning the relationship between interrogative suggestibility, confidence, and hypnotizability [142].

Two recent investigations assessed both levels of interrogative suggestibility and (pretested) hypnotizability. In one study [146] these two assessments were conducted in separate experimental contexts, while in the second study [147] some subjects received a hypnotic induction during GSS testing.

In the Gwynn, Spanos, Nancoo, and Chow [146] study, 120 subjects who had been pretested on the Carleton University Responsiveness to Suggestion Scale (the CURSS [148]) were contacted to participate in a study on memory (the GSS). Subjects were not told of any connection between the hypnotic responsiveness testing session and the GSS session; the sessions were held in different laboratories and conducted by different experimenters. The CURSS yields objective as well as subjective indexes of hypnotizability.

Subjects' objective and subjective CURSS scores failed to correlate signifi-cantly with intrusions, yielding, shifting, or total suggestibility scores on the GSS (all absolute r values less than .07). CURSS scores did not predict subjects' confidence scores for either their narrative recall or their interrogative question responses (all absolute r values less than .11). Further, GSS scores and CURSS scores were found to load on separate factors under a factor analysis. Taken together, these results indicate that, when tested in different contexts, sugges-tibility and confidence on the GSS are independent of hypnotizability.

A second recent study also involved subjects ($n = 120$) who had been pretested on the CURSS [147]. One half of the subjects were later tested on the GSS with no knowledge of a connection between the sessions. The other sixty subjects were administered a hypnotic induction with or without a suggestion for improved memory (based on the hypnotic memory enhancement techniques of Reiser [149]) on one of the recall trials. Results indicated no improvement in recall for subjects receiving the hypnotic versus nonhypnotic procedures. As in the Gwynn, Spanos et al. study, there were no significant correlations between hypnotizability and interrogative suggestibility among subjects who did *not* receive the hypnotic procedures [146]. Among the subjects in the hypnotic conditions, however, it was found that objective and subjective CURSS scores correlated significantly with the number of confabulations (errors of memory other than those suggested during misleading questioning) reported following the hypnotic induction ($r = .40$, $p < .01$ and $r = .30$, $p < .05$, respectively).

The results of the two studies taken together indicate support for Gudjonsson's contention that hypnotic and interrogative suggestibility are independent of each other; this was found to be true when the two testing sessions were conducted in different contexts [137]. When hypnotic procedures were incorporated into the GSS testing, however, a relationship emerged between hypnotic responsiveness and at least one measure of reported memory errors under interrogation. These findings are similar to those obtained by Spanos, Quigley et al. when examining context effects on the relationship between hypnotizability and confidence in incorrect mug shot identifications [115]. Together, the findings of these studies underscore the role of contextually generated expectations in influencing relation-ships between different indexes of suggestibility.

CONCLUSIONS

As is evident from this review, it is difficult to argue that suggestibility consists of a unitary trait. There are multiple dimensions of suggestibility, with varying degrees of interrelatedness, and the degree of such interrelatedness itself appears to vary as a function of implicit expectations and other situation specific variables. In areas like conformity research what once appeared to be stable relationships between gender and suggestibility turned out to be mediated by situation specific variables such as particular task demands, and role specific background knowledge. Relatedly, the oft touted stability of hypnotizability appears to be substantially influenced by contextual information that influences subjects' understandings of the test situation. Hypnotizability often correlates with response to tests of primary or direct suggestibility, but even here, the findings are not entirely consistent. Although there are some indications that hypnotizability is related to the amount of confidence displayed by subjects in false memories, it seems to be unrelated to tests of interrogative suggestibility which also assess confidence in false memories. Future research which varies the degree of perceived relatedness between testing procedures may provide answers to the questions of the effects of context on the relationships between different measures of suggestibility.

REFERENCES

1. G. W. Allport, The Historical Background of Modern Social Psychology, in *The Handbook of Social Psychology*, Vol. 1, G. Lindzey and E. Aronson (eds.), Addison-Wesley, Reading, Missouri, pp. 1-80, 1968.
2. W. MacDougall, *Introduction to Social Psychology*, Methuen, London, 1908.
3. H. J. Eysenck, W. J. Arnold, and R. Meili, *Encyclopedia of Psychology: Vol. 2, L to Z*, Herder and Herder, New York, 1972.
4. J. F. Schumaker, *Human Suggestibility: Advances in Theory, Research, and Application*, Routledge, New York, 1991.
5. H. M. Bernheim, *Hypnotisme et suggestion*, Doin et Fils, Paris, 1910.
6. J. Braid, The Power of the Mind over the Body, in *Foundations of Hypnosis: From Mesmer to Freud*, M. M. Tinterow (ed.), Thomas, Springfield, Illinois, 1846/1970. (Original work published in London by J. Churchill, 1846.)
7. A. Forel, *Hypnotism and Psychotherapy*, Allied Book Company, New York, 1907.
8. C. L. Hull, *Hypnosis and Suggestibility*, Appleton-Century-Crofts, New York, 1933.
9. B. Sidis, *The Psychology of Suggestion*, Appleton, New York, 1898.
10. G. Jahoda, Some Historical and Cultural Aspects of Suggestion, in *Suggestion and Suggestibility: Theory and Research*, V. Gheorghiu, P. Netter, H. J. Eysenck, and R. Rosenthal (eds.), Springer-Verlag, New York, pp. 255-262, 1989.
11. B. Franklin, S. Majault, J. B. LeRoy, J. S. Bailly, J. D'Arcet, G. De Bory, J. I. Guillotin, and A. L. Lavoisier, Report on Animal Magnestism, in *Foundations of Hypnosis from Mesmer to Freud*, M. M. Tinterow (ed.), Charles C Thomas, Springfield, Illinois, pp. 82-128, 1785/1970.
12. F. A. Mesmer, *Memoire sur la Decouverte du magnetisme animal*, 1779 (trans. *Mesmerism*, London: MacDonald, 1948).
13. N. P. Spanos and J. Gottlieb, Demonic Possession, Mesmerism and Hysteria: A Social Psychological Perspective on their Historical Interrelationships, *Journal of Abnormal Psychology, 88*, pp. 527-546, 1979.
14. N. P. Spanos and J. F. Chaves, History and Historiography of Hypnosis, in *Theories of Hypnosis: Current Models and Perspectives*, S. J. Lynn and J. W. Rhue (eds.), Guilford, New York, pp. 43-78, 1991.
15. P. Janet, *Psychological Healing*, Crowell-Collier and Macmillan, New York, 1925.
16. R. W. White and B. J. Shevach, Hypnosis and the Concept of Dissociation, *Journal of Abnormal and Social Psychology, 37*, pp. 309-328, 1942.
17. A. Binet, *La suggestibilite*, Schleicher Freres, Paris, 1900.

18. C. E. Seashore, Measurement of Illusions and Hallucinations in Normal Life, *Studies from the Yale Psychological Laboratories, 2,* pp. 1-67, 1895.
19. C. H. Cooley, *Human Nature and the Social Order,* Scribner's Sons, New York, 1922.
20. G. H. Mead, *Mind, Self, and Society,* University of Chicago Press, Chicago, 1934.
21. R. W. White, A Preface to the Theory of Hypnotism, *Journal of Abnormal and Social Psychology, 36,* pp. 477-505, 1941.
22. T. X. Barber, *Hypnosis: A Scientific Approach,* Van Nostrand Reinhold, New York, 1969.
23. T. X. Barber, Suggested ("Hypnotic") Behavior: The Trance Paradigm Versus an Alternative Paradigm, in *Hypnosis: Developments in Research and New Perspectives* (2nd Edition), E. Fromm and R. E. Shor (eds.), Aldine, New York, pp. 217-271, 1979.
24. T. R. Sarbin and W. C. Coe, *Hypnosis: A Social Psychological Analysis of Influence Communication,* Holt, Rinehart and Winston, New York, 1972.
25. N. P. Spanos, Hypnotic Behavior: A Social Psychological Interpretation of Amnesia, Analgesia, and Trance Logic, *Behavioral and Brain Sciences, 9,* pp. 449-467, 1986.
26. K. S. Bowers, *Hypnosis for the Seriously Curious,* Brooks/Cole, Monterey, California, 1967.
27. F. J. Evans, Suggestibility in the Normal Waking State, *Psychological Bulletin, 67,* pp. 114-129, 1967.
28. E. R. Hilgard, *Divided Consciousness: Multiple Controls in Human Thought and Action,* Wiley, New York, 1977.
29. M. T. Orne, The Construct of Hypnosis: Implications of the Definition for Research and Practice, *Annals of the New York Academy of Sciences, 296,* pp. 14-33, 1977.
30. M. J. Diamond, Hypnotizability is Modifiable, *International Journal of Clinical and Experimental Hypnosis, 25,* pp. 147-165, 1977.
31. N. P. Spanos and W. C. Coe, A Social Psychological Approach to Hypnosis, in *Contemporary Hypnosis Research,* E. Fromm and M. R. Nash (eds.), Guilford Press, New York, pp. 102-130, 1992.
32. N. P. Spanos, Interpretational Sets, Hypnotic Responding, and the Modification of Hypnotizability, in *Suggestion and Suggestibility: Theory and Research,* V. Gheorghiu, P. Netter, H. J. Eysenck, and R. Rosenthal (eds.), Springer-Verlag, New York, pp. 169-176, 1989.
33. F. Aveling and H. Hargreaves, Suggestibility With and Without Prestige in Children, *British Journal of Psychology, 11,* pp. 53-75, 1921.
34. C. Bird, *Social Psychology,* Appleton-Century, New York, 1940.
35. B. A. Gheorghiu, Relationship between Suggestion and Hypnosis: A Critical Survey, in *Third European Congress of Hypnosis in Psychotherapy and Psychosomatic Medicine,* G. Guantieri (ed.), Padavo, Italy, pp. 107-117, 1984.
36. H. J. Eysenck and W. D. Furneaux, Primary and Secondary Suggestibility: An Experimental and Statistical Study, *Journal of Experimental Psychology, 35,* pp. 485-503, 1945.
37. V. A. Gheorghiu, G. Meiu, A. Onofrei, and G. Timofte, Experimental Investigation on Suggestibility: Effects of Direct and Indirect Suggestion, *Revue Roumaine des Sciences Sociales, Serie de Psychologie, 10,* pp. 163-174, 1966.
38. A. G. Hammer, F. J. Evans, and M. Bartlett, Factors in Hypnosis and Suggestion, *Journal of Abnormal and Social Psychology, 67,* pp. 15-23, 1963.
39. M. A. Otis, A Study of Suggestibility of Children, *Archives of Psychology, 11:*70, 1924.

40. W. Brown, Individual and Sex Differences in Suggestibility, *University of California Publications in Psychology, 2,* pp. 291-430, 1916.
41. G. H. Estabrooks, Experimental Studies in Suggestion, *Journal of Genetic Psychology, 36,* pp. 120-139, 1929.
42. F. V. Grimes, An Experimental Analysis of the Nature of Suggestibility and of its Relation to Other Psychological Factors, *Studies in Psychology and Psychiatry at the Catholic University of America, 7:*4, 1948.
43. A. L. Benton and A. Bandura, "Primary" and "Secondary" Suggestibility, *Journal of Abnormal and Social Psychology, 48,* pp. 336-340, 1953.
44. A. J. Yates, Abnormalities of Psychomotor Functions, in *Handbook of Abnormal Psychology,* H. J. Eysenck (ed.), Pitman Medical, London, pp. 32-61, 1960.
45. H. J. Eysenck, Suggestibility and Hysteria, *Journal of Neurology and Psychiatry, 36,* pp. 349-354, 1943.
46. J. D. Duke, Intercorrelational Status of Suggestibility Tests and Hypnotizability, *The Psychological Record, 14,* pp. 71-80, 1964.
47. K.-G. Stukat, *Suggestibility: A Factorial and Experimental Model,* Almqvist and Wiksell, Stockholm, 1958.
48. V. A Gheorghiu, The Development of Research on Suggestibility: Critical Considerations, in *Suggestion and Suggestibility: Theory and Research,* V. A. Gheorghiu, P. Netter, H. J. Eysenck, and R. Rosenthal (eds.), Springer-Verlag, Berlin, 1989.
49. H. H. L. Abraham, The Suggestible Personality: A Psychological Investigation of Susceptibility to Persuasion, *Acta Psycholgica, 20,* pp. 167-184, 1962.
50. T. X. Barber, Hypnotizability, Suggestibility, and Personality: V. A Critical Review of Research Findings, *Psychological Reports, 14* (Monograph Supplement 3), 1964.
51. L. Berkowitz and R. M. Lundy, Personality Characteristics Related to Susceptibility to Influence by Peers or Authority Figures, *Journal of Personality, 25,* pp. 306-316, 1957.
52. L. W. Ferguson, An Analysis of the Generality of Suggestibility to Group Opinion, *Character and Personality, 12,* pp. 237-243, 1944.
53. J. R. Hilgard, *Personality and Hypnosis: A Study of Imaginative Involvement,* University of Chicago Press, Chicago, 1970.
54. S. J. Ceci, D. F. Ross, and M. P. Toglia, Are Differences in Suggestibility: Narrowing and Uncertainties, in *Children's Eyewitness Memory,* S. J. Ceci, M. P. Toglia, and D. F. Ross (eds.), Springer, New York, pp. 79-91, 1987.
55. T. E. Coffin, Some Conditions of Suggestion and Suggestibility: A Study of Certain Attitudinal and Situational Factors Influencing the Process of Suggestion, *Psychological Monographs, 53,* pp. 1-121, 1941.
56. B. Latané and S. W. Wolfe, The Social Impact of Majorities and Minorities, *Psychological Review, 88,* pp. 438-453, 1981.
57. S. Moscovi and B. Personnaz, Studies in Social Influence. V. Minority Influence and Conversion Behavior in a Perceptual Task, *Journal of Experimental Social Psychology, 16,* pp. 270-282, 1980.
58. I. L. Janis and P. B. Field, Sex Differences and Personality Factors Related to Persuasibility, in *Personality and Persuasibility,* C. I. Hovland and I. L. Janis (eds.), Yale University Press, New Haven, pp. 55-68, 1959.
59. W. J. McGuire, Personality and Susceptibility to Social Influence, in *Handbook of Personality Theory and Research,* E. F. Borgatta and W. W. Lambert (eds.), Rand McNally, Chicago, pp. 1130-1187, 1968.
60. M. Sherif and C. Sherif, *Reference Groups: Explorations into Conformity and Deviation in Adolescents,* Harper and Row, New York, 1964.

61. A. Maass and R. D. Clark, III, Internalization versus Compliance: Differential Processes Underlying Minority Influence and Conformity, *European Journal of Social Psychology, 13,* pp. 197-215, 1983.
62. P. R. Nail, Toward an Integration of Some Models and Theories of Social Responses, *Psychological Bulletin, 100,* pp. 190-206, 1986.
63. W. O. Bearden, R. G. Netemeyer, and J. E. Teel, Measurement of Consumer Susceptibility to Interpersonal Influence, *Journal of Consumer Research, 15,* pp. 473-481, 1989.
64. B. L. Cutler and R. N. Wolfe, Construct Validity of the Concern for Appropriateness Scale, *Journal of Personality Assessment, 49,* pp. 318-323, 1985.
65. A. L. Porterfield, F. S. Mayer, K. G. Dougherty, K. E. Kredich, M. M. Kronberg, K. M. Marsee, and Y. Okazaki, Private Self-consciousness, Canned Laughter, and Responses to Humorous Stimuli, *Journal of Research in Personality, 22,* pp. 409-423, 1988.
66. F. Sistrunk, Two Processes of Conformity Demonstrated by Interactions of Commitment, Set, and Personality, *Journal of Social Psychology, 89,* pp. 63-72, 1973.
67. G. H. Gudjonsson, Historical Background to Suggestibility: How Interrogative Suggestibility Differs from Other Types of Suggestibility, *Personality and Individual Differences, 8,* pp. 347-355, 1987.
68. E. P. Hollander and R. H. Willis, Some Current Issues in the Psychology of Conformity and Nonconformity, *Psychological Bulletin, 68,* pp. 62-76, 1967.
69. C. I. Hovland and I. L. Janis, *Personality and Persuasibility,* Yale University Press, New Haven, Connecticut, 1959.
70. R. K. Moore, Susceptibility to Hypnosis and Susceptibility to Social Influence, *Journal of Abnormal and Social Psychology, 68,* pp. 282-294, 1964.
71. S. Schachter, *The Psychology of Affiliation; Experimental Studies of the Sources of Gregariousness,* Stanford University Press, Stanford, California, 1959.
72. M Sherif, A Study of Some Social Factors in Perception, *Archives of Psychology, 27:*187, 1935.
73. A. Patel and J. Gordon, Some Personal and Situational Determinants of Yielding to Influence, *Journal of Abnormal and Social Psychology, 61,* pp. 411-418, 1960.
74. H. Reitan and M. Shaw, Group Membership, Sex, Composition of the Group, and Conformity Behavior, *Journal of Social Psychology, 64,* pp. 45-51, 1964.
75. J. Whittaker, Sex Differences and Susceptibility to Interpersonal Persuasion, *Journal of Social Psychology, 66,* pp. 91-94, 1965.
76. T. F. Pettigrew, The Measurement and Correlation of Category Width as a Cognitive Variable, *Journal of Psychology, 26,* pp. 532-544, 1958.
77. A. H. Eagly and L. L. Carli, Sex of Researchers and Sex-typed Communications as Determinants of Sex Differences in Influencibility: A Meta-analysis of Social Influence Studies, *Psychological Bulletin, 90,* pp. 1-20, 1981.
78. F. L. Fink, L. D. Rey, K. W. Johnson, K. I. Spenner, D. R. Morton, and E. T. Flores, The Effects of Family Occupation Type, Sex, and Appeal on Helping Behavior, *Journal of Experimental Social Psychology, 11,* pp. 43-52, 1975.
79. R. T. Santee and S. F. Jackson, Identity Implications of Conformity: Sex Differences in Normative and Attributional Judgments, *Journal of Personality and Social Psychology, 42,* pp. 690-700, 1982.
80. W. L. Nord, Social Exchange Theory: An Integrative Approach to Social Conformity, *Psychological Bulletin, 71,* pp. 174-208, 1969.
81. F. Sistrunk and J. W. McDavid, A Comparison of the Socially Influenced Behavior of College Students and College Dropouts, *Psychonomic Science, 15,* pp. 411-418, 1971.

82. A. M. Weitzenhoffer and E. R. Hilgard, *The Stanford Scale of Hypnotic Suscep-tibility, Forms A and B,* Consulting Psychologists Press, Palo Alto, California, 1959.
83. M. L. Shames, Hypnotic Susceptibility and Conformity: On the Mediational Mechanism of Suggestibility, *Psychological Reports, 49,* pp. 563-566, 1981.
84. H. Spiegel, An Eye-roll Test for Hypnotizability, *American Journal of Clinical Hypnosis, 14,* pp. 25-28, 1970.
85. N. P. Spanos and T. X. Barber, Behavior Modification and Hypnosis, *Progress in Behavior Modification, 3,* pp. 1-44, 1976.
86. G. F. Wagstaff, *Hypnosis, Compliance, and Belief,* St. Martin's Press, New York, 1981.
87. R. J. Miller, The Harvard Group Scale of Hypnotic Susceptibility as a Predictor of Nonhypnotic Suggestibility, *International Journal of Clinical and Experimental Hypnosis, 28,* pp. 46-52, 1980.
88. G. W. Farthing, S. W. Brown, and M. Venturino, Effects of Hypnotizability and Mental Imagery on Signal Detection Sensitivity and Response Bias, *International Journal of Clinical and Experimental Hypnosis, 30,* pp. 289-305, 1982.
89. K. R. Graham and L. M. Schwartz, Suggested Deafness and Auditory Signal Detectability, *Proceedings of the 81 Annual Convention of the American Psychological Association, 8,* pp. 1091-1092, 1973.
90. B. Jones and N. P. Spanos, Suggestions for Altered Auditory Sensitivity, the Negative Subject Effect and Hypnotic Susceptibility: A Signal Detection Analysis, *Journal of Personality and Social Psychology, 43,* pp. 637-647, 1982.
91. B. Wallace, J. B. Garrett, and S. P. Anstadt, Hypnotic Susceptibility, Suggestion, and Reports of Autokinetic Movement, *American Journal of Psychology, 87,* pp. 117-123, 1974.
92. P. Hajek and J. Spacek, Territory, Hypnotic Susceptibility, and Social Influence: A Pilot Study, *British Journal of Experimental and Clinical Hypnosis, 4,* pp. 115-117, 1987.
93. J. R. Council and D. Loge, Suggestibility and Confidence in False Perceptions: A Pilot Study, *British Journal of Experimental and Clinical Hypnosis, 5,* pp. 95-98, 1988.
94. K. R. Graham and L. D. Green, Hypnotic Susceptibility Related to an Independent Measure of Compliance—Alumni Annual Giving: A Brief Communication, *International Journal of Clinical and Experimental Hypnosis, 29,* pp. 66-76, 1981.
95. J. M. Malott, A. L. Bourg, and H. J. Crawford, The Effects of Hypnosis upon Cognitive Responses to Persuasive Communication, *International Journal of Clinical and Experimental Hypnosis, 37,* pp. 31-40, 1989.
96. L. D. Bertrand, The Assessment and Modification of Hypnotic Susceptibility, in *Hypnosis: The Cognitive Behavioral Perspective,* N. P. Spanos and J. F. Chaves (eds.), Prometheus, Buffalo, 1989.
97. N. P. Spanos, Hypnosis and the Modification of Hypnotic Susceptibility: A Social Psychological Perspective, in *What is Hypnosis?,* P. L. N. Naish (ed.), Open University Press, Philadelphia, pp. 85-120, 1986.
98. N. P. Spanos, N. J. Gabora, L. Jarrett, and M. I. Gwynn, Contextual Determinants of Hypnotizability and Relationships between Hypnotizability Scales, *Journal of Personality and Social Psychology, 46,* pp. 688-696, 1989.
99. J.-R. Laurence and C. Perry, Hypnotically Created Memories among Highly Hypnotizable Subjects, *Science, 222,* pp. 523-524, 1983.
100. J.-R. Laurence and C. Perry, *Hypnosis, Will, and Memory: A Psycho-legal History,* Guilford, New York, 1988.

101. N. P. Spanos and E. Bures, Pseudomemory Responding in Hypnotic, Task-motivated and Simulating Subjects: Memory Distortion or Reporting Bias, *Imagination, Cognition and Personality, 13,* pp. 303-310, 1994.
102. N. P. Spanos and J. McLean, Hypnotically Created Pseudomemories: Memory Distortions or Reporting Biases, *British Journal of Experimental and Clinical Hypnosis, 3,* pp. 155-159, 1986.
103. A. J. Barnier and K. M. McConkey, Reports of Real and False Memories: The Relevance of Hypnosis, Hypnotizability, and Test Control, *Journal of Abnormal Psychology, 101,* pp. 521-527, 1992.
104. P. W. Sheehan, D. Statham, and G. A. Jamieson, Pseudomemory Effects Over Time in the Hypnotic Setting, *Journal of Abnormal Psychology, 100,* pp. 39-44, 1991.
105. P. W. Sheehan, D. Statham, and G. A. Jamieson, Pseudomemory Effects and Their Relationship to Level of Susceptibility to Hypnosis and State Instruction, *Journal of Personality and Social Psychology, 60,* pp. 130-137, 1991.
106. N. P. Spanos, M. I. Gwynn, S. L. Comer, W. J. Baltruweit, and M. de Groh, Are Hypnotically Induced Pseudomemories Resistant to Cross-examination?, *Law and Human Behavior, 13,* pp. 271-289, 1989.
107. P. W. Sheehan, *Memory Bias in Hypnosis,* paper presented at the 10th International Congress of Hypnosis and Psychosomatic Medicine, Toronto, Canada, August 1985.
108. P. W. Sheehan and L. Grigg, Hypnosis, Memory, and the Acceptance of an Implausible Cognitive Set, *British Journal of Clinical and Experimental Hypnosis, 3,* pp. 5-12, 1985.
109. P. W. Sheehan and J. Tilden, Effects of Suggestibility and Hypnosis on Accurate and Distorted Retrieval from Memory, *Journal of Experimental Psychology: Learning, Memory, and Cognition, 9,* pp. 283-293, 1983.
110. P. W. Sheehan and J. Tilden, The Consistency of Occurrences of Memory Distortion Following Hypnotic Induction, *International Journal of Clinical and Experimental Hypnosis, 34,* pp. 122-137, 1986.
111. J. R. Council, I. Kirsch, and L. P. Hafner, Expectancy versus Absorption in the Prediction of Hypnotic Responding, *Journal of Personality and Social Psychology, 50,* pp. 182-189, 1986.
112. H. P. de Groot, M. I. Gwynn, and N. P. Spanos, The Effects of Contextual Information and Gender on the Prediction of Hypnotic Susceptibility, *Journal of Personality and Social Psychology, 50,* 1988.
113. S. D. Drake, M. R. Nash, and G. N. Cawood, Imaginative Involvement and Hypnotic Susceptibility: A Re-examination of the Relationship, *Imagination, Cognition and Personality, 10,* pp. 141-155, 1991.
114. N. P. Spanos, M. Arango, and H. P. de Groot, Context as a Moderator of the Relationship between Attribute Variables and Hypnotizability, *Personality and Social Psychology Bulletin, 19,* pp. 71-77, 1993.
115. N. P. Spanos, C. A. Quigley, M. I. Gwynn, R. L. Glatt, and A. H. Perlini, Hypnotic Interrogation Pretrial Preparation, and Witness Testimony during Direct and Cross-examination, *Law and Human Behavior, 15,* pp. 639-653, 1991.
116. G. H. Gudjonsson, Suggestibility, Intelligence, Memory Recall and Personality: An Experimental Study, *British Journal of Psychiatry, 142,* pp. 35-37, 1983.
117. G. H. Gudjonsson, A New Scale of Interrogative Suggestibility, *Personality and Individual Differences, 5,* pp. 303-314, 1984.
118. G. H. Gudjonsson, Interrogative Suggestibility: Comparison between 'False Confessors' and 'Deniers' in Criminal Trials, *Medicine, Science and the Law, 24,* pp. 56-60, 1984.

119. G. H. Gudjonsson and N. K. Clark, Suggestibility in Police Interrogation: A Social Psychological Model, *Social Behaviour, 1,* pp. 83-104, 1986.
120. W. Stern, *General Psychology: From the Personalistic Standpoint,* Macmillan, New York, 1938.
121. H. E. Burtt, *Applied Psychology,* Prentice-Hall, New York, pp. 291-321, 1949.
122. E. F. Loftus, *Eyewitness Testimony,* Harvard University Press, London, 1979.
123. R. L. Cohen and M. A. Harnick, The Susceptibility of Child Witnesses to Suggestion, *Law and Human Behavior, 4,* pp. 201-210, 1980.
124. P. A. Powers, J. L. Andriks, and E. F. Loftus, Eyewitness Accounts of Males and Females, *Journal of Applied Psychology, 64,* pp. 339-347, 1979.
125. P. C. Young, Intelligence and Suggestibility in Whites and Negroes, *Journal of Comparative Psychology, 9,* pp. 339-355, 1929.
126. G. H. Gudjonsson and J. Gunn, The Competence and Reliability of a Witness in Criminal Court, *British Journal of Psychiatry, 141,* pp. 624-627, 1982.
127. G. H. Gudjonsson, Interrogative Suggestibility and Perceptual Motor Performance, *Perceptual and Motor Skills, 58,* pp. 671-672, 1984.
128. G. H. Gudjonsson, The Relationship between Interrogative Suggestibility and Acquiescence: Empirical Findings and Theoretical Implications, *Personality and Individual Differences, 7,* pp. 195-199, 1986.
129. G. H. Gudjonsson, A Parallel Form of the Gudjonsson Suggestibility Scale, *British Journal of Clinical Psychology, 26,* pp. 215-221, 1987.
130. K. K. Singh and G. H. Gudjonsson, The Internal Consistency of the "Shift" Factor on the Gudjonsson Suggestibility Scale, *Personality and Individual Differences, 8,* pp. 265-266, 1987.
131. G. H. Gudjonsson, The Relationship of Intelligence and Memory to Interrogative Suggestibility: The Importance of Range Effects, *British Journal of Clinical Psychology, 27,* pp. 185-187, 1988.
132. G. H. Gudjonsson and S. Lister, Interrogative Suggestibility and its Relationship with Perceptions of Self-concept and Control, *Journal of the Forensic Science Society, 24,* pp. 99-110, 1984.
133. G. H. Gudjonsson and J. A. C. MacKeith, Retracted Confessions: Legal, Psychological, and Psychiatric Aspects, *Medicine, Science and the Law, 28,* pp. 185-187, 1988.
134. E. Haraldsson, Interrogative Suggestibility and its Relationship with Personality, Perceptual Defensiveness and Extraordinary Beliefs, *Personality and Individual Differences, 6,* pp. 765-767, 1985.
135. G. H. Gudjonsson and K. K. Singh, Interrogative Suggestibility and Delinquent Boys: An Empirical Validation Study, *Personality and Individual Differences, 5,* pp. 425-430, 1984.
136. G. H. Gudjonsson, Compliance in an Interrogative Situation: A New Scale, *Personality and Individual Differences, 10,* pp. 535-540, 1989.
137. G. H. Gudjonsson, The Relationship of Intellectual Skills to Suggestibility, Compliance and Acquiescence, *Personality and Individual Differences, 11,* pp. 227-231, 1990.
138. P. Tata and G. H. Gudjonsson, Some Effects of Stress and Feedback on Interrogative Suggestibility, *Personality and Individual Differences, 11,* pp. 1079-1085, 1990.
139. G. H. Gudjonsson, Interrogative Suggestibility: Its Relationship with Assertiveness, Social-evaluative Anxiety, State Anxiety and Method of Coping, *British Journal of Clinical Psychology, 27,* pp. 159-166, 1988.
140. K. K. Singh and G. H. Gudjonsson, Interrogative Suggestibility, Delayed Memory, and Self-concept, *Personality and Individual Differences, 5,* pp. 203-209, 1984.

141. G. H. Gudjonsson, The Effects of Suspiciousness and Anger on Suggestibility, *Medicine, Science and the Law, 29,* pp. 229-232, 1989.
142. P. A. Register and J. F. Kihlstrom, Hypnosis and Interrogative Suggestibility, *Personality and Individual Differences, 9,* pp. 549-558, 1988.
143. I. Hansdottir, H. S. Thornsteinsson, H. Kristinsdottir, and R. S. Ragnarsson, The Effects of Instructions and Anxiety on Interrogative Suggestibility, *Personality and Individual Differences, 11,* pp. 85-87, 1990.
144. K. Smith and G. H. Gudjonsson, Investigation of the Responses of 'Fakers' and 'Non-fakers' on the Gudjonsson Suggestibility Scale, *Medicine, Science and the Law, 26,* pp. 66-71, 1986.
145. E. C. Hardarson, *Sambað daleidslu-og yfirheyrslu naemis og fylgni with personuleika og namsarangur,* B.A. thesis, University of Rekjavik, 1985.
146. M. I. Gwynn, N. P. Spanos, S. Nancoo, and L. Chow, *Interrogative Suggestibility, Hypnotizability, and Persuasibility: Are They Related?,* manuscript submitted for publication, 1995.
147. E. Gordon, M. I. Gwynn, and N. P. Spanos, *Effects of Hypnosis, Suggestion, and Delay on Interrogative Suggestibility and Confidence,* unpublished master's thesis, Carleton University, Ottawa, 1993.
148. N. P. Spanos, H. L. Radtke, D. C. Hodgins, H. J. Stam, and L. D. Bertrand, The Carleton University Responsiveness to Suggestion Scale: Normative Data and Psychometric Properties, *Psychological Reports, 53,* pp. 523-535, 1983.
149. M. Reiser, *Handbook of Investigative Hypnosis,* LEHI, Los Angeles, 1980.

[The preparation of this chapter was supported in part by a Social Sciences and Humanities Research Council of Canada Postdoctoral Fellowship to the first author and a grant from the Social Sciences and Humanities Research Council to the second author.]

CHAPTER 9

Conviction Management: Lessons from Hypnosis Research about How Self-Images of Dubious Validity Can Be Willfully Sustained

DONALD R. GORASSINI

[There is an] ease with which people can come to believe whatever is convenient to believe, however ludicrous it may be [1, p. 201].

Who we think we are affects how we feel. Therefore, if we could regulate self-reflection, we would, thereby, regulate affect. Rid ourselves of some self-knowledge, that which demonstrates such traits as incompetence or callousness, and we escape anxiety and guilt. Bring forth other self-knowledge, that which implies good characteristics like intelligence and caring, and we gain a sense of pride. It is an unfortunate fact of life that things we would rather not know about ourselves are true, and things we wish *were* self-descriptive are, sadly, false. Therein lies the incentive to cheat, to ignore painful self-reflection and create conviction in pleasurable self-images, images that an unbiased analysis would reveal to be invalid.

This chapter concerns people's ability to engage in the ostensibly paradoxical activity of telling convincing lies to themselves about who they are. It is argued that people can indeed, as Chomsky asserts, easily convince themselves of ludicrous propositions. A model is presented to show how people succeed at manufacturing conviction in pre-selected self-definitions, even when the definitions are clearly invalid. Perhaps nowhere is the ability to lie effectively to the self about the self more clearly demonstrated than in hypnosis research. After presenting the self-deception model, which was spawned by my observations of unhypnotizable subjects role-playing hypnotizable ones, hypnotic research that bears on the model is reviewed.

178 / HYPNOSIS AND IMAGINATION

SEEKING A CHANGE IN SELF-DEFINITION
BY ILLEGITIMATE MEANS

Some selves that we do not possess we would nonetheless like to have. Only some of these desired selves are, however, pursuable. Pursuable selves (e.g., gardener) can be sought and achieved whereas unpursuable selves (e.g., math genius) are imposed or bestowed by forces acting outside of our control. There is usually no hope of achieving unpursuable selves by legitimate means. But even if we do not possess a desired, unpursuable self, there is another way, albeit illegitimate, of attaining it: pretending it is true.

Consider pursuable self-definitions like gardener and doctor. In each case, the specified self can be thought of as a goal composed of a series of sub-goals. It is only through a conscious planning process that each of the sub-goals in the progression can be achieved. Successfully executing the acts serving as means to the overarching goal result in valid application of the self-label. To be sure, pursuable selves vary in difficulty of attainment, with gardener being substantially easier than doctor, but no matter how difficult achievement is, the end can at least be sought, and it will be attained only if there is conscious planning and effort.

Some selves we cannot seek; they become part of our identity without any attempt on our parts to bring them about. These unpursuable selves result from internal (frequently medical) conditions that alter experience or behavior (e.g., migraine, schizophrenia); external events that subtly change our preferences (e.g., mere exposure, classical conditioning) (see, e.g., [2, 3]); or assignment by nature (e.g., male, math genius), other people (e.g., the religion of childhood as assigned by one's parents), or circumstance (e.g., citizenship) before the opportunity to choose and pursue alternatives presents itself.

Consider as an example of an unpursuable self-definition that of a migraine sufferer. An individual having a migraine attack, which occurs due to the constriction of cranial arteries on one side of the head, has unusual experiences (which can include an experience of detachment, partial blindness, numbness facially and in a hand, and the inability to form sentences) followed by extreme head pain. To be defined a migraine sufferer, you must have the disorder that causes the aforementioned syndrome to appear periodically. The process that controls the nature and course of symptoms operates on its own, interfering with consciously governed activity. The condition can be controlled somewhat, with medication, but is nonetheless impervious to direct and decisive conscious control.

The only self-definitions we can hope to attain, therefore, are the pursuable types, but even here attainment usually takes time, with success not always assured. Unpursuable self-definitions, we cannot even hope to attain through our own efforts because they depend on decisive forces operating completely, or almost so, beyond our control. But sometimes strong incentives to claim a particular self, whether the self applies validly or not, are present and demand an immediate response. For those who do not possess the desired definition, there is something to be gained by claiming the self in question nonetheless. Frequently the incentive is affect management: the acquisition of the good feeling that results when flattering information about the self is believed.

To illustrate, consider the richly detailed case study by Festinger, Riecken, and Schachter [4] of a doomsday cult in the United States in which one of the group's leaders, pseudonymed Marion Keech by the investigators, makes what in our terms is an invalid self-claim [4]. She has others believe that beings not of this world communicate through her by controlling what she writes. Keech, in describing her first discovery of the ability, is quoted as saying:

> I felt a kind of tingling or numbness in my arm, and my whole arm felt warm right up to the shoulder. . . . I had the feeling that someone was trying to get my attention. Without knowing why, I picked up a pencil and a pad that were lying on the table near by bed. My hand began to write in another handwriting. I looked at the handwriting and it was strangely familiar, but I knew it was not my own. I realized that somebody else was using my hand, and I said: "Will you identify yourself?" And they did. I was much surprised to find that it was my father, who had passed away [4, p. 33].

A number of different entities communicated in this fashion through Keech, principal among them an outer space creature named Sananda, who made several testable predictions about visits to earth by space beings, incipient cataclysms that earth would undergo, and when believers would be rescued by spaceships. None of the predictions came true and the cult ultimately broke up in disarray.

Admittedly, the case study methodology makes it impossible to rule out completely that communication from outer space beings occurred, but the evidence that does exist suggests the messages were untrue. The case study is used here for its expository and heuristic value—to show the possibility and conditions of successfully lying to the self about the self. More definitive, experimental evidence concerning self-deceptive ability will be presented in the third major section of this chapter.

Consider what the above example suggests: First it illustrates that affect-change incentives for believing in invalid self-definitions can be powerful. As Festinger et al. put it:

> We can only imagine the awe, the reverence, with which the Armstrongs [other leading members of the doomsday cult] and Mrs. Keech received these momentous pronouncements [from outer space]. Here, in the hands of three fairly ordinary people (by the world's standards) had been placed the most important news of our time, if not of all recorded history. A grave responsibility, an incomparable privilege had been thrust upon them [4, p. 57].

Incentives to Mrs. Keech to lie knowingly—to others but not to herself—about mediumship were weak in comparison to the pay-off for her to deceive herself. In fact, public knowledge of her and the group's beliefs brought nothing but trouble, including vicious practical jokes, national ridicule, and attention from the police. The only apparent reason for her to press on in the face of such difficulty, with the courage and conviction she displayed, was to maintain a particular kind of self-image, one that brought with it great inner meaning.

Second, the case study illustrates what I mean by a self-claim. Such an assertion need not literally be a statement of the form, "I am ____," but can be, and usually is, nonverbal. Mrs. Keech repeatedly engaged in the behavior of mediumship, which served to reinforce and elaborate her own and the group's knowledge of her apparent gift.

Third, self-conviction takes place in a social setting, usually involving the support of like-minded accomplices [4]. Keech was part of a group of doom-sayers whose members refrained from questioning each other's claims and cooperated for the most part in building and reinforcing the group's belief system.

Fourth, the example also sets out the nature of the lie to be told to the self. On one hand, Mrs. Keech in some sense knows she is not a medium, for she deliberately acts out behaviors and deliberately engenders experiences that, if they were authentic, would occur involuntarily. On the other hand, she seems able to avoid consciously registering knowledge of her active role-playing, with the result being conviction that she really is a medium.

Finally, the lie that is told to the self is a blatant one: Sananda, the mediumship, and all the other core assumptions on which the group operated were false. Lies are always blatant when told about unpursuable selves. If the unpursuable self has not been bestowed or imposed, there is little or nothing the person can do voluntarily to achieve the definition by legitimate means. (Shades of truth are, however, possible when it comes to pursuable selves. In the case of pursuable self-definitions, a lie can be minor, as when a person refers to herself as a doctor after she has completed all her medical training but has three days to go before being admitted to the College of Physicians officially; or the lie can be blatant, as when someone calls herself a doctor even though she has had no medical education at all.)

Summary and Conclusion

We can experience pressure to claim self-definitions we do not possess. Unfortunately for us, attainment of some desirable selves is beyond our control. The dilemma faced by the individual in these cases is either forego the definition and suffer disappointment and anxiety or convince the self that the definition applies (even though, in reality, it doesn't apply) and, in so doing, bring more meaning to life.

In this chapter, I will focus mainly on lies about the possession of unpursuable self-definitions. Given that these are always the most blatant of lies, it should be that they are the most difficult to tell successfully to the self. If one can sustain these, then upholding lies of a less blatant nature (often the case with pursuable selves) should be a relatively easy task.

Some research in hypnosis bears nicely on the question of how lying to the self about the self takes place. I will present a model of the process in the next section. In the section after that I will present hypnotic research that addresses aspects of the model.

MANUFACTURING CONVICTION

Assume you are asked a question about yourself—"Are you a migraine sufferer?" or "Are you a gardener?" or some such—and the identity is indeed true of you. A truthful "Yes, I am" response will have associated with it a high degree of conviction. Underlying the certainty with which the answer is given is the recall of pertinent events, a large proportion of which support the crucial elements of the self-definition in question; or perhaps a previous confident "Yes, I am" assertion, which itself was prefaced by the analysis of supporting evidence, is recalled and serves as the source of conviction. Directly or indirectly, then, event recall is the identity judgment's ultimate source. If you actually are a gardener, you have literally gotten dirty, and seen, smelled, and perhaps tasted the results of your labor; have spoken to other gardeners; and are referred to and treated by friends as a gardener. If you actually are a migraine sufferer, you have had intimate experience with the condition's symptoms, have been diagnosed by a physician, and are known to intimates as a migraine sufferer. Against a background of such richly detailed supporting experiences, self-definitions that are actually possessed come to be held with virtual certainty.

By contrast, invalid identity claims—for example, saying you possess a self-definition (even though you do not)—are apt to be recognized by the actor for the lies that they are. This is because there are few or no supporting experiences to recall. If conviction is to be manufactured at all, a strategy would be needed to circumvent the usually very effective reality testing process. Assume, then, that someone wants to manufacture conviction in the validity of (untrue) assertions about the self. (As I have argued above, there are frequently strong incentives for doing so.) How might one go about it? One way would be to create event memories from imagination, but somehow define the information as having originated from the physical world. While memory may be subject to some degree of distortion, in which events only imagined are remembered as real [5], it would be a tall order for someone to imagine the many and detailed events necessary for supporting an identity claim and then make it seem that the events really happened.

An alternative method of manufacturing conviction in an identity claim would be to create the very perceptual experiences on which the claim is to be based. One tactic within this strategy would be to hallucinate the events that comprise the self-definition. Hallucinations are internally generated images that are mistakenly judged to be originating from external stimulation. This approach, if successfully implemented, would serve to implant the experiences necessary for making future (invalid) identity claims believable. Like memory creation, though, hallucinating is difficult. It has been proposed that members of a highly select group—less than 5 percent of the population—do have the ability to imagine events "as real as real" [6, 7]. It was once thought certain conditions, especially hypnosis [8], could enhance the ability to hallucinate. For instance, in the nineteenth century, Bernheim proposed that, in hypnosis, there is "exaltation of the ideo-sensorial excitability, which affects the unconscious transformation of thought into sensation, or into sensory image" [9, p. 137]. Today, there is skepticism that hypnosis has this facilitating effect [10, 11], and even though it is apparent that certain teachable cognitive skills are instrumental in facilitating imagery vividness [11], it is doubtful that very many people could construct from nothing, through hallucination, the experiences necessary for supporting an identity claim.

Another perceptually related tactic, one that has a much better chance of being effective, is insuring that many of the physical events that support the existence of a desired, target self-definition actually take place. With events that support the identity *actually having occurred,* the individual is in possession of the most convincing of information for backing up a claim. This approach has a far better chance of being successful than either memory creation or hallucination, is likely the tactic of choice of dedicated conviction managers, and is apparently what Marian Keech used to bring conviction to her claim of mediumship: she created, then used, real events as the foundation for her claims. This method of conviction management obviates the difficulties inherent in the hallucination and memory creation strategies. Hallucination is not a necessary component of the process because actual stimuli are used to bring about perceptual experiences. Nor does memory have to be relied on for the creation of event recollections. Memory is given the relatively easy task of lending particular interpretations to events actually being perceived. Therefore, my focus in the rest of the chapter will be on the method of physical event creation for managing conviction.

Controlling Perception

In his book, *Cognition and Reality,* Neisser describes perception as a cycle [12]. Involved are a *schema* or mental structure representing what the perceiver expects to perceive; *perceptual plans* that derive from the schema, orient the perceiver to the stimulus, and govern information search; and *information* itself, which will either confirm, contradict, or fail to inform the schema under test. A percept results when there is confirmation of what the perceiver expects to encounter. In other words, all the elements must be cycled through for there to be perception. If an expectation is held—for example, that you will hear Jingle Bells—but no Jingle Bells is playing, there will be no percept. If, on the other hand, the tune is actually playing, but there is no Jingle Bells schema in current operation, it will take time for one to be called forth to complete the cycle and create a percept of the tune.

The perceptual cycle is subject to control at many points. You can control which schemas you will think about, and you along with your associates can control the stimulus information to be picked up. These controllable sub-processes make it possible to make to order perceptions of self to be experienced.

Schema Control. It is possible for us to control, to some extent, what we think about, including what we think about ourselves. We can entertain certain hypotheses about who we are, and once under consideration, the definitions give us an idea of what we will do and feel in particular situations. If the hypotheses are confirmed in the situations specified, then certainty in the validity of the proposed self-definition is enhanced. Consider the self-definition, doctor. When a diagnosis is communicated to a patient, it is the doctor who gives the results, it is the patient who listens apprehensively to the news, and all occurs in an expected setting, such as a doctor's office or a hospital room. If the doctor and patient observe events that correspond to these expectations, then their respective self-definitions will be reinforced. If something as counter-expectational as the patient giving the test results to an apprehensive doctor, or the interview taking place in a circus ring with doctor and patient dressed in clown suits, there would be confusion, at the root of which is the failure of schema-based expectations to predict actual events.

The same sort of process applies to unpursuable self-definitions. For example, once a migraine attack begins, the sufferer knows what to expect: what will be experienced and when; what will be done to combat symptoms; that frustration at the interruption of planned activity will be experienced; and how one's close associates will react to the news of the attack. Events will either confirm or contradict these expectations and affect conviction in the self-schema accordingly.

Stimulus Control. It is also possible to control the events that our self-definitions lead us to expect will happen, which gives us flexibility and power in determining whether self-definitions are confirmed or contradicted. And stimuli we cannot control, our associates can; so that, with help, it is possible to insure that only expectation-confirming events occur.

Consider the simulation set up by Janis and Mann in their study of emotional role-playing and its influence on smoking cessation [13]. University students who were smokers participated in the study. Each subject played the role of a patient receiving lung cancer test results from a doctor. In each case, the doctor, played by the experimenter, broke the bad news that the test was positive. The physical setting of the exchange was similar to that of a physician's office.

Consider what the actor playing the role of patient would observe during the simulation and note the fact that the observations match those a real patient in such a setting would have. These include what the patient observes her- or himself doing (e.g., looking apprehensive, showing concern at the bad news, requesting further information), how the doctor treats the patient (e.g., gives the bad news, displays concern for the patient, prescribes a course of treatment), and what the physical setting is like (e.g., a doctor's office, doctor wears white lab coat). Under the circumstances, a high degree of conviction in the validity of the self-definition, patient, can be manufactured, as Janis and Mann found:

> [R]ole players displayed considerable affect arousal during their performance including tremors, trembling, and flushing. These manifestations of fear impressed us as being far beyond the call of duty, even for whole-hearted adherents of the Stanislavsk method of acting. . . . Spontaneous comments made by almost every role-player at the end of the session indicated awareness of fear arousal: e.g., "You scared me to death"; "I was really getting scared"; "That just shook me up—it does scare me—it does! [13, p. 88].

There was, in reality, no cancer. The "doctor" was no doctor and the "patient" was no patient. Yet, on short notice and for the enactment's duration, subjects portraying patients were able to lie to themselves about themselves successfully.

Insuring Schema Confirmation. Some self-definitions are easier than others to confirm. The likelihood of a confirmation will be high when a *version* of the self, for which the actor and the actor's associates are able to provide confirming physical evidence, is defined. The doctor and patient identities described above were relatively easy to confirm because 1) no special skills were required of either role and 2) the three sources of supporting evidence—the actor's behavior, the behavior of the actor playing opposite, and the physical setting—were present. The actors were not given the onerous task, for example, of hallucinating the physical setting or the other actor. Similarly, aspects of a migraine sufferer's experience, the early part of the attack that involves relatively indistinct symptoms and little or no pain, could be simulated: the sufferer could take a pill and lie down, anticipate further symptoms, think about the plans the headache will be interrupting, and take note of concern expressed by others. Advanced stages of an attack, which can involve aphasia and usually involve intense head pain, would be extremely difficult to produce, and the failure to make them occur would undermine the experience of conviction in being a migraine sufferer. The same reasoning applies to someone playing a math genius. A number of elements (e.g., dress, mannerisms) that fit the stereotype can be fulfilled convincingly. The whole edifice of the managed identity would crumble, though, if math ability were actually tested by experts.

Note that hallucinated images need not be involved in the conviction manufacturing process. The self-schemas selected by the actor can be confirmed by actual events. This is not to say hallucination cannot be used to help supplement the experience. In fact, as noted, a small proportion of the population is said to be capable of hallucinating skillfully. These rare people are apt to supplement perceptions with hallucinated images and deepen their conviction as a result.

Meta-Knowledge

The conviction manager is in possession of two contradictory kinds of information at the same time. On one hand, there is the control structure that guides role-play behavior. If the actor is fully aware of this structure's nature, he or she will know the identity being projected is not real. If, for instance, an actor portraying a doctor has insight into the process, she will think of herself as *playing* a doctor, not *being* a doctor. On the other hand, the physical evidence, consisting of one's own behavior, the behavior of others, and the physical setting generally, supports the existence of the identity in question—according to this information, the person *is* a doctor. The goals of the conviction manager are (a) to purge from consciousness knowledge of the plan to manage conviction and (b) to think only about the target self-schema (i.e., doctor, gardener, or whatever).

This may not be that difficult a task. There is reason to believe that little conscious attention is demanded in acting a role because the process is over-learned: self-presentations occur on a frequent basis [14], as do attempts during self-presentations to construe the self in illusory ways [15]. The situation, too, can be constructed so that there are no reminders that an act may be in progress. With the combination of overlearning and the absence of cues necessary for stimulating insight into the conviction management process, the actor can remain unaware of his or her acting.

By contrast, the self-definition the actor is trying to become convinced of will produce a strong mental trace, partly because the conviction management process requires the actor to keep the targeted schema in mind. There is also much information that the actor observes as supporting the suppositions inherent in the self-schema. The net effect is a perceptual cycle, in which beliefs being entertained about the self receive immediate support. This cycling among schema, expectation, and available information brings with it a strong sense of conviction in the self-definition's validity.

Summary

Valid identity claims tend to be laden with conviction because they are based on richly detailed matching experiences. This perceptual matching process, ironically, can be used to cultivate conviction in assertions about identity, *even when the claims have no validity.* In this process, a version of the sought-after self-definition, capable of being confirmed, is considered; and events, including the behavior of the actor, the behavior of others, and the physical setting generally, that support the reality of the proposed self-definition, are made to occur. The result for actors is a sense that the identity in question is genuine. The perceptual system, usually so effective in separating fact from fiction, is thus used to insure the success of a lie to the self about the self.

CONVICTION MANAGEMENT IN HYPNOSIS

Suggestions of various sorts are given in the hypnotic situation. The suggestions call for "sleep," for motor responses, for perceptual distortion, and for failures—or feats—of memory, and it is implied by the hypnotist that these responses will occur involuntarily. It is therefore clear to the subject that the defining feature of hypnotically susceptible persons is that they exhibit suggested responses involuntarily.

Suppose that a subject sits and waits for the promised responses to occur, and nothing happens. This means that the psychological conditions necessary for involuntary responding are not present and that the subject is not hypnotically susceptible. Put another way, the unpursuable self-definition, hypnotizable person, fails to apply to the subject. The only way that such a person can claim to be hypnotically susceptible is by illegitimate means—by cheating. The hypnotic situation supports the conviction manufacturing process 1) by giving a detailed description of what hypnotized persons do and feel, and 2) by presenting stimuli that confirm the hypnotic self-schema. Let us examine the hypnotic situation more closely.

The Hypnotic Situation

Learning the Self-schema. Even someone with a barely articulated notion of what hypnosis is has little trouble gleaning from hypnotic procedures what a hypnotized person looks and acts like. A typical hypnotic session begins with a seated subject being requested by the hypnotist to relax with eyes closed. Next, a hypnotic induction procedure in which the hypnotist speaks continuously for several minutes on end, repeating phrases over and over, is administered. The main theme of the induction is that subjects are falling into a sleeplike state in which attention is to be paid exclusively to the hypnotist's speech and that, in hypnosis, responses occur involuntarily when merely mentioned by the hypnotist [16]. Following the induction, suggestions are made.

A suggestion is a description of behavior (e.g., a simple arm movement) or of a cognitive response (e.g., a hallucination, or failure or feat of memory) traditionally associated with the topic of hypnosis. Also specified are the times when each response is to occur and for how long it is to last. It is not unusual, for instance, for the hypnotist to trace with a steady stream of speech the response's course as it is to be occurring (e.g., "Your arm is slowly beginning to go up. It is slowly rising. More and more. More and more. . . ."). Although each suggestion focuses mainly on tracing one principal response, a number of other responses, which somehow relate to the focal act, are also usually described. If, for example, you are told that you hear a fly buzzing around you (principal response), you may also be told to swat at it (secondary response). It is also implied that the principal response is involuntary, as in the statement "an apple has appeared on the table in front of you," which implies that the apple has appeared without the viewer trying to make it appear. From listening to the hypnotist, then, the subject learns that a hypnotized person exhibits principal responses at the times and for the durations specified, and that these responses occur involuntarily.

Help in the Conviction Manufacturing Process. The hypnotic situation helps the subject sustain conviction in the idea that he or she is hypnotized. In the midst of describing what the various behaviors and experiences that characterize hypnosis are, the hypnotist also defines the responses as the *subject's own*: *"You are falling into a sleep . . .*"; *"You* feel your arm getting lighter . . ."; *"You* see a kitten on your lap . . ."; *"You* can no longer remember. . . ." This immediate social feedback defines the subject as hypnotized and as someone who is emitting hypnotic, involuntary responses. As argued above, the behavior of others has an impact on beliefs about the validity of a self-definition. In hypnosis, the actions of the hypnotist are strongly supportive of the idea that the subject is hypnotized. The physical setting, too, complements the presence of hypnosis in the subject, for it resembles places (e.g., a doctor's office, a university laboratory) in which hypnosis is "known" to occur.

At the same time as social and physical support for the reality of hypnosis is introduced, information supporting the chief rival explanation for the subject's behavior—that it's all an act—is withheld. Hypnotists tend, during a session, to refrain from making references to notions like role-playing, conviction management, cheating, game-playing and the like. Furthermore, cues that hint of stage notions, such as audiences, lights and sets, cameras, and so on are also usually absent.

Information about Pursuability. As indicated above, subjects of hypnosis are taught early in a session what hypnosis and hypnotizability are. One gets labeled as hypnotically susceptible, the hypnotist indicates, when certain involuntary responses—most notably, perceptual distortions and memory changes—occur. This information affects how subjects conduct themselves for the rest of the session, especially during the administration of hypnotic suggestions. A majority of subjects, comprised mostly of low hypnotizables, assume that, since principal responses will be involuntary, subjects must *wait* for the promised responses to occur on their own [17]. Doing the opposite (i.e., simulating principal responses) would undermine the chief purpose of the session, which is to measure the subject's propensity for hypnotic (translate as *involuntary*) responding.

To illustrate by way of analogy the low hypnotizable subject's reasoning, compare him or her to a patient who, in the midst of undergoing a physical examination, is given a test of the patellar reflex. The reflex is an involuntary jerk of the leg induced by the physician's tapping on the patellar ligament. During the test, the patient is expected to wait for the response to occur on its own. Simulating the knee jerk, which would cloud test results, is considered inappropriate and is thus avoided.

So, even though the typical low hypnotizable subject learns about how a person who is high in hypnotizability feels and acts, and even though a situation that supports conviction management is provided, the subject assumes that waiting for hypnosis and hypnotic responses to take hold is the most appropriate course of action; conviction management is not considered an option. In the next section, I will show that only a slight corrective is needed to change this way of thinking and launch low hypnotizable subjects on a campaign of successful conviction management.

Conviction Training

If we want to see how easily unhypnotized subjects are able to convince themselves they are actually hypnotized, we must insure that conviction management actually takes place. Low hypnotizables are unlikely to engage in the process because they believe that hypnosis and hypnotizability are unpursuable. To change these interpretations, the following conviction management instructions were given in two studies to subjects who pretested low in hypnotic susceptibility:

> We greatly appreciate your past participation in our research. Today I would like you to take part in a very interesting experiment that is quite different from any in which you have participated to date. The last time you were here you scored as low in hypnotic susceptibility. In today's session, you will be given the same susceptibility test as you were the first time you were here. However, your task today is totally different from last time. You will be given instructions that will easily enable you to increase your level of hypnotic susceptibility substantially (underlined in the original).
> A common misconception about hypnosis must be cleared up from the outset. Hypnosis cannot change your actions and thoughts. If you just sit and wait for suggested responses to happen on their own, NOTHING WILL HAPPEN. If the hypnotist suggests that your arm is rising, the arm will certainly *not* rise by itself. Likewise, if the hypnotist suggests that you are forgetting something, this cannot make you forget in the least! With this in mind, read the two instructions which follow. If you do you best to follow both instructions, you will be able to increase your susceptibility level greatly.
> INSTRUCTION 1: MAKE THE SUGGESTED RESPONSES HAPPEN AUTOMATICALLY. This simply means that you should make each of the responses that are suggested, but don't pay attention to the fact that you are making them. Automatic responses of this sort are commonly made in everyday life. For instance, when you are reading the newspaper, you might reach automatically for a cup of coffee and have a sip. Reaching for a coffee cup is usually something that you do with minimal attention because most of your attention is directed elsewhere to more interesting things (e.g., toward reading of the newspaper).
> Thus if a suggestion tells you to raise your arm, then lift your arm automatically; if a suggestion says that your arm can't bend, then automatically make the arm so stiff that it cannot bend; if a suggestion says you can see a butterfly, then automatically let some sort of image of a butterfly appear; if a suggestion says you cannot remember something, then automatically push the memories out of your mind. The last time you were here, you may not have realized that you were to make the responses. It is no wonder, then, that nothing happened in response to the suggestions!
> INSTRUCTION 2: DEVOTE ALL OF YOUR ATTENTION TO THE SUGGESTIONS. Suggestions can be thought of as little stories. Think of each suggestion as a little story that describes events that are happening to you. Your task is to concentrate as deeply as possible on the stories. Your very

deep and continuous attention to the stories is what enables you to achieve hypnotic experiences.

To summarize: Make the responses that are suggested, but pay no attention to the fact that you are making them. Instead, devote your full, undivided, and continuous attention to the stories [18, 19]

Several features are built into these instructions: First, subjects are asked to refrain from formulating unauthorized interpretations of their behavior (i.e., "don't pay attention to the fact you are making [the principal response]") and to stick strictly to the definition provided by the hypnotist (i.e., "Your task is to concentrate as deeply as possible on the stories"). Asking subjects to pay attention to suggestions also helps insure that little or no introspection occurs. When attention is directed outward, toward the environment, the inward thought necessary for thinking up definitions of self that compete with the one being offered by the hypnotist is prevented [20]. The net effect is uncritical acceptance of the hypnotist's definition of the subject as someone in whom involuntary responses are occurring.

Second, the requirement that subjects themselves make, or at least try making, the responses suggested by the hypnotist is an essential element of training. These behaviors serve as evidence in support of the hypnotic self-definition. A failure of suggested responses to occur would represent a glaring contradiction of the hypnotic self-schema and thereby undermine conviction.

Third, in referring to suggestions as stories, the instructions underscore the creative and make-believe nature of the task. The purpose of this was twofold. Subjects are more likely to cooperate when their task is couched in these positive terms than when it is described using terms like cheating or self-deception. Use of terms like creative and make-believe were also expected to reduce the likelihood that a process of critical evaluation of the hypnotist's suggestions would be embarked on.

Fourth, instructions are brief. Five minutes to read and study them are allotted. A minimum of guidance need be provided because 1) the hypnotic situation already provides much information about the hypnotic role and 2) people come into the situation with abundant life experience and know-how in conviction management [15].

Can such brief training lead subjects to believe they are hypnotized? In two recent investigations [18, 19], subjects were administered a test of hypnotic susceptibility, and, from the pretest group, low hypnotizable subjects were selected. Half of them were randomly assigned to conviction training and the other half to a no-training control group. After receiving their respective treatments, subjects in the training and control conditions were again administered the susceptibility scale that was used at pretest. A change score was computed by subtracting the pretest susceptibility score from the retest score. Positive changes exhibited in the training condition combined with no changes in the control condition would reflect successful conviction management by trained subjects.

At each testing, subjects were administered the Carleton University Responsiveness to Suggestion Scale (CURSS; [21]). The test's suggestions, listed by principal response are, 1 = right arm light and rising, 2 = outstretched arms moving apart, 3 = left arm too heavy to lift, 4 = left arm too stiff to bend, 5 = hallucination of *Jingle Bells,* 6 = hallucination of a kitten, and 7 = amnesia for specified experimental events. Each subject received all seven suggestions in the order shown.

The susceptibility index of primary importance in these investigations was the objective-involuntariness (OI) score. For a given suggestion, two elements were scored: 1) whether or not evidence that the principal response was observed, and 2) the degree of involuntariness the subject reported having felt in response to the suggestion. If both elements occurred, the subject was assigned a point for that suggestion. The subject's OI score for a given test was the sum, over suggestions, of individual OI points (range, 0 to 7). As noted above, subjects were selected for the experiments if they obtained relatively low scores at pretest. Of all the subjects participating in the two studies ($n = 116$), most ($n = 62$) received an OI-score of 0 at pretest, 113 scored low by scale conventions (i.e., either 0, 1, or 2) [21], and the remaining three scored 3. No one obtaining a pretest OI-score in the 4 to 7 range was selected.[1]

Change score distributions are given in Figure 1. The change data are collapsed across studies because the methods involved and the results obtained in the two instances were very similar. Mean susceptibility increased substantially from before training to afterward ($p < .001$) but remained stable when no training was given. In the training condition, changes of one or more points were observed in approximately three-quarters of cases and substantial changes, i.e., of four or more points, occurred in 20 percent. In the control condition, scores tended to remain stable, with modal change equal to zero and all change scores, save one, distributed symmetrically within two points of the mode.

The effectiveness of training is even more impressive when it is considered that not all subjects complied with the request to use the self-imaging strategy. Several items, designed to assess the subject's vigor in implementing the conviction management strategy (e.g., "I held myself back from making the responses that were suggested."; "I held myself back from full concentration."), were administered. The items intercorrelated highly and were combined to form an effort score. The Pearson correlation between degree of effort (with higher scores indicating

---

[1] Subject selection for such an experiment, which tests for the ability to believe in an invalid self-claim, is important for insuring that the targeted self-definition is not already possessed, i.e., that actors are not authentically hypnotizable. Someone who is hypnotizable is thought to respond involuntarily to suggestions for alterations in perception and memory. So if subjects who are not pretested respond as hypnotizable after conviction training, it might be because they really do possess the features of the self-definition. However, if subjects are known before training to be low in hypnotizability, and they exhibit high levels of involuntary responding after training, we can be confident that the increase is attributable to the conviction management for which they were trained.

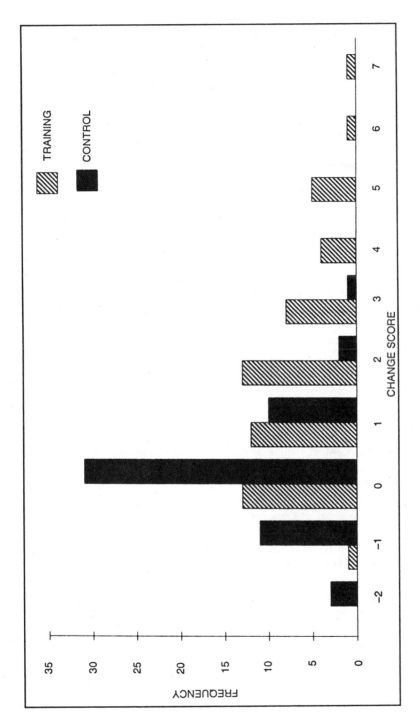

Figure 1. Distributions of change scores. The higher the score, the more that our index of conviction, CURSS-OI, increased from pretest to post-test.

more effort) and CURSS-*OI* was significant, $r(28) = .49$, $p < .01$. To further illustrate the relationship between effort and success, we broke subjects in the training condition into two groups, compliant and non-compliant, on the basis of their effort scores. CURSS-*OI* gains were exhibited by 93.8 percent of compliers but by only 42.9 percent of non-compliers. Almost one-third (31.3%) of compliers gained 4 or more points whereas the maximum gain exhibited by a non-complier was 3 points. Thus, it was common for those who used the conviction management strategy to show dramatic improvement.

Hypnotic depth ratings were also elicited in one of the studies [18]. Subjects rated the deepest level of hypnosis reached as well as the percentage of the session in which hypnosis was experienced. Subjects in the training condition made higher depth and longer time ratings than did controls. In other words, the hypnotic depth data were consistent with the hypnotic susceptibility findings, with both showing the frequent presence of hypnotic experiences among trained subjects.

In an effort to test the validity of self-reports, we led half the subjects in each of the training and control conditions to believe that their involuntariness reports were completely anonymous, whereas, the other half were led to expect that the reports and the identities of those making them would become known to the experimenter [19]. Compared to subjects in the public condition, those in the private condition were under relatively little pressure to report what they believed the experimenter expected them to report—namely, that responses felt involuntary. If training brings about an increase in reported, but not actual, experiential changes, then gains in susceptibility among trained subjects would be evident in the public condition but not in the private condition. If, however, involuntariness is really felt after training, and public impression management is of little concern to subjects, then susceptibility gains would occur among trained subjects whether self-reports were made publicly or anonymously.

CURSS-*OI* scores rose significantly after training in both the public *and* private conditions, and to equal degrees, suggesting that experiential self-reports were valid. As further evidence of a lack of relationship between the two variables, beliefs that involuntariness reports would indeed be kept anonymous (also measured in the investigation) and CURSS-*OI* gains failed to correlate in the training condition, $r = .03$ (or, for that matter, in the control condition). This finding supports the contention that experiences reported by subjects who are asked to use the conviction management strategy validly represent experiences they actually have.

Summary and Conclusions

In the typical hypnotic situation, the hypnotist's expectations are stated clearly: hypnotizable individuals respond involuntarily to suggestions. However, what subjects are not advised of, typically, is that it is *they personally* who are to produce suggested principal responses and associated experiences of involuntariness. When, through conviction training, this corrective is given, subjects exhibit significant and often large increases in hypnotic susceptibility. In short, subjects persuade themselves, for a time, that they are hypnotized and hypnotizable.

The hypnosis modification research has some interesting implications: First, it demonstrates the ease and extent to which conviction can be managed intentionally by the actor. The unpursuable self-definition, hypnotically susceptible, did not apply to our subjects. They failed to exhibit involuntary responses when pretested, and, given the high reliability of the susceptibility test used [21], were unlikely to exhibit them in the future. However, after being instructed to produce the experiences characteristic of hypnotized persons, and on being given the opportunity to role-play, subjects were able to convince themselves that they were hypnotized and responding to suggestions involuntarily. Subjects were, in other words, readily able to sustain lies to themselves about their identities.

In a related vein, the results suggest that the ability to manage conviction successfully is close to universal. Almost all of our subjects who complied with the training protocol were able to experience more suggestions as involuntary after training than they did before training, and several subjects exhibited dramatic changes. Our low susceptibles were able, without hypnosis, to exhibit a skill that is thought to be restricted to high susceptibles under hypnosis. The latter are thought to be able to undergo a dissociation in cognition, one in which the versions of self provided by the hypnotist occupy consciousness while knowledge of the self as the manager of conviction stays outside consciousness [22]. The fact that even low susceptibles produced "dissociation" tends to support the idea that creating illusions about the self is a normal function of cognition [15]. The skill is not necessarily restricted to the few (e.g., high hypnotizables or vivid imagers) or to highly unusual circumstances (e.g., hypnosis).

A further implication of the findings reported above concerns beliefs about control. Human beings tend to exhibit what is known as the illusion of control: "perception of uncontrollable events as subject to one's control or as more controllable than they are" [23, p. 121]. The illusion that characterizes hypnosis, what can be called the *illusion of being controlled,* reflects two variations on the illusion of control theme: First, it is possible to underestimate or deny completely personal control over events, if doing so serves to further the actor's goals. (Denial served Mrs. Keech well, as it did the trained subjects in the experiments described previously, and as it sometimes does persons attempting to avoid responsibility for questionable behavior.) Second, illusions about source of control can extend to something as intimate as one's own motor and cognitive responses. Apparently, a sense of personal agency is an extremely weak internal cue and is quite easy to distort.

Finally, these data contribute to discussions about the nature of the self, particularly with respect to its degree of malleability [24]. The conviction management research indicates that the self is in one sense changeable and in another sense stable. The fact that conviction in a fictitious self can be created relatively easily shows the self to be potentially mercurial. However, there is a stable side to the self, an executive that selects, using stable criteria (e.g., affect management), the self-definitions to be believed in.

Hallucination Requirement

In the studies described previously [18, 19], hallucinating was the principal response required in two different suggestions: suggestion number 5, hearing Jingle Bells, and suggestion number 6, seeing a kitten. People with the ability to imagine "as real as real" [7] should be able to use their skills to hallucinate the tune or the kitten. For the vast majority of people who fail to possess such acute imaginative skills, a hallucination requirement should undermine conviction management because the crucial evidence (i.e., the tune, the kitten) necessary for supporting suggested versions of the self (i.e., someone hearing the tune, someone seeing the animal) would not be perceived. Only the few subjects capable of hallucinating the stimulus would be able to produce the requisite evidence and, as a consequence, come to believe in the reality of the selves being suggested.

Figure 2 gives the proportion of subjects, at post-test, passing each hallucination suggestion. Pretest results in the training and control conditions (which are not given in Figure 1) were very similar to post-test results in the control condition (which are given in Figure 1). It is evident that, in the post-test training condition, the least frequently passed item was one of the hallucination suggestions, seeing the kitten. The other hallucination suggestion, hearing Jingle Bells, was also quite infrequently passed. The auditory hallucination was experienced as easier than the visual, possibly because background "noise" is typically greater in auditory than in visual hallucination tasks; which would result in more false positive identifications of the auditory stimulus.

It is also true, however, that there was an increase over baseline in the rate at which the two hallucination suggestions were passed ($ps < .05$), and passes were more frequent (at post-test) in the training condition than in the control condition ($ps < .05$). This indicates that being required to hallucinate important identity-supportive evidence is a very difficult task and one likely to undermine conviction management in everyone except a few, appropriately disposed individuals.[2]

---

[2] It should be noted that, in this research, it is not precisely clear what a positive hallucination rating really means. It is possible that an image took on the quality of a percept. However, imagery ability, measured in one of the studies [19], failed to correlate with increases in susceptibility. A second possibility is that subjects interpreted conviction instructions as requiring a weak test of the to-be-hallucinated stimulus, which resulted in more false positives than would have occurred had a more stringent reality testing criterion been used. A third possibility is that the rating questionnaire was interpreted as a test of how much the subject *felt like a person* hearing Jingle Bells (as opposed to whether or not the song itself was actually heard). Since some stimuli (e.g., the reactions of others, one's own head-bobbing behavior) underlying the experience of someone hearing Jingle Bells were present, the experience was at least partially replicated, which could easily result in a positive hallucination rating being made even if the song was not actually heard.

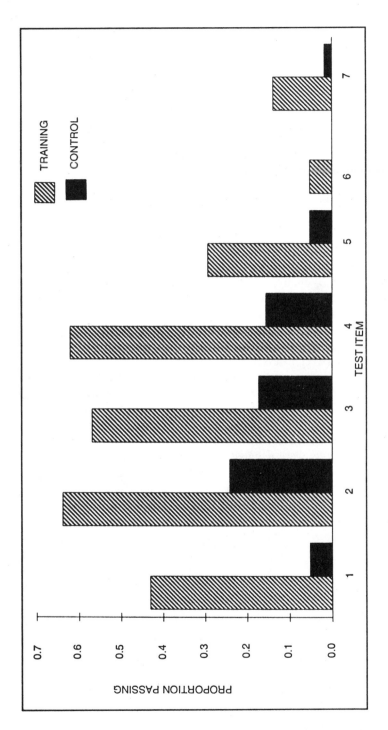

Figure 2. Proportion of subjects who passed each post-test suggestion. The suggestions administered were: 1 = right arm light and rising, 2 = outstretched arms moving apart, 3 = left arm too heavy to lift, 4 = left arm too stiff to bend, 5 = hallucination of *Jingle Bells*, 6 = hallucination of a kitten, 7 = amnesia for specified experimental events. Each subject received all seven suggestions in the order shown.

GENERAL CONCLUSIONS

This chapter began with Chomsky's bold assertion that we can, when motivated, easily convince ourselves of ludicrous propositions. A model was presented to show how this might occur with respect to beliefs about the self. From the hypnosis research that was described, it is apparent that people can be very good at quickly manufacturing conviction in pre-selected self-definitions, even if the definitions are clearly invalid.

There are two basic skills involved in the process. First, the conviction manager must pick a self for which supporting evidence can be produced and in relation to which contradictory evidence is unlikely to emerge. In other words, a sustainable version of the self must be chosen. Second, the identity must receive support from three sources: the conviction manager's own behavior, the behavior of others, and the physical setting. Exercise of the two skills results in a perceptual cycle in which expectations deriving from the targeted self-schema are well-supported by physical evidence that is observed. It is in the operation of this process that a strong sense of conviction in the validity of the self-schema develops. And as the anecdotal reports and experimental research reviewed above suggest, conviction managers are remarkably adept at quickly convincing themselves of their identity claims, this despite the fact the assertions have no basis in reality.

The hallucination findings indicate that some versions of the self are more easily conviction managed than others. Success goes down, not surprisingly, when crucial portions of supporting evidence must be hallucinated. By contrast, a sense of involuntariness is easy to bring to a behavioral performance because personal agency is a weak internal cue and thus easy to distort.

The identities subjects were required to take on in the experimental studies discussed above were temporary, lasting only one hypnotic session. As reported, subjects were able, on short notice, with minimal training, and for the duration required, to convince themselves that the (fictitious) identities were real. A question unanswered by this research is, could subjects have maintained their credulity over a relatively long period of time if they were required to do so? Here again the doomsday cult case study is suggestive (also see [25, 26]). It served Mrs. Keech well to persist in believing that the space beings were real and using her as an instrument of communication; these beliefs brought continued deep meaning to her life. What is more, it is likely that once conviction management was practiced for a time, pressures to justify the foregone behavior became strong; leading to a cycle in which conviction management would beget more conviction management. Under the circumstances, it would have been very difficult for Mrs. Keech to stop her act abruptly and admit to dissimulation (provided that moments of doubt in which she questioned her self-claims even arose). Owning up would have resulted in heavy affective costs, in the form of cognitive dissonance, loneliness (after ostracism from the group), and a loss of meaning. In dropping her facade, Mrs. Keech would have gone from a figure of cosmic importance to just another earthling.

The hypnosis research, I believe, illuminates the beginnings of a slide down a slippery slope, showing just how quickly the sleigh can accelerate; that is, the research shows how remarkably quickly and easily conviction can be produced. And once a lie to the self about the self is told, it may already be too late to stop a self-deceptive slide. This is because conviction management often takes place in a social system containing stable incentives and consistent support for believing in (invalid) self-claims and because conviction management produces its own self-justification pressures.

REFERENCES

1. N. Chomsky, *Deterring Democracy,* Hill and Wang, New York, 1991.
2. M. Gazzaniga, *The Social Brain: Discovering the Networks of the Mind,* Basic Books, New York, 1985.
3. R. B. Zajonc, Feeling and Thinking: Preferences Need No Inferences, *American Psychologist, 35,* pp. 151-175, 1980.
4. L. Festinger, H. W. Riecken, and S. Schachter, *When Prophesy Fails,* Harper Torchbooks, New York, 1964. (Originally published in 1956.)
5. M. K. Johnson and C. L. Raye, Reality Monitoring, *Psychological Review, 88,* pp. 67-85, 1981.
6. S. C. Wilson and T. X. Barber, The Fantasy-prone Personality: Implications for Understanding Imagery, Hypnosis, and Parapsychological Phenomena, in *Imagery: Current Theory, Research, and Application,* A. A. Sheikh (ed.), Wiley, New York, 1983.
7. S. J. Lynn and J. W. Rhue, Fantasy Proneness: Hypnosis, Developmental Antecedents, and Psychopathology, *American Psychologist, 43,* pp. 35-44, 1988.
8. T. R. Sarbin, Attempts to Understand Hypnotic Phenomena, in *Psychology in the Making,* L. Postman (ed.), Knopf, New York, 1962.
9. H. Bernheim, *Suggestive Therapeutics,* Putnam, New York, 1890. (Originally published in 1880.)
10. N. P. Spanos, Imagery, Hypnosis and Hypnotizability, in *Mental Imagery,* R. G. Kunzendorf (ed.), Plenum Press, New York, 1990.
11. B. Wallace, Hypnotic Susceptibility, Imaging Ability, and Information Processing: An Integrative Look, in *Mental Imagery,* R. G. Kunzendorf (ed.), Plenum Press, New York, 1990.
12. U. Neisser, *Cognition and Reality: Principles and Implications of Cognitive Psychology,* W. H. Freeman, San Francisco, 1976.
13. I. L. Janis and L. Mann, Effectiveness of Emotional Role-playing in Modifying Smoking Habits and Attitudes, *Journal of Experimental Research in Personality, 1,* pp. 84-90, 1965.
14. E. E. Jones and T. S. Pittmann, Toward a General Theory of Strategic Self-presentation, in *Psychological Perspectives on the Self,* Vol. 1, J. Suls (ed.), Erlbaum, Hillsdale, New Jersey, 1982.
15. S. E. Taylor, *Positive Illusions: Creative Self-Deception and the Healthy Mind,* Basic Books, New York, 1989.
16. J. Haley, An Interactional Explanation of Hypnosis, *American Journal of Clinical Hypnosis, 1,* pp. 41-57, 1958.
17. D. R. Gorassini, The Relationship between Planned and Actual Responses to Hypnotic Suggestions, *Imagination, Cognition and Personality, 8,* pp. 283-284, 1988-89.

18. D. R. Gorassini, D. Sowerby, A. Creighton, and G. Fry, Hypnotic Suggestibility Enhancement through Brief Cognitive Skill Training, *Journal of Personality and Social Psychology, 61,* pp. 289-297, 1991.
19. D. R. Gorassini, *Conviction Management in Hypnosis,* unpublished manuscript, University of Western Ontario, 1992.
20. R. A. Wicklund and D. Frey, Self-awareness Theory: When the Self Makes a Difference, in *The Self in Social Psychology,* D. M. Wegner and R. R. Vallacher (eds.), Oxford University Press, New York, 1980.
21. N. P. Spanos, H. L. Radtke, D. C. Hodgins, H. J. Stam, and L. D. Bertrand, The Carleton University Responsiveness to Suggestion Scale: Normative Data and Psychometric Properties, *Psychological Reports, 53,* pp. 523-535, 1983.
22. J. F. Kihlstrom and I. P. Hoyt, Hypnosis and the Psychology of Delusions, in *Delusional Beliefs,* T. F. Oltmanns and B. A. Maher (eds.), Wiley, New York, 1988.
23. D. G. Myers, *Social Psychology* (3rd Edition), McGraw-Hill, New York, 1990.
24. H. Markus and Z. Kunda, Stability and Malleability of the Self-concept, *Journal of Personality and Social Psychology, 51,* pp. 858-866, 1986.
25. C. Haney, C. Banks, and P. Zimbardo, A Study of Prisoners and Guards in a Simulated Prison, in *Readings about the Social Animal* (6th Edition), E. Aronson (ed.), Freeman, New York, 1992. (Originally published in 1973.)
26. N. Osherow, Making Sense of the Nonsensical: An Analysis of Jonestown, in *Readings about the Social Animal* (6th Edition), E. Aronson (ed.), Freeman, New York, 1992.

[I thank Karen Fields for her helpful comments on an earlier version of the manuscript. Preparation of this chapter was supported, in part, by research grants from the Social Sciences and Humanities Research Council of Canada.]

CHAPTER 10

Hypnotic Negative Hallucinations: A Review of Subjective, Behavioral, and Physiological Methods

ARTHUR H. PERLINI,
NICHOLAS P. SPANOS,
AND BILL JONES

Since its inception, the concept of hypnosis has been associated with the idea of profound alterations in perception, and since the middle of the nineteenth century "deeply hypnotized" subjects have been viewed as experiencing such alterations following suggestions delivered by the hypnotist [1]. For the most part, the profound perceptual alterations purportedly experienced by hypnotic subjects have been inferred solely on the basis of verbal reports or other responses under subjects' voluntary control. Erickson, for example, concluded that hypnotically suggested deafness was indistinguishable from neurological deafness because his hypnotically deaf subjects failed to exhibit startle responses when presented with an unexpected sound, failed to raise their voice when reading aloud, and so on [2].

The use of verbal reports and other voluntary responses as the sole criteria for inferring profound sensory alterations in hypnotic subjects engendered a good deal of early skepticism concerning the validity of such criteria [e.g., [3-6]). These early critics were aware that the hypnotic situation contains what are today labeled strong demands for compliant responding, and that hypnotic subjects were motivated to respond in terms of those demands [7]. Sutcliffe, in fact, categorized investigators of hypnotic phenomena as either skeptical or credulous depending upon their willingness to infer actual changes in perception following suggestions solely on the basis of verbal reports and other voluntary responses [5].

In most of the studies in this area, the perceptual phenomenon of interest involved suggested negative hallucinations. This term refers to a suggestion-induced failure of perception. For example, when exposed to a loud tone following a suggestion for deafness, some subjects report that the tone sounds much less loud than it did before they received the suggestion, and a few subjects report that they can no longer hear the tone [8]. Most subjects, however, report that the loudness of the tone was not appreciably affected by the suggestion. In other words, negative hallucination suggestions are difficult, and most subjects fail them (i.e., most subjects report having the perceptual experiences despite the suggestion). Those subjects who"pass" negative hallucination suggestions (i.e., report the perceptual decrements called for) tend to attain relatively high scores on standardized hypnotizability scales. From the perspective of credulous investigators these findings suggest that high hypnotizability involves cognitive abilities that enable subjects to dampen their sensory experiences (e.g., [9]). More skeptical investigators suggest instead that highly hypnotizable subjects develop a strong investment in the hypnotic role, and thereby are particularly likely to alter their perceptual reports in line with the social demands of the test situation in order to maintain their self-presentation as "deeply hypnotized" [10-11]. Two major research avenues have been developed to examine negative hallucination responding without relying on subjects' verbal reports as valid indexes of perceptual experience. One avenue involves the use of objective behavioral criteria to infer suggestion-induced perceptual change (or the lack of such change), or the use of paradigms that allow for the assessment of suggestion-induced reporting biases independently of perceptual change. A second avenue involves assessing the electrophysiological correlates of negative hallucination responding.

BEHAVIORAL RESEARCH METHODS AND NEGATIVE HALLUCINATIONS

In order to bypass the problem of compliance, a number of investigators have assessed hypnotically induced negative hallucinations by using objective behavioral indexes of perceptual responding that cannot be faked as easily as verbal reports (see [12] for a review). For example, in one line of research, hypnotic subjects were administered suggestions for deafness and then tested in a delayed auditory feedback paradigm [6, 13, 14]. In the delayed auditory feedback (DAF) paradigm subjects wear headphones while they read aloud. Subjects are tape-recorded as they read, and their voice is played back to them over the headphones. When a slight delay is introduced between what subjects are reading and what they are hearing over the headphones, subjects with normal hearing begin to pause and stutter. Deaf subjects, of course, are not affected by DAF. Hypnotic subjects who are given deafness suggestions, and who claim not to hear, stutter during DAF in the same way as subjects with normal hearing.

A related line of research has been conducted with the Ponzo illusion [15]. This illusion involves a series of radiating background lines upon which are superimposed two vertical lines. One vertical line is placed near the intersection of the background lines and the other is placed in a parallel location distant from the intersection of the radiating lines. When the vertical lines are the same length, their imposition on the radiating background creates the compelling illusion that one line is longer than the other. By varying the length of one of the vertical lines until the two lines appear to be subjectively equal, it is possible to measure the magnitude of the illusion.

Miller et al. administered the Ponzo illusion to hypnotic subjects who had been instructed to no longer see the radiating background lines that produce the illusion [15]. Subjects exhibited the illusion even when they reported not seeing the background lines.

These studies [6, 13, 15], and a large number of others that also assessed perceptual responding independently of verbal report [12, 16], have consistently obtained findings which call into question the validity of negative hallucination responding. Thus, despite verbal reports to the contrary, hypnotic subjects given negative hallucination suggestions continue to exhibit normal perceptual responding on objective behavioral indexes of perceptual functioning.

Studies that assessed perception with objective behavioral indicators indicate that negative hallucination responses do not involve the automatic suppression by suggestion of normal perceptual processes. On the other hand, these studies have revealed relatively little about the processes that do mediate the verbal reports elicited by negative hallucination suggestions. A number of recent studies have employed newly developed behavioral paradigms designed to cast light on the psychological mediators of negative hallucination responding, and the next section reviews this work.

Reporting Bias and Negative Hallucination

Although skeptical investigators have long been aware that the perceptual reports elicited by negative hallucination suggestions were contaminated by demand-induced reporting biases [16], paradigms for assessing reporting bias independently of perceptual change have only rarely been employed in this area [17]. A recent series of studies has, however, employed such a paradigm [18-22]. In several of these experiments subjects were exposed to a loud tone for thirty seconds. A few seconds after termination of the tone subjects rated its loudness. Subjects were then administered an hypnotic induction procedure followed by a suggestion for deafness and a readministration of the same tone. After termination of the second presentation of the tone subjects again rated its loudness. The hypnotic induction and suggestion were then canceled, and subjects were presented the same tone a third time. However, in the interval after termination of the third tone but before it was rated for loudness, subjects in one condition were given an instruction designed to induce compliance. These subjects were told that they had probably slipped back into hypnosis and therefore heard the third tone less loudly than they otherwise would have. Following this demand instruction these subjects rated the loudness of the third tone. Control subjects rated the loudness of the third tone without the intervention of the demand instruction.

In order to understand the logic of this paradigm it is important to keep in mind that, up until the termination of the trial 3 tone, subjects administered the demand instruction and control subjects were treated identically. For this reason any differences between these two groups in loudness ratings for the trial 3 tone could not reflect actual differences in the loudness with which that tone had been perceived on trial 3. Instead, a reduction in rated loudness for subjects given the demand instruction would reflect a reporting bias.

Studies that used this paradigm consistently found that control subjects reported that the tones were equally loud on trials 1 (before suggestion) and 3, and less loud on trial 2 (during the suggestion period) than on trials 1 and 3. In other words, control subjects exhibited a standard negative hallucination response. They reported that the tone was perceived as less loud during the period when they were responding to the deafness suggestion than before they had received the suggestion or after the suggestion had been canceled. Subjects given the demand instruction exhibited a different pattern of responding. These subjects reported that the tone was less loud on both trial 2 (deafness) and trial 3 (demand instruction) than on trial 1. Moreover, subjects given the demand instruction rated the trial 3 tone as lower in loudness than did the control subjects [18, 20, 21]. These studies indicate that hypnotic subjects given negative hallucination suggestions bias their perceptual reports independently of any actual change in their perceptual experiences.

Importantly, the methodology used in these studies enables the investigator to obtain an individual differences measure of the extent to which subjects who are given the demand instruction bias their perceptual reports. Extent of reporting bias is assessed by subtracting trial 3 (demand) loudness ratings from trial 1 loudness ratings. In two studies, the extent of reporting bias exhibited on trial 3 was almost as large as the extent to which subjects reported hypnotic deafness on trial 2 [20, 21].

The fact that subjects frequently bias their reports on trial 3 does not necessarily indicate that the reductions in rated loudness shown on trial 2 (hypnotic deafness) also reflect biased responding. Perhaps, for example, trial 2 loudness reductions involve some combination of real perceptual change and bias, or perhaps only a small subset of the subjects who exhibit hypnotic deafness on trial 2 also bias their responses on trial 3.

These ideas suggest that the psychological processes that lead subjects to bias their responses on trial 3 (e.g., compliance) differ from the psychological processes that lead to lowered loudness ratings on trial 2 (e.g., diminished perceptual sensitivity). If the psychological processes that led to decrements on these two trials were substantially different, then performance on these two trials would be unlikely to correlate highly. After all, there is little reason to suppose that an actual suggestion-induced reduction in perceptual sensitivity should correlate highly with reporting bias that occurs in the absence of any real perceptual change.

Contrary to this "different processes" hypothesis, the extent to which subjects reported hypnotic deafness on trial 2 was found to correlate very substantially with the degree of reporting bias shown on trial 3. In addition, the correlation between trial 3 deafness scores and hypnotizability did not differ in magnitude from the correlation between trial 2 bias scores and hypnotizability. Thus, subjects who exhibit large bias scores following a demand instruction tend to be the same people who report high levels of hypnotic deafness, and it is highly hypnotizable subjects who tend to report both high levels of hypnotic deafness and who bias their reports independently of perceptual change. These findings suggest that the psychological processes that lead subjects to bias their perceptual reports on trial 3 also exert a strong influence on the loudness reductions that they report during hypnotic deafness testing.

The demand instruction paradigm has also been used to examine hypnotically suggested pain reduction and hypnotically suggested color change by replacing the tone on the three trials with a pain stimulus or with a color stimulus [19, 22, 23]. Regardless of the nature of the stimulus, the results were the same. Subjects given a demand instruction exhibited significant levels of bias on trial 3, and those who exhibited large bias effects on trial 3 also reported large perceptual decrements following hypnotic negative hallucination suggestions on trial 2.

Spanos et al. assessed both hypnotic deafness and hypnotic blindness in the same experiment [20]. In an initial session, hypnotic subjects were given the suggestion that they would be unable to see a word that was clearly printed on a page. After responding to the suggestion, subjects rated the extent to which they had used various strategies in an attempt to distort their vision (e.g., unfocusing their eyes, creating an image to "cover" the printed word). Although all of the subjects reported using one or more of the strategies to distort their vision, there was no significant correlation between strategy usage and degree of reported blindness.

In a second session, subjects were tested in the deafness/demand instruction paradigm. The extent to which subjects biased their trial 3 loudness reports correlated with their session 1 reports of hypnotic blindness as well as their session 2 reports of hypnotic deafness. Thus, as in earlier studies, subjects who were willing to bias their auditory reports independently of any real perceptual change in order to meet experimental demands, tended to be the same people who reported perceptual decrements in response to hypnotic suggestions for blindness as well as for deafness.

It is likely that the subjects in the Spanos et al. study did carry out various strategies in an attempt to induce perceptual distortion during the hypnotic blindness suggestion period [20]. However, the extent to which any resultant perceptual alteration was defined by subjects as blindness was unrelated to strategy use. Instead, the extent to which subjects reported themselves as experiencing hypnotic blindness was related to their willingness to bias their perceptual reports in line with situational demands but independently of any actual perceptual change.

Spanos et al. assessed the extent to which instruction-induced reporting bias correlated with response to a wide range of difficult hypnotic suggestions [19]. Highly hypnotizable subjects were administered a variant of the demand instruction paradigm that allowed them to be dichotomized into those who biased their responses following the instruction (i.e., biasers) and those who did not (nonbiasers). In a separate session these subjects were tested on a wide range of difficult hypnotic test suggestions. Biasers responded to significantly more of the difficult suggestions than nonbiasers. In addition, biasers reported higher levels of subjective response to suggestions than did nonbiasers. Taken together, the findings of studies that employed the demand instruction paradigm indicate that the tendency of subjects to bias their responses in terms of situational demands is a pervasive characteristic of hypnotic responding.

The tendency of subjects in the demand instruction paradigm to bias their trial 3 responses is open to two interpretations [24]. The most parsimonious interpretation holds that trial 3 reporting biases reflect compliant responding. According to this interpretation, for example, subjects in a deafness experiment who report reduced loudness following the instruction on trial 3 deliberately mis-describe their experience; they report that the tone was less loud than they knew it to be in order to convey the impression that the suggestion "worked." Subjects in psychology experiments frequently lie in order to conform with normative pressures [25, 26], and they frequently respond to the requests of authority figures by carrying out behaviors that they find personally distasteful [27]. Consequently, it should not be surprising if it turns out that some hypnotic subjects also knowingly exaggerate their degree of perceptual responding in order to meet experimental demands.

An alternative to the compliance hypothesis suggests that the demand instruction may lead some subjects to reinterpret their experience [24]. According to this idea, subjects in a deafness experiment who are given the demand instruction following the trial 3 tone may reinterpret or reclassify their experience of the tone so that they now remember it as less loud than they initially perceived it to be. Both the compliance and the interpretation hypothesis assume that subjects are motivated to respond in terms of situational demands, and both hypotheses acknowledge that subjects' perceptual reports are inaccurate. However, the compliance hypothesis holds that subjects' inaccurate perceptual reports reflect purposeful deception whereas the reinterpretation hypothesis does not imply purposeful deception. It is worth noting that the compliance and reinterpretation hypothesis are not mutually exclusive, and both processes may occur in the same subject. For instance, a subject who initially lies and reports the trial 3 tone as less loud than he knows it to have been may, on further reflection, come to convince himself that "I guess it really wasn't all that loud after all" [24].

Although the reporting biases outlined in the demand instruction paradigm cannot be unambiguously classified as compliance as opposed to reinterpretation, another recently developed paradigm allows for the unambiguous assessment of compliance during negative hallucination responding.

Compliance and Negative Hallucinations

Spanos, Flynn, and Gabora gave highly hypnotizable subjects an hypnotic induction procedure [28]. While their eyes remained closed these subjects were told that they would be shown a blank piece of paper. This suggestion informed them repeatedly that the paper was blank and had nothing on it. In fact, the piece of paper had printed on it a large and easily visible number 8. Subjects were asked to open their eyes and look at the paper. During this period subjects were asked several times what was on the paper. The large majority of subjects reported seeing a number 8. However, fifteen subjects reported on each probe that the paper was completely blank and had nothing on it. The paper was then removed from subjects' view and the hypnotic procedure and blindness suggestion were canceled. The fifteen subjects who had consistently claimed blindness were then interviewed by a second experimenter who administered preliminary instructions designed to elicit a confession from subjects that they, in fact, had seen the number that they denied seeing. These subjects were told that people who attempted to fake hypnosis always insisted that they saw nothing on the paper, whereas real subjects see a figure that gradually fades. Subjects were further told that the experimenter was interested in determining how the figure on the paper faded over the one-minute exposure interval, and subjects were asked to draw what they had seen of the figure during each fifteen second segment of the interval.

It is important to keep in mind that the experimenter never told the subjects what figure had been on the paper. Consequently, subjects who produced a figure "8" as being present during one or more of the fifteen-second intervals must have seen the figure on the page during the suggestion period but lied at that time about having done so. Because subjects were asked about what was on the paper as they looked at it, their reports of seeing nothing cannot be interpreted in terms of retrospective reinterpretation or memory failure [29].

All but one of the fifteen subjects who claimed to see nothing on the paper during the suggestion period drew an "8" during the interview period. These findings provide strong support for the hypothesis that subjects who report the perceptual distortions called for by negative hallucination suggestions purposely exaggerate the extent of any distortion they experience in order to meet experimental demands.

The negative visual hallucination suggestion used by Spanos et al. [28] was very similar to the one used by Spanos, Burgess et al. [20]. Because blindness scores in the Spanos, Burgess et al. [20] study correlated significantly with trial 3 reporting bias scores, the finding that blindness reports in the Spanos et al. [28]

study involved substantial levels of compliance suggests that trial 3 reporting bias also is likely to consist largely of compliant responding [29].

In order to examine these ideas Burgess et al. conducted a two session study [29]. In the first session, subjects were tested for color change hallucination using the three trial demand instruction paradigm. In session 2 subjects were exposed to the negative visual hallucination suggestion used by Spanos et al. [28]. Subjects who reported seeing nothing on the page were once again interviewed about their experiences. Half of these subjects were given the interview described above which encouraged them to draw the figure that had been on the page (confession interview). However, the other half were given an interview which reinforced the idea that good hypnotic subjects see nothing on the page (compliance interview).

As in the Spanos et al. study almost all of the subjects given the confession interview drew a number "8" [28]. On the other hand, only one subject given the compliance interview drew an "8." The remainder continued to report that they had seen nothing on the page. Because subjects given the confession interview and those given the compliance interview were assigned at random to their respective interview conditions (after insisting during the suggestion that nothing was on the page), it is safe to assume that the subjects in these two groups had similar experiences during the negative hallucination suggestion period. The fact that almost all of those given the confession interview acknowledged having seen the "8," indicates that those in the compliance interview had also seen the "8" during the suggestion period but lied about doing so when given an interview that encouraged such lying.

Recall that subjects in the Burgess et al. experiment had been initially tested in the demand instruction paradigm. Subjects who had denied seeing the "8" during the suggestion period of session 2 but later drew an "8" during the confession interview were classified as "compliers." Subjects who failed this suggestion by reporting during the suggestion period that they had seen the "8" were classified as noncompliers. These two groups were then compared on the extent to which they had biased their responses to the trial 3 suggestion when administered the session 1 demand instruction paradigm. Compliers exhibited significantly higher trial 3 bias scores than noncompliers. In short, these findings provide strong support for the hypothesis that trial 3 reporting bias, to a large extent, reflects compliance. Subjects who bias their reports consciously exaggerate the magnitude of their experiences in order to meet suggested demands. Moreover, because trial 3 reporting bias correlates with standardized hypnotizability test scores as well as with response to particularly difficult suggestions, these findings support the hypothesis that compliance is a central component of hypnotic responding [11, 29-31].

Taken together, behavioral studies on hypnotic negative hallucinations indicate that suggestions do not interfere in any profound, substantial or automatic way with the ability of subjects to process sensory information. Despite what subjects might say following such suggestions, the objective evidence indicates that they do not become deaf or blind in the usual sense of those terms. On the other hand, these findings do not preclude the possibility that subjects may use voluntary oculomotor and/or attentional-cognitive strategies that produce perceptual alterations. For example, by unfocusing their eyes, subjects can easily blur the image of a number or word that is presented on a page or computer screen. Such de-focusing can occur either as a voluntary strategy, or as a more or less automatic accompaniment of voluntary attention diversion strategies. As indicated by the findings of the Spanos et al. study, however, subjects perceive such stimuli well enough to later identify them, despite any such alterations [28]. Relatedly, a large literature on selective attention indicates that subjects often fail to perceive messages presented to one ear when they focus attention to different messages presented in the other ear. However, it is the subjects who control their own attentional processes and who voluntarily shift attention from one focus to the next as a function of task demands [32].

The behavioral studies further indicate that the reports of dampened perceptual experience given by subjects following negative hallucination suggestions are social products. These reports do not appear to reflect altered perceptions in any direct way, and instead are strongly influenced by contextual demands and by the impressions subjects are attempting to convey.

NEUROPHYSIOLOGICAL RESEARCH: EVOKED POTENTIAL METHODS

The development of electrophysiological recording procedures gave investigators tools for studying physiological markers of experience. For hypnosis researchers such tools seemed to provide an objective and relatively direct means for assessing the validity of the dramatic phenomenological report changes elicited by negative hallucination suggestions. The recording of phasic evoked potentials (EPs) became the primary electrophysiological tool for examining these issues.

EP procedures involve the summation and averaging of the brain's ongoing electrical activity (i.e., EEG), as well as the brain's electrical response to a periodic external stimulus. The EEG activity is random; sometimes it is negative and sometimes it is positive. In theory, when averaged over a large number of samples, this random activity approximates zero electrical potential. In contrast, an external stimulus presented at a constant rate and intensity (e.g., a flashing light) evokes an electrical response which, when averaged over many samples, results in a clearly identifiable signal that is greater than zero. The signal which emerges from this averaging process is the evoked potential [33].

The evoked potential (EP), if recorded at the cortex or skull surface, is thought to reflect both a sensory component and higher level processing components. Cognitive psychophysiologists consider the EP waveform to be composed of a number of smaller component waves, each identified by their polarity (P or N for positive or negative) and peak latency (100 msec, 200 msec, etc.). For example, N100 refers to the first negative wave (also known as N1) which occurs at approximately 100 milliseconds. Responses occurring prior to approximately 100 second are generally designated by their polarity followed by Roman numerals I-VI. The earlier components of the waveform are thought to reflect different processes than the later components of the waveform [34].

The early components (approximately 0-100 msec following stimulus onset) are called exogenous components and are considered to be dependent on the physical qualities of the stimulus, such as its intensity, frequency, and rate of presentation. Changes in these parameters, for example dimming the intensity of a light stimulus, are reflected in changes (e.g., decreases) in the amplitude of the early EP components. The psychological condition of the subject has little bearing on these early components. It is irrelevant whether subjects are attending to the stimulus or not, or even if they are unconscious (e.g., during sleep). On the other hand, the later components of the waveform (i.e., those greater than 100 msec following stimulus onset) are influenced by the manner in which the information is processed. These later components, called endogenous components, are affected by higher level psychological processes (e.g., attention, decision strategies, memory) [34].

Contemporary researchers have attempted to associate individual EP components with specific aspects of information processing in order to identify the functional significance of specific EP components. For example, a distinct negative-positive complex, commonly called N1-P2, has been linked to an early stage of stimulus selection for distinct and conspicuous physical properties (e.g., selective attention), while P3 has been linked to the psychological event of analyzing these physical properties for significance and meaning [35]; in other words, stimulus evaluation. A late negative wave, N400 or N4, has been associated with a number of verbal processing constructs that depend on expectancy (e.g., lexical decision making, word recognition, etc.). It is important to note that as yet, no EP component has been shown to bear a one-to-one correspondence with any specific psychological process. Thus, while P3 has been linked to stimulus evaluation, it has also been variously attributed to uncertainty resolution, orientation to unexpected input, the activation of attention, the amount of stimulus information, activation of specific response systems appropriate to processed information, stimulus-independent perceptual decisions, the detection of monitored events, matching of neural templates, and the amount of utilization of cortical information processors [36]. In addition to these specific factors, EP components are strongly influenced by such general factors as instructional set, task difficulty (e.g., simple versus complex discrimination) and task demands (e.g., no response, motor response, or cognitive decision).

The application of EP methodologies to the study of negative visual hallucinations was designed to assess whether suggestion-induced reports of failing to see (or hear or smell) an objectively presented visual (or auditory or olfactory) stimulus were associated with EP changes. The assumption underlying the use of these methodologies was that if subjects' reports of not perceiving supraliminal stimuli were accurate, then the potentials ordinarily evoked by the stimulus would change in correspondence with such reports. For instance, there might be an attenuation in the amplitude of select components in the EP waveform, that reflected a change in the way the stimulus information was processed.

Early applications of EP methodology to the study of negative hallucinations lacked both statistical and methodological sophistication. Methodological developments played an important role in improving the sensitivity of EP methods for assessing information processing and the research to be reviewed will be classified accordingly. Refer to Table 1 for a summary of these findings.

Early Research:
Visual Analyses of Wave Morphology

Early studies in this area employed small samples of clinical patients with temporarily implanted electrodes in various cortical and subcortical sites. Both Hernandez-Peon and Donoso [37] and Guerrero-Figueroa and Heath [38] exposed their subjects to an unspecified number of 1 msec light flashes of constant intensity under two conditions: 1) baseline, 2) nonhypnotic suggestions of brighter and dimmer light. In these studies, the magnitude of the waveform was positively related to each suggestion. However, since the samples consisted of clinical patients with severe impairments (e.g., schizophrenia), it is possible that biochemical and/or neurological anomalies were present in these samples. More recent research (e.g., [39]) indicates that these types of clinical samples are characterized by unusual EP patterns. For these reasons an interaction of selection and treatment factors may have threatened the internal validity of these studies.

Suggestions for increased and decreased visual acuity that were preceded by an hypnotic induction procedure were employed in several early EP studies that used single-case experimental designs with normal (i.e., nonclinical) subjects. For example, Clynes, Kohn, and Lifshitz [40] exposed a single subject to repeated flashes of light and found that the amplitude of the EP waveform decreased following hypnotic suggestions for blindness. Unfortunately, these investigators could not replicate their findings on a second subject. Clynes et al. [40] also described an unpublished report by another team of investigators [41] who first obtained and then failed to replicate a similar pattern of EP change. Beck and Barolin [42] performed an exact replication of the procedures used by Clynes et al. [40], but found no EP changes. Serafinides also found no overall waveform changes in response to hypnotic suggestions for blindness [43].

Other early research used nonvisual evoking stimuli on larger samples. For example, Halliday and Mason tested hypnotic suggestions for analgesia and deafness with repeated shocks and clicks [44]. Although their subjects' verbal reports were consistent with the suggestions, there were no accompanying

Table 1. Methods and Results of Evoked Potentials—Suggestion Studies

Study	Scale	N	Stimulus	EP Index	Change	Comment on Methods
Hernandez-Peon and Donoso, 1959	None	2	Visual	Overall wave	Yes	Nonhypnotic: brightness and dimness Subjects: neurological patients
Guerrero-Figueroa and Heath, 1964	None	3	Visual	Overall wave	Yes	Nonhypnotic: brightness and dimness Subjects: schizophrenic patients
Clynes, Kohn, and Lifshitz, 1964	D & H	1	Visual	Overall wave	Yes	Hypnotic: blindness; unreplicated on second subject
Beck and Barolin, 1965	D & H	2	Visual	Overall wave	No	Hypnotic: blindness; failed to replicate Clynes, Kohn and Lifshitz, 1964
Serafinides, 1968	None	1	Visual Auditory	Overall wave Overall wave	No No	Hypnotic and nonhypnotic blindness Hypnotic and nonhypnotic deafness
Halliday and Mason, 1964	None	9	Pain/ Auditory	Overall wave	No	Hypnotic analgesia and deafness; Subjects: clinical pain patients
Beck and Barolin, 1965	D & H	8	Visual	N1-N4, P1-P3	No	Hypnotic brightness and dimness
Beck et al., 1966	D & H	10	Visual	N1-N4, P1-P3	No	Hypnotic brightness and dimness

Study	Scale	N	Modality	Components	Significant	Comments
Amadeo et al., 1975	None	4	Pain/Auditory	P2	No	Hypnotic and nonhypnotic increase and decrease; attention controls
Andreassi et al., 1976	None None	12 6	Visual Visual	P1 N2 P2 P1 N2 P2	No No	Hypnotic brightness and dimness; attention controls Hypnotic and nonhypnotic dimness; attention controls
Zakrzewski and Szelenberger, 1981	D & H	5	Visual	N1-N4, P1-P3	Yes (N2) No	Hypnosis versus hypnotic blindness Baseline versus hypnotic blindness; Ss were three medium and two low hypnotizables
Spiegel, Cutcomb, Ren, and Pribram, 1985	HGSHS	18	Visual	N1 N2, P1-P3	Yes (P3)	Hypnotic obstruction versus enhancement only Subjects: six high, six low, six attention controls
Perlini, Lorimer, Campbell, and Spanos, 1993	CURSS	9	Visual	N1-N4, P1-P3 amplitude latency	No Yes (P1, P3) Yes (P1)	Overall ANOVA: failed to replicate Spiegel et al., 1985 Post-hoc t-tests: support Spiegel et al., 1985 Post-hoc t-tests: fail to replicate Spiegel et al., 1985; Ss were 9 highs
Barabasz and Lonsdale, 1983	SSHS:C	9	Olfactory	P3	Yes (highs) No (lows)	Hypnotic anosmia > baseline
Spiegel, Bierre, and Rootenberg, 1989	SSHS:C	20	Somato-sensory	N1-N4, P1-P3	Yes (highs) No (lows)	Hypnotic obstruction versus baseline at P100 and P300

amplitude changes in the EP waveform. Findings of this kind are consistent with the hypothesis that subjects reported inaccurately about their experiences to meet the demands of the experimental situation. Halliday and Mason did not test their subjects with standardized hypnotizability scales and, consequently, it can be argued that their results may have been different if they had selected only highly hypnotizable subjects [44]. On the other hand, the fact that Halliday and Mason's [44] subjects reported the decrements called for by the suggestions indicates that a lack of suggestibility was not the cause of their negative EP findings [44].

Taken together, the early search for visually apparent changes in EP waveforms did not prove promising; studies when replicated did not yield the same findings. Selection and individual difference factors may account for some of these inconsistent findings, but this is unclear. Of course, the practice of visually inspecting waveform morphology, in the absence of quantitative analysis, lends itself to the problem of subjective and unreliable interpretations. There is the possibility of imagining patterns in data when there is nothing there [45]. Moreover, because EPs are multidimensional, visual inspection makes it difficult to determine how two or more responses are different. The responses may have identical wave shapes but different amplitudes, or alternatively some components may differ while others may be identical [46]. Potential problems of these kinds made even more suspect the few findings in the early EP literature that did suggest a relationship between suggested perceptual changes and EP changes.

Quantitative EP Component Analyses

The research which followed the early studies involved 1) relatively large samples without neurological impairments, 2) statistical rather than visual comparisons of the EP waveforms, 3) the use of suggestions that were always preceded by hypnotic instructions, and 4) with only two exceptions, the use of visual stimuli and standardized tests of hypnotizability.

Beck and Barolin recorded bilateral visual evoked potentials (VEPs) in response to trains of 150 light flashes under baseline and hypnotic conditions of stimulus brightness and dimness [42]. Seven of the eight subjects were highly hypnotizable. No changes were found in either the amplitude or latency of the EPs between hypnotic and baseline conditions. An insensitive signal averaging procedure prompted Beck, Dustman, and Beier to repeat the experiment on another sample [47]. An experimental group of seven high hypnotizables, two medium hypnotizables, and one low hypnotizable were exposed to 100 light flashes delivered during periods of 1) hypnosis-no suggestion, 2) hypnotic suggestions of bright light and dim light, and 3) two baseline (nonhypnotic) conditions. A control group of ten subjects unselected for hypnotizability received the flash stimuli under actual light intensity changes. For the experimental subjects analysis of the latency and amplitude of seven EP components (N1, P1, N2, P2, N3, P3, N4) indicated no differences between periods. In contrast, the group exposed to actual light intensity changes showed differences at N3 and P3. Taking both Beck studies together, it appears that amplitude changes occurred concomitantly with actual, but not suggested changes in brightness.

Other research comparing baseline, hypnosis alone, and hypnotically-suggested blindness trials also found no amplitude differences between trials, but obtained evidence for latency differences; that is, N2 latency was the same across the hypnosis conditions, but both were longer than N2 latency in the baseline condition (e.g., [48]). Increases in N2 latency have been linked to increased difficulty of stimulus detection; in other words, a slower stimulus evaluation process [35]. The investigators did not speculate on the relation of hypnosis or hypnotizability to these psychological processes. Interestingly, however, the findings were obtained from subjects who were low to medium in hypnotizability.

Several studies using visual evoking stimuli compared hypnotic and nonhypnotic conditions while controlling for attentional state. Recall that attentional variables play a critical role in endogenous components of the EP waveform. When comparing hypnotic and nonhypnotic procedures, it is important to keep all other variables (e.g., attention) constant between conditions. Attempts to do this usually involve the use of some task that directs subjects' attention toward or away from the stimulus (e.g., having the subject press a key or count in response to a given stimuli). Using such a procedure Andreassi, Balinsky, Gallichio, DeSimone, and Mellers exposed twelve subjects to 100 light flashes following hypnotic suggestions for brightness and dimness, as well as following hypnotic induction without suggestions [49]. Each condition was presented twice. During each condition subjects' attention was controlled by requiring them to count the number of light flashes. An analysis of amplitudes and latencies of P1, N2, and P2 indicated no differences across the three hypnotic conditions. In a second experiment, six additional subjects were exposed to the same stimuli under both baseline and hypnotic conditions of suggested dimness. Analysis of the VEP components again failed to show any amplitude or latency differences between hypnotic suggestion and baseline. It appears that when attention was engaged by counting the flash stimuli, neither hypnotic induction alone nor hypnotic suggestions altered EPs.

Andreassi et al. failed to assess hypnotizability in their sample, leaving open the possibility that their null findings were due to a preponderance of unhypnotizable subjects [49]. To examine this hypothesis, Spiegel, Cutcomb, Ren, and Pribram conducted a similar study using twelve subjects (6 highs, 6 lows) pretested on hypnotizability [50]. The task required that subjects manually respond to target colors in a pattern evoking stimulus. This task was completed under three hypnotic conditions: 1) enhanced (bright and interesting), 2) diminished (dull and uninteresting), and 3) disappeared. The latter condition required subjects to hallucinate an opaque box blocking their view of the stimulus pattern. High hypnotizables but not low hypnotizables, showed a decrease in P300 amplitude throughout the cortex, and N200 and P300 amplitudes in the occipital region. An interpretation in terms of group inequality of motor response (i.e., lows pressed the target button more than highs) was dismissed by including a group of non-hypnotic subjects who completed the discrimination task during alternative conditions of button pressing to all targets and also none of the targets. The authors interpreted the amplitude decrements as a result of attentional diversion from the stimulus to the hallucinated image. This interpretation of P300 amplitude decrement is consistent with much contemporary research linking P300 amplitude to attentional factors. Nevertheless, an alternative hypothesis suggests that Spiegel et al.'s findings may have resulted from subjects shifting the focus of their gaze from the visual stimuli to in front of the visual stimuli when they were instructed to imagine a box that blocked their view of the stimuli [50]. Since subjects imagined a box in front of the stimuli they may have shifted their eyes to focus at the point of subjective location of their image rather than focusing directly at the stimuli.

Spiegel et al. also concluded that the EP amplitude decrements shown by their subjects indicated that these subjects were reporting accurately when they claimed to no longer see the visual stimuli [50]. This conclusion, however, is unwarranted regardless of the validity of their attentional shift hypothesis. EP amplitude decrements may, as Spiegel et al. suggest, indicate that subjects expended cognitive effort in an attempt to attend away from the visual stimulus [50]. Nevertheless, such attending away is no guarantee that subjects succeeded in not seeing the stimuli. For example, many of the subjects in the Spanos, Burgess et al. study reported attempting to attend away from the visual stimulus during the suggestion period [20]. Nonetheless, the use of this strategy failed to correlate with subjects' reports of blindness.

With the intent of conceptual replication, Perlini, Lorimer, Campbell, and Spanos measured the VEPs of nine high hypnotizables who were required to perform a visual discrimination task [51]. Unlike the task employed by Spiegel et al. [50], Perlini et al. [51] used a semantic task (i.e., lexical decision). Following baseline, subjects were administered the same task under four hypnotic hallucination conditions: (a) imagining an opaque box blocking their view of the letter strings, (b) imagining a transparent box superimposed but not blocking their view of the letter strings, (c) hallucinating a dimming and ultimate disappearance of the letter strings, and (d) imagining the letter strings as incomprehensible. The obstructive (a) and stimulus diminution (c) suggestions mimicked those of Spiegel et al. [50]. Perlini et al. found that the overall ANOVA on amplitudes yielded no significant conditions effects [51]. Nevertheless, more liberal multiple t-tests predicated on Spiegel et al.'s findings indicated a decrease of P300 amplitude in the obstructive imagery condition, but only at the parietal site. To examine the possibility that subjects focused their view away from the stimulus while generating their obstructive images, P100 latency was compared between the obstructive imagery and baseline conditions. P100 latency was increased in the obstructive imagery conditions compared to baseline, a finding consistent with the hypothesis that subjects were de-focusing their view of the stimulus [52].

Perlini et al.'s [51] findings of P300 decrements were consistent with those of Spiegel et al. [50], and consistent with the hypothesis that subjects divert attention (and perhaps re-focus their eyes) away from a visual stimulus and toward their images in an attempt to create perceptual distortions. It is important to note that these preliminary reports found amplitude attenuation only when subjects were asked to create an obstructive image (i.e., see a box that is not really there). When the task suggested a decreases in the intensity of the stimulus, there were no P300 changes.

Subjects in the Perlini et al. study rated the vividness with which they saw the visual stimuli in each condition. Although P300 decrements were obtained only in the obstructive imagery condition, equivalent decreases in ratings of stimulus vividness occurred in all of the suggestion conditions. Moreover, even in the obstructive imagery condition subjects reported decreases in stimulus intensity but not a failure to see the stimuli. In short, it should not be assumed that changes in the late components of the VEP indicate a failure to see stimuli.

In both the Perlini et al. [51] and Spiegel et al. [50] studies hypnotic procedures were confounded with suggestions. Consequently, it is unclear that hypnotic procedures played any role in the EP changes that were observed. Any procedure which requires that subjects divert their attention from a stimulus may produce similar changes in the endogenous components of the EP wave. Along these lines, Edmonston suggested that the Spiegel et al. study would have benefitted from the inclusion of control subjects who simply shifted their focus point from the target stimuli to a point in front of the target [53]. The Perlini et al. study is subject to a similar criticism [51].

Somatosensory and Auditory. In addition to visual stimuli, pain and auditory stimuli have been employed to examine the electrophysiological effects of hypnotic suggestions. For example, Amadeo and Yanovski exposed five clinical patients to bursts of shock and clicks under nonhypnotic and hypnotic conditions [54]. The subjects were exposed to these treatments under conditions in which they were required to respond manually to one or the other stimulus (i.e., attention conditions), and neither stimulus (i.e., rest condition). In addition, the hypnotic treatment was followed by a series of conditions involving suggested increase or decrease in the intensity of each of the two evoking stimuli. Subjects were not required to produce a motor response in the latter conditions. There were no differences between the hypnotic and nonhypnotic treatments on the EP index (amplitude of peak between 120-230 msec, approximately P200), during either rest or attention conditions. Furthermore, all subjects failed to show any changes in the EP amplitude to either the click or shock stimuli in the hypnotic suggestion conditions. These null findings are consistent with those of Halliday and Mason [44].

Spiegel, Bierre, and Rootenberg also employed attention-control procedures to compare hypnotic and nonhypnotic responses to somatosensory stimuli; however, a nonclinical sample was used [55]. Ten high and ten low hypnotizable subjects performed a shock-discrimination task under baseline conditions of attention or inattention, and two hypnotic conditions: 1) suggestion to redefine the shock as pleasant and interesting, and 2) suggestions to imagine the arm as numb and insensitive. Only the highly hypnotizable subjects showed increased P100 amplitudes during the hypnotic redefinition condition and decreased P100 and P300 amplitudes during the hypnotic-imagery condition compared to baseline. The latter findings are consistent with those of Spiegel et al. [50] and Perlini et al. [51], who both used visual rather than somatosensory tasks. Once again, however, the failure of Spiegel et al. [50] to employ nonhypnotic-suggestion conditions precludes any firm conclusions about whether the alterations in EP amplitudes were related to the use of hypnotic procedures.

   Olfactory.   Only one published study attempted to examine hypnotic alterations of P300 to stimuli in the olfactory modality. Barabasz and Lonsdale exposed four high hypnotizables and five low hypnotizables to repeated puffs of weak and strong odors, under waking and hypnotic anosmia conditions [56]. During the hypnotic anosmia conditions, high hypnotizables but not lows showed increases in temporal region P300s for both weak and strong odors. These findings are opposite to those obtained by Spiegel et al. [50] and Perlini et al. [51] for visual stimuli, and they contradicted the author's predictions that there would be an attenuation in P300 during the anosmia conditions for high hypnotizable subjects.

   Spiegel and Barabasz argued that these findings reflected subjects' response to novel stimuli [57]. Novelty of stimulus has been found to be related to P300 increments [36]. The anosmia suggestion informs subjects not to expect the odors; any violation of this expectation (i.e., detection of the odor) produces a "surprise" effect, according to this hypothesis. Of course, this hypothesis also predicts that suggestions which inform subjects that a visual stimulus will disappear will also lead to P300 increments. As shown by Perlini et al. [51] and Spiegel et al. [50] this is clearly not the case. Thus, while it is true that task demands are important variables to consider, this particular hypothesis of Spiegel and Barabasz [57] cannot adequately explain the data. One speculation is that tasks which invite subjects to actively engage in a distracting task (e.g., generate, and focus on an image that will compete with the evoking stimulus) will be accompanied by decreases in the P300 components of the EP. In contrast, instructions which inform subjects that a stimulus will disappear (e.g., the anosmia suggestion told subjects that they would no longer smell anything) may not involve the same attentional demands, and thus may not alter the P300 of the evoking stimulus. This explanation highlights the importance of implicit and explicit task demands in determining subjects' electrophysiological response to stimuli. However, it does not account for the enhancement in P300 responding obtained by Barabasz and Lonsdale [56].

   Taken together the EP findings and the behavioral findings concerning negative hallucinations suggest that no simple and straightforward relationship is likely to emerge between EP changes, the subjective experience of perceptual distortion, and verbal reports of perceptual distortion. Each of these effects may be related to different variables, and the occurrence of experiential distortions is particularly difficult to document. Unfortunately, neither EP changes nor verbal reports can be assumed to accurately or directly reflect the occurrence or degree of distortions in perceptual experience.

CONCLUSION

Reports by hypnotic subjects which indicate that they are blind, deaf, or otherwise sensorially impaired following suggestions are highly dramatic, and are consistent with the view that hypnotic responding involves highly unusual properties that enable subjects to transcend normal functioning. Such reports have been obtained from hypnotic subjects since the nineteenth century, and depending upon the theoretical orientation of investigators have been accepted uncritically or subjected to skeptical examination. By and large, those who endorse the reality of negative hallucinations have accepted subjects' verbal reports or other affirming voluntary behaviors at face value. According to these investigators (e.g., [9]) subjects' statements that they cannot see a number on a page constitutes good evidence that they actually are unable to see the number. Skeptical investigators, on the other hand, have been wary about accepting the uncorroborated testimony of hypnotic subjects and, instead, have devised a number of paradigms designed to assess negative hallucination responding independently of subjective reports.

Our review indicates that skeptical researchers have been justified in their suspicions concerning the validity of subjects' verbal reports. The behavioral evidence indicates that sensory functioning is not appreciably interfered with by negative hallucination suggestions, whereas verbal reports are greatly influenced by social demands and compliance pressures independently of any change in perceptual functioning.

Most of the electrophysiological evidence concerning negative hallucinations has also yielded negative results. Although much of this evidence is flawed methodologically, it is consistent in demonstrating that the early components of the EP are not affected by suggestions. Actually dimming a light and suggesting that a light will look dimmer does not produce equivalent electrophysiological effects even when subjects given the suggestion insist that the light looks dimmer. These findings are consistent with the behavioral ones which indicate that basic sensory processing is uninfluenced by suggestion. The electrophysiological evidence concerning the role of late component EP activity in negative hallucination responding is mixed and contradictory. Most of this research, however, has yielded negative results. The reasons for the contradictory findings remain unclear and require new research involving larger subjects samples, the random assignment of subjects to both hypnotic and nonhypnotic conditions, more systematic use of standardized hypnotizability measures, systematic variation in both the nature of the suggestions employed (e.g., suggestions to directly dampen experience vs. suggestions to shift attention) and the nature of the stimulus conditions.

Unfortunately, interpretive problems concerning the meaning of late component EP changes may remain even with improved methodologies. Although there appears to be general agreement in the EP literature that late components are influenced by attentional and other cognitive activity, the inferences that can be made about subjects' phenomenological experiences on the basis of late component EP changes are far from clear.

REFERENCES

1. T. R. Sarbin, Attempts to Understand Hypnotic Phenomena, in *Psychology in the Making: Histories of Selected Research Problems*, L. Postman (ed.), Alfred A. Knopf, New York, pp. 745-785, 1962.
2. M. H. Erickson, A Study of Clinical and Experimental Findings on Hypnotic Deafness: I. Clinical Experimentation and Findings, *Journal of General Psychology, 19*, pp. 127-150, 1938.
3. E. Hart, *Hypnotism, Mesmerism, and the New Witchcraft*, Appleton, New York, 1898.
4. F. A. Pattie, A Report of Attempts to Produce Uniocular Blindness by Hypnotic Suggestion, *British Journal of Medical Psychology, 15*, pp. 230-241, 1935.
5. J. P. Sutcliffe, "Credulous" and "Skeptical" Views of Hypnotic Phenomena: A Review of Certain Evidence and Methodology, *International Journal of Clinical and Experimental Hypnosis, 8*, pp. 73-101, 1960.
6. J. P. Sutcliffe, "Credulous" and "Skeptical" Views of Hypnotic Phenomena: Experiments in Esthesia, Hallucination, and Delusion, *Journal of Abnormal and Social Psychology, 62*, pp. 189-200, 1961.
7. M. T. Orne, The Nature of Hypnosis: Artifact and Essence, *Journal of Abnormal and Social Psychology, 58*, pp. 277-299, 1959.
8. N. P. Spanos, B. Jones, and A. Malfara, Hypnotic Deafness: Now You Hear It—Now You Still Hear It, *Journal of Abnormal Psychology, 91*, pp. 75-77, 1982.
9. H. S. Zamansky and S. P. Bartis, The Dissociation of an Experience: The Hidden Observer Observed, *Journal of Abnormal Psychology, 94*, pp. 243-248, 1985.
10. N. P. Spanos, Hypnotic Behaviour: A Social-psychological Interpretation of Amnesia, Analgesia, and "Trance Logic," *Behavioural and Brain Sciences, 9*, pp. 449-467, 1986.
11. G. F. Wagstaff, *Hypnosis, Compliance and Belief*, St. Martin's Press, New York, 1981.
12. B. Jones and D. M. Flynn, Methodological and Theoretical Considerations in the Study of "Hypnotic" Effects in Perception, in *Hypnosis: The Cognitive-behavioural Perspective*, N. P. Spanos and J. F. Chaves (eds.), Prometheus, Buffalo, pp. 149-174, 1989.
13. T. X. Barber and D. S. Calverley, Experimental Studies in Hypnotic Behaviour: Suggested Deafness Evaluated by Delayed Auditory Feedback, *British Journal of Psychology, 55*, pp. 439-446, 1964.
14. M. V. Kline, H. Guze, and A. D. Haggerty, An Experimental Study on the Nature of Hypnotic Deafness: Effects of Delayed Speech Feedback, *International Journal of Clinical and Experimental Hypnosis 2*, pp. 145-156, 1954.
15. R. J. Miller, R. T. Hennessy, and H. W. Leibowitz, The Effects of Hypnotic Ablation of the Background on the Magnitude of the Ponzo Perspective Illusion, *International Journal of Clinical and Experimental Hypnosis, 21*, pp. 180-191, 1973.

16. T. X. Barber, *Hypnosis: A Scientific Approach*, Van Nostrand Reinhold, New York, 1969.
17. B. Jones and N. P. Spanos, Suggestions for Altered Auditory Sensitivity, the Negative Subject Effect and Hypnotic Susceptibility: A Signal Detection Analysis, *Journal of Personality and Social Psychology, 43*, pp. 637-647, 1982.
18. C. A. Burgess, S. C. DuBrueil, B. Jones, and N. P. Spanos, Compliance and the Modification of Hypnotizability, *Imagination, Cognition and Personality, 10*, pp. 293-304, 1991.
19. N. P. Spanos, C. A. Burgess, L. Coco, and N. Pinch, Reporting Bias and Response to Difficult Suggestions in Highly Hypnotizable Subjects, *Journal of Research in Personality, 27*, pp. 270-284, 1993.
20. N. P. Spanos, C. A. Burgess, P. Cross, and G. McCleod, Hypnosis, Reporting Bias and Negative Hallucinations, *Journal of Abnormal Psychology, 101*, pp. 192-199, 1992.
21. N. P. Spanos, C. A. Burgess, and A. H. Perlini, Compliance and Suggested Deafness in Hypnotic and Nonhypnotic Subjects, *Imagination, Cognition and Personality, 11*, pp. 211-223, 1992.
22. N. P. Spanos, A. H. Perlini, L. Patrick, S. Bell, and M. I. Gwynn, The Role of Compliance in Hypnotic and Nonhypnotic Analgesia, *Journal of Research in Personality, 24*, pp. 433-453, 1990.
23. N. P. Spanos, C. A. Burgess, and A. Gardin, *Reporting Bias, Dissociation and Expectancy in Hypnotic Analgesia*, unpublished manuscript, Carleton University, 1993.
24. N. P. Spanos, Compliance and Reinterpretation in Hypnotic Responding, *Contemporary Hypnosis, 9*, pp. 7-15, 1992.
25. S. E. Asch, *Social Psychology*, Prentice Hall, Englewood Cliffs, 1952.
26. L. H. Levy, Awareness, Learning and the Beneficient Subject as Expert Witness, *Journal of Personality and Social Psychology, 6*, pp. 365-370, 1967.
27. S. Milgram, *Obedience to Authority*, Harper and Row, New York, 1974.
28. N. P. Spanos, D. M. Flynn, and N. Gabora, Suggestive Negative Visual Hallucinations in Hypnotic Subjects: When No Means Yes, *British Journal of Experimental and Clinical Hypnosis, 6*, pp. 63-67, 1989.
29. C. A. Burgess, N. P. Spanos, J. Ritt, T. Hordy, and S. Brooks, *Compliant Responding in High Hypnotizables: An Experimental Demonstration*, unpublished manuscript, Carleton University, 1993.
30. N. P. Spanos and W. C. Coe, Hypnosis: A Social Psychological Perspective, in *Contemporary Perspectives in Hypnosis Research*, E. Fromm and M. Nash (eds.), Plenum, New York, pp. 102-130, 1992.
31. G. F. Wagstaff, Hypnosis as Compliance and Belief, in *What is Hypnosis?*, P. Naish (ed.), Open University Press, Philadelphia, pp. 59-84, 1986.
32. D. Kahneman, *Attention and Effort*, Prentice-Hall, Englewood Cliffs, 1973.
33. K. B. Campbell, D. Deacon-Elliott, and G. Proulx, Electrophysiological Monitoring of Closed Head Injury. I: Basic Principles and Techniques, *Cognitive Rehabilitation, 4*, pp. 26-32, 1986.
34. D. Regan, *Evoked Potentials in Psychology, Sensory Physiology, and Clinical Medicine*, Chapman and Hall, London, 1972.
35. S. A. Hillyard and M. Kutas, Electrophysiology of Cognitive Processing, *Annual Review of Psychology, 34*, pp. 33-61, 1983.
36. E. R. John and E. L. Schwartz, The Neurophysiology of Information Processing and Cognition, *Annual Review of Psychology, 29*, pp. 1-29, 1978.
37. R. Hernandez-Peon and M. Donoso, Influence of Attention and Suggestion upon Subcortical Evoked Electrical Activity in the Human Brain, in *First International*

Congress of Neurological Sciences, Vol. 3, L. van Bogaert and J. Radermecker (eds.), Pergamon Press, London, pp. 385-396, 1959.

38. R. Guerrero-Figueroa and R. G. Heath, Evoked Responses and Changes during Attentive Factors in Man, *Archives of Neurology, 10,* pp. 74-84, 1964.

39. J. Baribeau-Braun, T. W. Picton, and J. Y. Gosselin, A Neurophysiological Evaluation of Abnormal Information Processing, *Science, 219,* pp. 874-876, 1983.

40. M. Clynes, M. Kohn, and K. Lifshitz, Dynamics and Spatial Behaviour of Light Evoked Potentials, Their Modification under Hypnosis, and On-line Correlation in Relation to Rhythmic Components, *Annals of the New York Academy of Sciences, 112,* pp. 468-509, 1964.

41. J. B. Satterfield, R. Hicks, W. E. Edmonston, and H. Davis, Dynamics and Spatial Behaviour of Light Evoked Potentials, Their Modification under Hypnosis, and On-line Correlation in Relation to Rhythmic Components, in *Annals of the New York Academy of the Sciences, 112,* M. Clynes, M. Kohn, and K. Lifshitz, (J. H. Satterfield, Discussant), pp. 468-509, 1964.

42. E. C. Beck and G. S. Barolin, The Effect of Hypnotic Suggestion on Evoked Potentials, *Journal of Nervous and Mental Disease, 140,* pp. 154-161, 1965.

43. E. A. Serafinides, Electrophysiological Responses to Sensory Stimulation under Hypnosis, *American Journal of Psychiatry, 125,* pp. 150-151, 1968.

44. A. M. Halliday and A. A. Mason, Cortical Evoked Potentials during Hypnotic Anaesthesia, *Electroencephalography and Clinical Neurophysiology, 16,* p. 314, 1964.

45. P. Diaconis, Magical Thinking in the Analysis of Scientific Data, in The Clever Hans Phenomenon: Communication with Horses, Whales, Apes, and People, T. A. Sebeok and R. Rosenthal (eds.), *Annals of the New York Academy of the Sciences, 364,* pp. 236-244, 1981.

46. E. C. Beck, Electrophysiology and Behaviour, *Annual Review of Psychology, 26,* pp. 233-261, 1975.

47. E. C. Beck, R. E. Dustman, and E. G. Beier, Hypnotic Suggestions and Visually Evoked Potentials, *Electroencephalography and Clinical Neurophysiology, 20,* pp. 397-400, 1966.

48. K. Zakrzewski and W. Szelenberger, Visual Evoked Potentials in Hypnosis: A Longitudinal Approach, *International Journal of Clinical and Experimental Hypnosis, 29,* pp. 77-86, 1981.

49. J. C. Andreassi, B. Balinsky, J. A. Ballichio, J. J. DeSimone, and B. W. Mellers, Hypnotic Suggestion of Stimulus Change and Visual Cortical Evoked Potential, *Perceptual and Motor Skills, 42,* pp. 371-378, 1976.

50. D. Spiegel, S. Cutcomb, C. Ren, and K. Pribram, Hypnotic Hallucination Alters Evoked Potentials, *Journal of Abnormal Psychology, 94,* pp. 140-143, 1985.

51. A. H. Perlini, A. L. Lorimer, K. B. Campbell, and N. P. Spanos, An Electrophysiological and Psychophysiological Analysis of Hypnotic Visual Hallucinations, *Imagination, Cognition and Personality, 12,* pp. 301-312, 1993.

52. S. Sokol and A. Moskowitz, Effect of Retinal Blur on the Peak Latency of the Pattern Evoked Potential, *Vision Research, 21,* pp. 1279-1286, 1981.

53. W. E. Edmonston, Conceptualization and Clarification of Hypnosis and its Relationship to Suggestibility, in *Suggestion and Suggestibility: Theory and Research,* V. A. Gheorghui, P. Netter, H. J. Eysenck, and R. Rosenthal (eds.), Springer-Verlag, Berlin, pp. 69-78, 1989.

54. M. Amadeo and A. Yanovski, Evoked Potentials and Selective Attention in Subjects Capable of Hypnotic Analgesia, *International Journal of Clinical and Experimental Hypnosis, 23,* pp. 200-210, 1975.

55. D. Spiegel, P. Bierre, and J. Rootenberg, Hypnotic Alteration of Somatosensory Perception, *American Journal of Psychiatry, 146,* pp. 749-754, 1989.

56. A. E. Barabasz and C. Lonsdale, Effects of Hypnosis on P300 Olfactory-evoked Potential Amplitudes, *Journal of Abnormal Psychology, 92,* pp. 520-523, 1983.

57. D. Spiegel and A. E. Barabasz, Effects of Hypnotic Instructions on P300 Event-related Potential Amplitudes: Research and Clinical Implications, *American Journal of Clinical Hypnosis, 31,* pp. 11-17, 1988.

CHAPTER 11

Presence vs. Absence of a "Hidden Observer" during Total Deafness: The Hypnotic Illusion of Subconsciousness vs. the Imaginal Attenuation of Brainstem Evoked Potentials

ROBERT G. KUNZENDORF
AND PATRICIA BOISVERT

In this chapter, the appearance of a "hidden observer" in some hypnotically deafened subjects, but not in others, is explained without recourse to Hilgard's theory that the former subjects manifest a "temporary personality created in hypnosis [and engaged in] hearing at the covert level" [1, p. 236]. Hilgard discovered the "hidden observer" while working with a hypnotically deafened subject who denied any conscious perception of a test sound, but who had "subconscious" knowledge of the sound [1-3]. At the time of this discovery, Wilson and Barber were describing how vivid imagers, with or without hypnosis, "can 'block out' [a sound] or object from their perceptual field by fantasizing . . . something else in the place of the [sound] or object they are not to perceive" [4, p. 376]. We take the view that Wilson and Barber still provide the best explanation for total deafness in the *absence of a hidden observer,* and in this chapter we show that vivid images of deafening sensations physiologically "mask" brainstem auditory evoked potentials (BSAEPs) and effectively "muffle" perceptual sensations. The *presence of a hidden observer,* in our view, can occur only when deafening imagery is not vivid enough to prevent perceptual sensations from being heard, but is hypnoidal enough to prevent them from being registered as perceptual in source. The resulting sensations of "sourceless" sound can be misattributed to imaginal sources during the hypnotic suggestion of deafness, and can be misattributed to subconscious sources during the further suggestion of a hidden observer. Based on this bipartite thesis, and bolstered by the evidence in this

224 / HYPNOSIS AND IMAGINATION

chapter, we conclude that the hidden observer is not a "cognitive substructure" "denied conscious expression [and] accessible only through automatic writing" [1, pp. 219, 233-234], but is an illusory attribution sustained within hypnotic consciousness.

ABSENCE OF A HIDDEN OBSERVER IN NEGATIVE HALLUCINATORS: BLOCKING OF PERIPHERAL SENSATION IN VIVID IMAGERS

The first premise of the above theses—that *vividly imaged* sensations occlude perceptual sensations, and preclude a hidden observer—is consonant with the results of recent psychophysiological experiments. In one experiment, Deehan and Robertson found that auditory evoked potentials (AEPs) were flattened when deeply hypnotized subjects negatively hallucinated [5]. In another study, Kunzendorf, Jesses, Michaels, Caiazzo-Fluellen, and Butler found that brainstem auditory evoked potentials (BSAEPs) were dampened when unhypnotized children and adult musicians imaged deafening music, and were augmented when unhypnotized children imaged the evoking clicks "sounding much louder than they really are" [6, p. 161]. Anatomical studies confirm the existence of centrifugal pathways to the cochlea, where the sensory components of AEPs and BSAEPs originate [7, 8]. Such evidence suggests that the vividly imaged sensations of a juvenal, musical, or hypnotizable mind can centrifugally mask dissimilar ones.

To the extent that any auditory percept is masked peripherally and totally by deafening imagery, that percept may not be recovered through the "hidden observer" technique or through any other technique. By implication, subjects who exhibit total hypnotic deafness in the absence of a "hidden observer" should be subjects who possess auditory imagery vivid enough to attenuate BSAEPs. This is the first implication tested by the empirical study described later in this chapter.

PRESENCE OF A HIDDEN OBSERVER IN NEGATIVE HALLUCINATORS: ATTENUATION OF SOURCE MONITORING IN HYPNOTIC VIRTUOSOS

The second premise of our thesis—that auditory percepts during *faintly hallucinated* music are not masked, but are misattributed either to imaginal sources or to subconsciously "hidden" sources—is consonant with Kunzendorf's theory and research on source monitoring. According to Kunzendorf's theory, both the peripheral source of perceptual sensations and the central source of imaginal sensations are neurally monitored during normal self-consciousness [9-11]. During hallucinatory episodes when such self-conscious monitoring is attenuated, however, both percepts and images are immediately experienced as "sourceless" sensations, and are subsequently interpreted in accordance with contextual mediators [11-14].

By implication, in the context of "deafening" musical hallucinations that are too faint to mask BSAEPs, perceptual sensations of sound should be immediately experienced as sourceless, and should be mediately interpreted as "consciously imaged during deafness" or "subconsciously heard during deafness" (but not "consciously heard during deafness"). If hypnotists suggest that a "hidden observer" may have been present during negative hallucinating, as Hilgard suggests in his research, then faint hallucinators should interpret their "sourceless" auditory percepts as "subconsciously heard during deafness." But if hypnotists suggest that auditory imagery may have been present during negative hallucinating, as we suggest in the following investigation, then faint hallucinators should interpret their "sourceless" percepts as "consciously imaged during deafness." Thus, from the standpoint of monitoring theory, the hidden observer is neither a subconscious "personality" nor an unconscious "cognitive substructure," but an illusion resulting from the interaction of monitoring functions and contextual factors [1, pp. 219, 236].

INVESTIGATING THE PRESENCE/ABSENCE
OF A HIDDEN OBSERVER

In empirically investigating our bipartite thesis, we only tested subjects who reported total hypnotic deafness—for two reasons. First, for our "no hidden observer" group, we wanted subjects whose musical imagery was vivid enough to muffle other sounds completely, thus vivid enough to mask BSAEPs maximally. Relevant research by Kunzendorf has confirmed that the centrifugal effects of visual imagery on retinal activity are maximized in vivid imagers [15-16]. Second, for our "hidden observer" group, we wanted subjects whose negative hallucinosis was delusory enough to render percepts totally "sourceless," also dramatic enough to eclipse pure demand characteristics. In the latter regard, research by Spanos and Hewitt has shown that, for negative hallucinators who report partial perception rather than total negation, demand characteristics can induce either a "hidden observer" who reports slightly more perception or a "reverse hidden observer" who reports slightly less perception [17]. We agree that contextual demands contribute to the illusion of a "hidden observer," in both partial and total deafness; but as noted above, we believe that hypnotic demands interact dramatically with *the loss of source monitoring* in totally deafened subjects.

Also, in order to induce negative hallucinosis in our subjects, we explicitly instructed them to image deafening music "so powerful that . . . hearing will be blocked out, totally blocked out by this powerful music." Justification for this particular instruction comes not only from Wilson and Barber's imagistic theory of hypnotic deafness, but also from Hilgard's empirical observation that many hypnotic subjects "supplement the hypnotist's suggestions . . . by producing a competing sound to make it more difficult to hear" [1, p. 179].

For totally deafened subjects with no hidden observer, our bipartite theory predicts that vivid images of deafening music are occluding BSAEPs and are precluding auditory percepts, "hidden" or otherwise. Conversely, for totally deafened subjects with a hidden observer, our theory predicts that faint hypnotic hallucinations of musical sound are shutting down self-conscious "source monitoring" and are allowing other sounds to be misattributed either to subconscious sources or to imaginal sources, depending on suggested context.

METHOD

Apparatus: Brainstem Auditory Evoked Potentials

Brain potentials (EEGs) were recorded at the vertex from a miniature disc electrode, referenced to one ear-clip electrode and grounded by another ear-clip electrode. EEG recordings between 0.3 Hz and 3 kHz were amplified with a Grass Instruments 7P511 AC Amplifier.

In order to evoke brain potentials for computer averaging, an 8000 Hz click lasting .25 msecs was generated 500 times in succession—once every 200 msecs—by a computer-interfaced Coulbourn Instruments signal generator and audio amplifier. The individual clicks were transmitted through air-conduction earphones and, 11.0 msecs after their generation, were presented to both ears at 55 dB SPL.

Upon every presentation of the evoking click, amplified EEGs were sampled 100 times, once every 0.1 msec, and were digitized with a Tecmar PC-Mate Lab Master. If any of the 100 sampled digits for a particular click was below the digital floor (−2047) or above the digital ceiling (2048), then all 100 sampled digits were rejected by computer.

After each bout of 500 successive clicks, all unrejected 100-digit EEGs were stored in an IBM personal computer. During the entire experiment, 100-digit EEGs were stored for ten different bouts—one 500-click practice bout, plus three 500-click bouts in each of three within-subject conditions. Ultimately, for the three bouts (1500 evoking clicks) in each within-subject condition, all unrejected 100-digit EEGs were computer-averaged, and the resulting BSAEP for each condition was plotted on an IBM graphics printer.

Procedure: Hypnotic Suggestions

Hypnosis was preceded by the Vividness of Auditory Imagery Questionnaire (VAIQ), for which sixteen sounds are imaged auditorily and rated on a 5-point scale from "1 = as vivid as normal hearing" to "5 = no image" [18]. Hypnosis was induced with the "induction by hand levitation" from the Revised Stanford Profile Scales of Hypnotic Susceptibility, Forms I and II [19]. Thereafter, via the "music hallucination" suggestion from Form I and the "heat hallucination" suggestion from Form II, hypnosis was confirmed.

Via the next two hypnotic suggestions, negative auditory hallucinating was elicited on two successive trials, and the "hidden observer" was tested with two different within-subject treatments. Each trial's negative auditory hallucination was elicited by the following instruction:

> Very soon, you are going to imagine some very powerful music, not just loud but powerful. This imaginary music will be so powerful that you will not be able *to hear anything,* not even my voice—until I tap you on both shoulders. When I tap you on both shoulders, the powerful music will dissipate completely and will no longer block your hearing. Very soon, I am going to ask you to begin imaging some music, and I am going to tap your left shoulder three times. With each tap on your left shoulder, the music will sound more powerful. After the third tap, your hearing will be blocked out, totally blocked out by this powerful music—until I tap you on both shoulders. You can begin imaging some music now.

The subject's left shoulder was tapped three times. In the standard treatment condition for uncovering "subconscious" observation, the following version of the classic "hidden observer" suggestion was read aloud:

> Can you hear me? Follow the yellow brick road.
> Follow the yellow brick road.
> (. . . Both shoulders are tapped . . .)
> The powerful music is gone, completely gone. Can you hear me now? Moments ago, I recited part of a rhyme for children. Can you identify the rhyme or tell me some of the words?
> (. . . If not identified, suggestion is continued . . .)
> Even if you did not consciously hear the recited rhyme, your subconscious mind might have heard it. Starting right now, your subconscious mind is taking over the hand that you write with. Pick up your pen or pencil, and let's see whether or not your subconscious mind heard words from a children's rhyme. If such words were heard, even subconsciously, your hand will automatically write them down—quite possibly, without your conscious knowledge.
> (. . . A response of time of one minute is observed . . .)
> Now, put your pen or pencil down. Both of your hands are, once again, under the control of your conscious mind.

In the experimental treatment condition, which was designed to reveal "unmonitored" observation (rather than "subconscious" observation), the following modification of the above suggestion was read instead:

> Can you hear me? The bear went over the mountain. The bear went over the mountain.
> (. . . Both shoulders are tapped . . .)
> The powerful music is gone, completely gone. Can you hear me now? Moments ago, I recited part of a rhyme for children. Can you identify the rhyme or tell me some of the words?
> (. . . If not identified, suggestion is continued . . .)

Even if you did not consciously hear the recited rhyme, you might have imagined hearing words from a children's rhyme. Try to remember if you imagined hearing any rhyme during the powerful music. Pick up your pen or pencil, and write down all the rhymes that you imagined hearing while you were unable to hear sounds outside of your own mind.

(. . . A response time of one minute is observed . . .)

Now, put your pen or pencil down.

The order of these two within-subject treatment conditions was counterbalanced across subjects.

Finally, brainstem auditory evoked potentials (BSAEPs) were sampled under three within-subject conditions of suggestion: 1) a control suggestion to *"listen for clicks* and notice how loud [the evoking clicks] really are," 2) the above suggestion of "powerful music," powerful enough to *block out clicks,* and 3) a suggestion to *"image louder clicks,* much louder than they really are." The nine 500-click bouts of BSAEP sampling—three "listen for clicks" bouts, three "block out clicks" bouts, and three "image louder clicks" bouts—were randomly ordered for every subject. After each "blocking out clicks" bout, an inability to hear the 500 clicks was confirmed. Prior to the first bout, the 500-click practice bout was presented, and following the ninth bout, hypnosis was terminated.

Subjects

The above suggestions for negative hallucinating through deafening musical imagery were hypnotically administered to subjects who previously scored 11-12 out of 12 on the Stanford Hypnotic Susceptibility Scale, Form C [20], until *complete "blocking out"* was obtained in eight subjects. In response to the classic "hidden observer" suggestion, four subjects disclosed a "subconscious" observation of the completely blocked-out song, and four subjects exhibited no "hidden observer" of the completely blocked-out song. Even with four subjects per group, some theoretically and statistically significant differences emerged between the "hidden observer" group and the "no hidden observer" group.

RESULTS

One significant difference between groups emerged prior to hypnosis, when the VAIQ (Vividness of Auditory Imagery Questionnaire) was completed. In imaging the sixteen sounds on the VAIQ and rating their vividness from "1 = as vivid as normal hearing" to "5 = no image," the "no hidden observer" group gave an average rating of 1.6 to each imaged sound ($SD = 0.4$). In contrast, the "hidden observer" group averaged a significantly less vivid rating of 2.5 ($SD = 0.4$)—$t(7) = 3.41, p < .025$.

A comparable difference emerged during hypnosis, when the 55 dB clicks evoking the BSAEPs (brainstem auditory evoked potentials) were *imaged louder* by both groups. As the tracings in Figure 1 illustrate, and as the means in Table 1 corroborate, BSAEP amplitudes increased if the evoking clicks were *imaged louder* by vivid imagers in the "no hidden observer" group. However, BSAEP amplitudes did not increase if the evoking clicks were *imaged louder* by less vivid imagers in the "hidden observer" group.

This group-specific effect of image vividness on BSAEP amplitude emerged, also, when music powerful enough to *block out clicks* was imaged. BSAEP amplitudes decreased if deafeningly powerful music was imaged by vivid imagers in the "no hidden observer" group, as Figure 1 and Table 1 reveal. In contrast, BSAEP amplitudes did not decrease if such music was imaged by less vivid imagers in the "hidden observer" group.

An Analysis of Variance for the dependent variable, BSAEP amplitude, confirms that the "hidden observer" and "no hidden observer" groups interact significantly with the three suggestions in Table 1—to *block out clicks,* to *listen for clicks,* and to *image louder clicks*—$F(2,12) = 13.84$, $p < .001$. Because amplitude shifts only in the imaged direction are expected, given both logical expectation and past evidence, the *t*-tests in Table 1 are one-tailed comparisons.

Finally, definitive differences between the groups emerged when the experimental suggestion for breaching negative hallucinations was employed, as well as when the standard "hidden observer" technique was employed. As Table 2

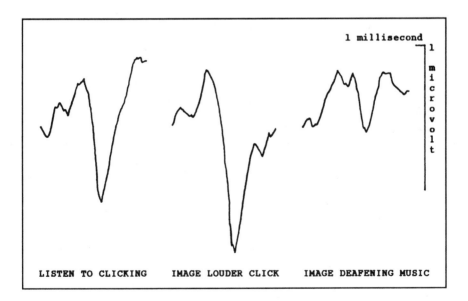

Figure 1. BSAEP tracings from one of the hypnotic virtuosos with "no hidden observer." (The long negative deflection approximately 7 msecs after click onset is Wave 5P-5N, which originates in the inferior colliculus of the brainstem, and which corresponds to the magnitude of the evoking sensation [21, 22].)

Table 1. Amplitude of Hypnotic Virtuosos' BSAEP (Wave 5P-5N) When Blocking Out Clicks *versus* Listening for Clicks *versus* Imaging Louder Clicks

	Between-Subject Groupings	
Within-S Condition of Suggestion	Group with a "Hidden Observer"	Group with "no Hidden Observer"
Suggestion of music powerful enough to block out clicks	$M = .32\ \mu V$ $SD = .15$	$M = .23\ \mu V^{a,c}$ $SD = .07$
Suggestion to listen for clicks, notice real loudness	$M = .29\ \mu V$ $SD = .12$	$M = .35\ \mu V^{a,b}$ $SD = .04$
Suggestion to image louder clicks	$M = .24\ \mu V$ $SD = .11$	$M = .45\ \mu V^{b,c}$ $SD = .11$

[a]Matched within "no hidden observer" Ss, $t(3) = 3.05$, $p < .05$
[b]Matched within "no hidden observer" Ss, $t(3) = 2.55$, $p < .05$
[c]Matched within "no hidden observer" Ss, $t(3) = 3.60$, $p < .025$

Table 2. Probability of Virtuosos Disclosing a Subconsciously "Hidden" Observation of the Blocked-Out Rhyme (P_{subc}) *versus* Probability of Virtuosos Disclosing an Imaginary Observation of the Blocked-Out Rhyme (P_{imag})

	Between-Subject Groupings	
Within-S Treatment Conditions	Group with a "Hidden Observer"	Group with "no Hidden Observer"
Standard condition for uncovering a "subconscious" observation of blocked rhyme	$P_{subc} = 1$	$P_{subc} = 0$
Experimental condition for uncovering an "imaginary" observation of blocked rhyme	$P_{imag} = 1$	$P_{imag} = 0$

indicates, the "hidden observer" group breached the negative hallucination of deafening music, not only in response to the standard suggestion—to disclose any subconsciously "hidden" awareness of hearing a rhyme during the music—but also in response to the experimental suggestion—to disclose any conscious awareness of imagining a rhyme during the music. Conversely, the "no hidden observer" group did not breach the negative hallucination when either technique was employed, presumably because the latter group's imagery of deafening music was vivid enough to drown out rhymes (and their BSAEPs), just like clicks and their BSAEPs.

DISCUSSION

Although subjects with total hypnotic deafness are quite scarce and our groups are consequentially small, the results of our current study are significant statistically. Furthermore, these results are consistent with our bipartite theory of the "hidden observer"—as well as with Barrett's bifurcation of the "hypnotic virtuoso" population into "fantasizers" and "dissociaters" [23, 24] and Hall's bifurcation of the hypnotic population into "vivid imagers" exhibiting physiological effects and "faint hallucinators" experiencing psychological effects [25].

First, in accordance with our theoretical premise explaining the *absence of a hidden observer*, our study indicates that totally deafened subjects with no "hidden observer" can image sounds more vividly on the VAIQ, can amplify their BSAEPs by vividly imaging the evoking percepts as "louder," and can mask their BSAEPs by vividly fantasizing percept-muffling music. Given these results, we conclude that negative hallucinators with no "hidden observer" are *vivid fantasizers* who can imaginally mask perceptual sensations in the peripheral nervous system and cannot possibly retrieve these totally masked sensations, not even through Hilgard's "hidden observer" technique. Given the results of other recent studies, we further conclude that *unhypnotized* vivid imagers, also, can imaginally mask BSAEPs and irretrievably muffle auditory percepts. In particular, Kunzendorf's recent developmental study of click-evoked brainstem potentials has confirmed that, without hypnosis, eidetic children and collegiate musicians can amplify BSAEPs by fantasizing louder clicks and can mask BSAEPs by imaging click-muffling music [6]. In addition, Spanos' recent study of the peripheral effects of hypnoidal and imaginal healing has demonstrated that, with or without hypnosis, vivid imagers tend to be more successful at imaginally healing warts [26]. Indeed, a series of studies reviewed both by Kunzendorf and by Spanos has shown that hypnosis does not increase the vividness of mental imagery [9, 27].

Second, our current study indicates that totally deafened subjects with a "hidden observer" cannot hallucinate vividly enough to mask the BSAEPs of auditory percepts, and yet, can only remember such percepts as "consciously imaged during deafness" or "subconsciously perceived during deafness" (but not "consciously perceived during deafness"). This latter finding is consonant with our second theoretical premise: that external sounds during faintly hallucinated deafness are not self-consciously "monitored" as perceptual in source, and are consequently misinterpreted either as imaginal in source or as subconscious in source, depending on contextual mediation. Of course, it could be argued that even the basic failure to monitor "consciously perceived" sound is mediated by social context (notwithstanding the rare *totality* of conscious deafness in this study), but other recent studies show that "source monitoring" failures are associated with cognitive states and traits, rather than contextual factors. In particular, recent studies by Kunzendorf and by Rader, Kunzendorf, and Carrabino demonstrate that the self-conscious monitoring of imaginal sources is reduced in the hypnotic state, even though the vividness of images is not simultaneously increased [12, 28]. In the study by Rader, Kunzendorf, and Carrabino, "source monitoring" failures are also observable outside the hypnotic state, but are associated with the trait of getting less than a normal amount of sleep. Finally, another recent study by Kunzendorf shows that the posthypnotic inability to discriminate hypnotic images from hypnotic percepts is an irreversible state-induced amnesia (even though the posthypnotically suggested inability to recall such images and percepts is easily reversed by context—any context that shifts the criterion for overt recall from an "awareness of source" to a "feeling of familiarity") [13].

The presence of a hidden observer is thus an illusion, when it is theoretically reduced to the absence of self-conscious "source monitoring," plus a context attributing unmonitored sensations to subconsciously "hidden" sources. It is not that hypnosis does not entail subconsciousness, but that subconsciousness does not entail hidden observations by a "temporary personality" or computer-like "cognitive substructure" [1, pp. 219, 236]. Indeed, when the pre-computational psychologist Prince theorized about dissociated hearing, subconscious pain, "automatic" writing; and other hypnotic experiences, he defined each sub-conscious experience as "consciousness occur[ring] without self-consciousness" [29, p. 94]—and without "a plurality of I's or selves" [30, p. 178]. Consistent with Prince's theoretical alternative to the "hidden observer" interpretation of subconsciousness, Kunzendorf's monitoring theory further defines "consciousness . . . without self-consciousness" as conscious sensation without any self-awareness *that one is imaging the sensation* or *that one is perceiving the sensation* [31-33]. In our current chapter, this "source monitoring" interpretation of subconsciousness, as it interacts with contextual demands and fantasizing abilities, provides new insights into the illusory presence of a hidden observer.

REFERENCES

1. E. R. Hilgard, *Divided Consciousness: Multiple Controls in Human Thought and Action*, Wiley, New York, 1977.
2. H. J. Crawford, H. Macdonald, and E. R. Hilgard, Hypnotic Deafness: A Psychophysical Study of Responses to Tone Intensity as Modified by Hypnosis, *American Journal of Psychology, 92*, pp. 193-214, 1979.
3. E. R. Hilgard, Divided Consciousness and Dissociation, *Consciousness and Cognition, 1*, pp. 16-31, 1992.
4. S. C. Wilson and T. X. Barber, The Fantasy-prone Personality: Implications for Understanding Imagery, Hypnosis, and Parapsychological Phenomena, in *Imagery*, A. A. Sheikh (ed.), Wiley, New York, pp. 340-387, 1983.

5. C. Deehan and A. W. Robertson, Changes in Auditory Evoked Potentials Induced by Hypnotic Suggestion, in *Hypnosis in Psychotherapy and Psychosomatic Medicine*, M. Pamntar, E. Roskar, and M. Lavric (eds.), University Press, Ljubljana, pp. 93-95, 1980.
6. R. G. Kunzendorf, M. Jesses, A. Michaels, G. Ciazzo-Fluellen, and W. Butler, Imagination and Perceptual Development: Effects of Auditory Imaging on the Brainstem Evoked Potentials of Children, Adult Musicians, and Other Adults, in *Mental Imagery*, R. G. Kunzendorf (ed.), Plenum, New York, pp. 159-166, 1991.
7. R. Klinke and N. Galley, Efferent Innervation of Vestibular and Auditory Receptors, *Physiological Reviews, 54*, pp. 316-357, 1974.
8. M. D. Ross, Fluorescence and Electron Microscopic Observations of the General Visceral, Efferent Innervation of the Inner Ear, *Acta Oto-Laryngologica*, Supplement 286, pp. 1-18, 1971.
9. R. G. Kunzendorf, Self-consciousness as the Monitoring of Cognitive States: A Theoretical Perspective, *Imagination, Cognition and Personality, 7*, pp. 3-22, 1987-88.
10. R. G. Kunzendorf, Mind-Brain Identity Theory: A Materialistic Foundation for the Psychophysiology of Mental Imagery, in *Psychophysiology of Mental Imagery: Theory, Research, and Application*, R. G. Kunzendorf and A. A. Sheikh (eds.), Baywood, Amityville, New York, pp. 9-36, 1990.
11. R. G. Kunzendorf and D. Hoyle, Auditory Percepts, Mental Images, and Hypnotic Hallucinations: Similarities and Differences in Auditory Evoked Potentials, in *Imagery: Current Perspectives*, J. E. Shorr, P. Robin, J. A. Connella, and M. Wolpi (eds.), Plenum, New York, pp. 1-12, 1990.
12. R. G. Kunzendorf, Hypnotic Hallucinations as "Unmonitored" Images, *Imagination, Cognition and Personality, 5*, pp. 255-270, 1985-86.
13. R. G. Kunzendorf, Posthypnotic Amnesia: Dissociation of Self-concept or Self-consciousness?, *Imagination, Cognition and Personality, 9*, pp. 321-334, 1989-90.
14. R. G. Kunzendorf, S. M. Beltz, and G. Tymowicz, Self-awareness in Autistic Subjects and Deeply Hypnotized Subjects: Dissociation of Self-concept versus Self-consciousness, *Imagination, Cognition and Personality, 11*, pp. 129-141, 1991.
15. R. G. Kunzendorf, Centrifugal Effects of Eidetic Imaging on Flash Electroretinograms and Autonomic Responses, *Journal of Mental Imagery, 8*, pp. 67-76, 1984.
16. R. G. Kunzendorf, Afterimages of Eidetic Images: A Developmental Study, *Journal of Mental Imagery, 13*, pp. 55-62, 1989.
17. N. P. Spanos and E. C. Hewitt, The Hidden Observer in Hypnotic Analgesia: Discovery or Experimental Creation?, *Journal of Personality and Social Psychology, 39*, pp. 1201-1214, 1980.
18. R. G. Kunzendorf, Imagery and Consciousness: A Scientific Analysis of the Mind-Body Problem (doctoral dissertation, University of Virginia, 1979), *Dissertation Abstracts International, 40B*, (University Microfilms No. 8002505) pp. 3448-3449, 1980.
19. A. M. Weitzenhoffer and E. R. Hilgard, *Revised Stanford Profile Scales of Hypnotic Susceptibility, Forms I and II*, Consulting Psychologists Press, Palo Alto, California, 1967.
20. A. M. Weitzenhoffer and E. R. Hilgard, *Stanford Hypnotic Susceptibility Scale, Form C*, Consulting Psychologists Press, Palo Alto, California, 1962.
21. T. W. Picton, S. A. Hillyard, H. I. Krausz, and R. Galambos, Human Auditory Evoked Potentials. I: Evaluation of Components, *Electroencephalography and Clinical Neurophysiology, 36*, pp. 179-190, 1974.
22. J. R. Hughes, A Review of the Auditory System and Its Evoked Potentials, *American Journal of EEG Technology, 25*, pp. 115-158, 1985.

23. D. Barrett, Deep Trance Subjects: A Schema of Two Distinct Subgroups, in *Mental Imagery*, R. G. Kunzendorf (ed.), Plenum, New York, pp. 101-112, 1991.
24. D. Barrett, Fantasizers and Dissociaters: Two Types of High Hypnotizables, Two Different Imagery Styles, in *Hypnosis and Imagination*, R. G. Kunzendorf, N. P. Spanos, and B. Wallace (eds.), Baywood, Amityville, New York, pp. 123-139, 1996.
25. H. Hall, Imagery, Psychoneuroimmunology, and the Psychology of Healing, in *Psychophysiology of Mental Imagery: Theory, Research, and Application*, R. G. Kunzendorf and A. A Sheikh (eds.), Baywood, Amityville, New York, pp. 203-227, 1990.
26. N. P. Spanos, R. Stenstrom, and J. Johnston, Hypnosis, Placebo, and Suggestion in the Treatment of Warts, *Psychosomatic Medicine, 50*, pp. 245-260, 1988.
27. N. P. Spanos and H. L. Radtke, Hypnotic Visual Hallucinations as Imaginings: A Cognitive-Social Psychological Perspective, *Imagination, Cognition and Personality, 2*, pp. 195-210, 1982-83.
28. C. M. Rader, R. G. Kunzendorf, and C. Carrabino, The Relation of Image Vividness, Absorption, Reality Testing, and Synesthesia to Hypnotic States and Traits, in *Hypnosis and Imagination*, R. G. Kunzendorf, N. P. Spanos, and B. Wallace (eds.), Baywood, Amityville, New York, pp. 99-121, 1996.
29. M. Prince, The Subconscious—Part 5, in *Subconscious Phenomena*, H. Münsterberg, T. Ribot, P. Janet, J. Jastrow, B. Hart, and M. Prince (eds.), Gorham Press, Boston, Massachusetts, pp. 71-101, 1910.
30. M. Prince, Awareness, Consciousness, Co-consciousness and Animal Intelligence from the Point of View of the Data of Abnormal Psychology: A Biological Theory of Consciousness, *Pedagogical Seminary, 32*, pp. 166-188, 1925.
31. R. G. Kunzendorf, Subconscious Percepts as 'Unmonitored' Percepts: An Empirical Study, *Imagination, Cognition and Personality, 4*, pp. 367-375, 1984-85.
32. R. G. Kunzendorf and L. Montisanti, Subliminal Activation of Hypnotic Responses: Subconscious Realms of Mind *versus* Subconscious Modes of Mentation, *Imagination, Cognition and Personality, 9*, pp. 103-114, 1989-90.
33. R. G. Kunzendorf and W. Butler, Apperception Revisited: "Subliminal" Monocular Perception during the Apperception of Fused Random-dot Stereograms, *Consciousness and Cognition, 1*, pp. 63-76, 1992.

CHAPTER 12

Imagery, Hypnosis, and Hemispheric Laterality: An Examination of Individual Differences

BENJAMIN WALLACE
AND DEANNA D. TUROSKY

INTRODUCTION

For many years psychologists have been concerned with the concept of imagery, but few have been able to agree on a definition [1]. According to Pylyshin, mental images are at best subjective epiphenomena that play little or no functional role in significant processes of human thought [2]. On the other hand, Shepard cites many instances where people used imagery [3]. One such example was Albert Einstein who ". . . very rarely thought in words at all . . ." [4, p. 184], and that his ". . . .particular ability did not lie in mathematical calculation either, rather in visualizing effects, consequences and possibilities" [5, p. 110]. This example may be anecdotal, but it suggests that psychologists run the risk of missing something very important about human thinking if they believe that visual imagery holds no significant place in cognitive processing.

The controversy concerning mental imagery seems to center on several basic questions: 1) Is there physiological/neurological evidence to indicate that mental imagery exists or that there is hemispheric involvement in the use of images? 2) Do mental images play a functional role in our thinking, or are they merely epiphenomenal experiences as Pylyshin maintains? 3) Are there reliable and valid means for assessing imaging ability? 4) Is imagery utilization related to other measurable phenomena such as hypnotic susceptibility? We shall examine these issues in the course of this chapter.

IMAGERY AND PHYSIOLOGY

Hebb attempted to analyze imagery in physiological terms [6]. He believed that an image can be clearly understood in much the same way as phantom limb pain. After a limb is amputated, there is sometimes an hallucinatory awareness of the part that has been removed. When describing pain or feeling in the missing limb, the patient would in actuality be describing his/her mental processes through introspection. But Hebb maintained that this argument is faulty since we are really dealing with a mechanism of response to the environment, even though the mechanism is now functioning abnormally because part of it is missing. He believed that the ordinary image can be understood in much the same way. The central processes may be excited associatively (cell assemblies are excited by other assemblies instead of spontaneously firing afferent neurons), but in both cases we are dealing with a short-circuiting of the sensory-perceptual-motor pathway. Though there is no sensory input (in the case of imagery, one is not actually looking at an object, but is imaging it; with a missing limb, one does not actually feel the limb but does have some sensation of feeling it), the same central process is exciting the same motor response. It is the same outward-looking mechanism that is operative; it is not introspection.

Hebb also stipulated that it is important to note that one is not describing the image but the apparent object. He believed that the mechanism of imagery is an aberrant form of exteroception, not a form of looking inward to observe the operations of the mind. With this understood, the description of an imagined object has a legitimate place in objective psychology. Further, if Hebb is correct, there may be a physiological basis to mental imagery, a notion espoused earlier by Eccles [7].

A COMPUTATIONAL THEORY OF IMAGERY

In another respect, Kosslyn has provided a comprehensive, computational theory of imagery in adults [8]. He divides the imagery system into different types of information-bearing structures and information-manipulating processes. Within the information-bearing structures, Kosslyn maintains that images have two main components: *surface* representation and *deep* representation. The surface representation is the quasi-pictorial entity in memory that is accompanied by the experience of imaging. The deep representation is the information in long-term visual memory from which the image is derived. The visual buffer, a special visual short-term memory medium, is the structure in which we experience the quasi-pictorial image. The image that is experienced consists of a pattern of activation in the visual buffer. Kosslyn's theory also posits three basic information-manipulating processes which work together: one for generating images, one for evaluating or inspecting images, and another for transforming images. And some support for this approach exists [9].

ASSESSING IMAGING ABILITY

In addition to the contributions of Hebb and Kosslyn, current imagery theory identifies the effect of vividness as the very essence of the imagery experience. Imagery tests involving vividness ratings are aimed at being able to reliably predict a subject's ability to image. The tests that are most commonly used include the Sheehan [10] Questionnaire Upon Visual Imagery (QMI), the Marks [11] Vividness of Visual Imagery Questionnaire (VVIQ), and the Gordon [12] Test of Visual Imagery Control. If a person is rated a vivid imager, for example on the VVIQ, the most commonly employed test to assess imagery vividness, it is assumed that he/she would score approximately the same in a re-test situation. Thus, the reliability as well as the construct validity of a test such as the VVIQ is a crucial issue for imagery researchers who require a measure of imagery differences. Fortunately, a review of research findings indicates support for the reliability and construct validity of the VVIQ [13, 14].

However, such support is not universal. Ahsen found that imagery assessed on a standardized questionnaire is neither as reliable nor as stable as originally presumed and as a result, has introduced what is known as the Unvividness Paradox [15-17]. In his investigations using all three of the aforementioned imagery assessment tests, he found that in some cases a person can be considered a vivid imager, and in others, the person experiences weak or unvivid imagery. The instructions for the tests started with the request for subjects to produce an image of a relative or a friend. Certain items in the tests were then rephrased, replacing instructions to image a relative, a friend, or a car with instructions to image (the subject's) mother or father.

In one particular experiment by Ahsen, fifteen of the twenty-five subjects showed vivid imagery when "father" was inducted into the instructions and unvivid imagery when "mother" was inducted [15]. In twenty-two of the subjects, unvividness ratings with respect to using mother and father were at opposite ends of a continuum of vividness ratings. The test items showed vividness or unvividness ratings according to images involved, and it was obvious that responses to the mother and father images did not result in the same scores. According to Ahsen, consistency in the scores was absent. The vividness scores seemed to jump back and forth. Ahsen offered an important point due to these unexpected results: vividness of imagery changes depending upon which image is used.

In a study based on Ahsen's Unvividness Paradox, Wallace had vivid and poor imagers (based on scores obtained from the VVIQ) participate in a visual search where they were instructed to locate embedded objects within pictorial scenes [18]. Overall, vivid imagers were better at performing the task (locating more objects in a given period of time) because they used imagery in their performance. In this study, poor imagers were then trained to use the efficient search strategies of the vivid imagers (to use mental imagery). The performance of the poor imagers improved to levels comparable to those of the vivid imagers. It was

238 / HYPNOSIS AND IMAGINATION

concluded that imagery appears to play a role in processing information, and that poor imagers can be taught to be better imagers in a cognitive skill.

According to Ahsen, and supported by Wallace, unvividness or weak imagery is not a sign of the absence of imagery, but one of imagery's functional attributes. Their evidence has shown that unvividness is a separate effect of the imagery phenomenon, and its paradoxical role must be recognized. Ahsen considers unvividness to be a dynamic attribute involving the functional behavior of imagery, not a lack of ability [15].

IMAGERY AND ACTIVATION OF
INFORMATION-PROCESSING MECHANISMS

Finke considered the possibility that mental imagery also involves the activation of information-processing mechanisms at many levels of the visual system, some of which may also be independent of one's knowledge and expectations [19]. If these levels could be identified, one could speak of particular levels of equivalence between imagery and perception. Knowing the levels of equivalence between imagery and perception can help clarify the controversies about whether subjects differ in how vividly they can form images. One possibility is that the differences exist only because subjects differ in how confident they are when they rate their images or that they may differ in their interpretation of the instructions of vividness scales. Another possibility is that these differences are real and are due to differences in the extent to which mechanisms at a certain level of the perceptual system are activated when objects are imagined.

Finke's findings support the hypothesis that mental images can stimulate visual processing mechanisms directly. When mental images are formed, the mechanisms would respond in much the same way as they do when objects and events are observed, resulting in the sensation that an image can be seen, as if it were an actual object or event. And this interpretation has been supported by others [20, 21]. Finke's research also supported the hypothesis that these mechanisms show a larger effect for vivid imagers than for nonvivid imagers.

IMAGERY AND HEMISPHERIC LATERALITY

In much of the literature concerning imagery, there is an assumption that imagery is a product of the functioning of the right hemisphere of the brain. That is, imagery may be a lateralized process. This assumption is long-standing. More than 100 years ago, J. Hughlings Jackson noted an association between imagery and the known functions of the right hemisphere [22]. He believed that the posterior lobe of the right hemisphere was the seat of the revival of images. Unfortunately, this clinical observation provided little impetus for further study into right-hemisphere functions.

According to Ley, the earlier neglect of the functions of the right hemisphere was due largely to the interest in the cognitive activities of the left hemisphere [23]. The association between the right hemisphere and the processing of imagery preceded the accumulation of evidence which tested the presumed link. And Ley believes that the presumed link was an overgeneralization, perhaps inferred from studies associating visuospatial tasks to the right hemisphere. McGee also agreed that despite minimal empirical confirmation, an association between imagery and visuospatial abilities was formed [24]. As an example, he conveys the logic underlying the associational process through the following syllogism:

1. The right hemisphere subserves spatial perception
2. Imagery is integral to spatial perceptual abilities
3. Thus, the right hemisphere subserves imagery processes.

Much of the information that has accumulated on the relationship between imagery and right-hemisphere functioning has come from observations on split-brain patients, where the cortical pathway (corpus callosum) that connects the two hemispheres has been surgically severed; and from patients with neurological insults including stroke [25]. Special techniques now available make it possible to confine detailed sensory information to only one hemisphere, permitting investigators to also study hemispheric differences not only in split-brain and brain-damaged patients, but also in neurologically-normal subjects. A consequence of using the lateralization technique is speculation about what the asymmetries mean for everyday behavior.

Although the relationship between imagery and the right hemisphere began as an assumed one, evidence does suggest that the process of imaging is largely a right-hemisphere function. As an example, Humphrey and Zangwill described three cases where individuals had sustained mortar wounds to the right posterior parietal region [26]. All three individuals experienced a subjective loss in visual memory and had marked impairment on tests requiring visualization. One of the subjects reported that he had previously been a good visualizer, but at present, his visual images were ". . . very dim and hard to evoke" [26, p. 322]. It was concluded that visual thinking was significantly disturbed by the damage to the right posterior parietal area.

Further clinical evidence for the right hemisphere's role in imagery is demonstrated by Jones-Gotman and Milner [27]. They examined the performance of patients with right, temporal lobe lesions on a paired-associate learning task. The subjects were instructed to use imagery as a mnemonic aid in learning the word pairs. They found that a right, temporal lobectomy group was impaired when compared to normals in recalling image-lined pairs. They attributed the differences to the imagery component of the task because the right temporal group showed normal recall for abstract words linked by sentences, a condition in which they employed a verbal (left-hemispheric) mnemonic.

PSYCHOPHYSIOLOGICAL ASSESSMENTS
OF IMAGERY PROCESSES

In normal subjects, three experimental techniques, electroencephalography (EEG), galvanic skin response (GSR) recording, and conjugate lateral eye movement (CLEM) monitoring, have been used to study imagery processes. An association between alpha activity and visual imagery was found in studies examining the EEG characteristics of different types of mental imagery [28].

In addition, Morgan, McDonald, and MacDonald examined the possible relationship between alpha activity, hypnotic ability, and performance on various cognitive tasks [29]. While EEG activity was being monitored, subjects were asked to imagine scenes such as a child swinging in a swing or an individual sitting on a beach watching the waves roll in. These were examples of spatial activities. Subjects were also asked to perform analytic activities such as do arithmetic calculations and produce verbal responses. They found EEG alpha suppression over the right hemisphere during the performance of the spatial activities and suppression of alpha over the left hemisphere during the performance of analytic tasks. They concluded that the right hemisphere was involved in imaging, and the left was involved in processing arithmetic calculations and verbal responses.

Myslobodsky and Rattok recorded differences in the GSR of the left and right hands during imagery and the performance of visual and verbal tasks [30]. GSR is generally considered to be a nonspecific measure of arousal or emotional activity. Basically, it records the electrical conductivity of the skin. Because of the crossing of pathways for transmission of information in the sensorimotor system, a heightened GSR of the left hand or left side of the body is presumed to represent an increased activation of the right cerebral hemisphere. Greater left-hand, skin conductivity was found during the performance of tasks requiring visual activity such as holding an image of previously-presented artwork, landscapes, and sexual scenes; greater right-hand, skin conductivity was found when subjects were asked to perform a task requiring verbal activity (e.g., identify words, perform arithmetic calculations). Thus, their results offered support for the presumed link between the production of visual imagery and activation of the right hemisphere.

According to Springer and Deutsch, there have been negative consequences in spite of all of the discoveries made concerning hemispheric differences [30]. They believe that there is a tendency for investigators to interpret every behavioral dichotomy such as deductive versus imaginative thinking in terms of functioning of the left hemisphere and functioning of the right hemisphere. This tendency to classify behaviors as either right- or left-brain has important implications for the study of imagery. As mentioned earlier, the relationship between imagery and the functioning of the right hemisphere began through simple assumptions and broad generalizations. This may have been due to the focus on the abilities and processes of the left hemisphere. When the study of imagery came into vogue in psychology, reports of any left hemisphere involvement in such were virtually nonexistent. In recent years, however, some findings have shown that the left hemisphere also plays a vital role in the process of imagery. Thus, presumed support for the right hemisphere hypothesis is being strongly challenged. If the older literature is correct, imagery is a function of the right hemisphere. However, if the newer research is correct, imagery is a process involving both hemispheres.

As an example, Erlichman and Barrett believe that both hemispheres may be equally capable of constructing images, even though each hemisphere might differ in its ability to utilize or interpret images [32]. They define hemispheric specialization as existing when ". . . differences are found between hemispheres in a given task using a variety of converging methods. Thus, specialization of a function to one hemisphere implies a relative deficit of the other hemisphere" [32, p. 59].

Some evidence for the Erlichman and Barrett position is provided by Greenwood, Wilson, and Gazzaniga [33]. They studied three patients with partial or complete section of the corpus callosum and anterior commissure. They attempted to systematically investigate the hypothesis that there is an electro-physiological basis for right hemisphere dominance in dreaming. If it is assumed that visual dreaming (like visual imagery) is mediated in the right hemisphere, then callosum-sectioned patients exhibiting normal rapid eye movement (REM) episodes, and presumably normal visual dreams, may be unable to make a verbal report of at least the visual components of the dreams. This would be the case since the disconnected left hemisphere would have no access to the experience. Subjects were awakened at the outset of each REM episode and were asked to give a verbal report of dream content. Subjects were also awakened during non-REM sleep for control purposes. All subjects were able to recount some visual content. Thus, results failed to support a selective right hemisphere basis for visual dreaming and indicated a bilateral locus of mediation.

In another study, Seamon and Gazzaniga attempted to determine if varying coding strategies can produce differences which are consistent with the model of separate processing systems [34]. In particular, they were concerned with whether the left hemisphere will be faster than the right in a same-different recognition memory task when the information is verbally coded. They were also concerned with whether the right hemisphere is faster than the left when the same information is visually coded by the use of mental imagery. Subjects were exposed to coding strategies and memory probes which were presented laterally either to the left visual field or the right visual field. Subjects were then instructed to use either rehearsal instructions or relational imagery. When using the rehearsal strategy, subjects were instructed to rehearse two study words subvocally and continually during their presentation and during the blank period preceding the probe. When the picture probe was presented, the subjects were told to indicate if the picture represented one of the words in the two-word study set. When using the relational imagery strategy, subjects were instructed to generate an imaginal representation of each of the study words, and to put the two images together into a single interactive scene so that one image was always touching the other. The subjects were told to hold the imaginary scene by concentrating on it until the probe was presented, and to respond in the affirmative only if the probe represented one of the objects imagined in the scene. The relationship imagery data were consistent with the behavioral and neurological evidence from previous studies which showed a right-hemisphere superiority for visually-coded information. Instructions to produce verbal coding yielded a left-hemisphere superiority consistent with earlier reports for laterality effects and verbal information processing. These results would seem to support the hypothesis that mental imagery is a function of the right hemisphere.

However, Seamon and Gazzaniga offered an alternative explanation. They reasoned that the differences may be explained by the model that each hemisphere could process both informational codes; the differences would be interpreted as a reflection of efficiency differences between the hemispheres for verbal and visual information. This would suggest that verbal comparisons are performed faster in the left hemisphere and visual comparisons are performed faster in the right hemisphere. Therefore, they claim that their findings are at best ambiguous support for the right hemisphere hypothesis.

Lateral eye movements have also been hypothesized as being able to determine which hemisphere is activated during the performance of a task. Kinsbourne hypothesized that when the two hemispheres are equally active, orientation of the subject's eye gaze should be in the median plane [35]. When one hemisphere is primarily involved, head and eyes should turn to the opposite side. He predicted that right-handed individuals would look to the right during verbal activity (e.g., interpreting proverbs or defining words), and to the left when engaged in spatial thought (e.g., imagining a visual scene or mentally carrying out a spatial transformation). He also hypothesized that left-handed subjects would look either way in either case.

In Kinsbourne's experiment, subjects were videotaped while responding to three sets of twenty questions each (verbal, numerical, and spatial), while facing a wall covered by a floor-length black cloth which concealed the recording apparatus. Kinsbourne's hypotheses were supported when he found that, with verbal problems, right-handed subjects usually turned head and eyes to the right, whereas with numerical and spatial problems, subjects typically looked up and to the left. Left-handed subjects differed in all of these respects. These results suggested to Kinsbourne that the direction in which people look while thinking reflects the lateralization of the underlying cerebral activity. Unfortunately, serious doubts have been raised as to whether lateral eye movements can indicate cerebral activation. Several researchers have pointed out that there is little evidence that right- or left-hemisphere questions do in fact activate the hemispheres as they are intended [36-38]. Therefore, Kinsbourne's findings do not appear to unequivocally support a right-hemisphere dominance for mental imagery.

Robbins and McAdam also do not support the right-hemisphere hypothesis [39]. In their investigation, subjects were engaged in covert imagery of familiar material in three imagery modes: shapes and colors (forming a mental picture), words (subvocally describing a scene), or both. EEG waveforms were monitored throughout. The investigators hypothesized that when subjects were using the visuospatial mode that the interhemispheric distribution of alpha activity would reflect suppression over the right hemisphere, and that when the linguistic mode was used, the opposite relationship would be seen. An intermediate value of left-right activity was expected when both imagery modes were engaged. Comparisons of total integrated alpha brain-wave activity from both the left and the right hemispheres across imagery modes revealed no statistical differences in total alpha output as related to task activity.

Also in pursuit of information on hemispheric specificity during the performance of tasks, Corballis and Sergent tested a commissurotimized subject on several imagery tasks in which the stimuli were flashed tachistoscopically in the left or right visual half-field [40]. On tests requiring the generation of images or lowercase letters from their uppercase versions, or the generation of the positions of the hands on a clock face from digitally-presented times, there was a strong right half-field (left hemispheric) advantage in accuracy, but a left half-field (right hemispheric) advantage in reaction time (RT). On tests requiring mental rotation of letters or stick figures to the upright position, however, there was a strong left half-field advantage in accuracy and RT.

Although the aforementioned results suggest a strong right hemispheric advantage for mental rotation, the subjects were able to mentally rotate stimuli projected to the left hemisphere in the later sessions, although accuracy remained lower and RT longer than for the same stimuli projected to the right hemisphere. Once the left hemisphere produced a mental rotation, rates were comparable to those of the right hemisphere. Therefore, it cannot be argued that mental rotation occurs exclusively in the right hemisphere. These findings suggest the possibility that the left hemisphere adopts strategies for processing information that are different from those of the right hemisphere. These strategies may be more appropriate for tasks which require the generation of images than for those tasks requiring presented images to be transformed.

Farah also presented evidence against the right-hemisphere hypothesis for mental imagery [41]. In an investigation involving subjects with reports of loss of mental imagery ability following brain damage, she hypothesized that imagery is a faculty or system of the brain made up of identifiable subsystems, each having a direct neurological instantiation. With this system, the damaged imagery component could be inferred, such as generalization process deficit, long-term visual memory deficit, inspection process deficit, and associated cognitive deficit. The task most commonly used to assess imaging ability is to ask subjects to describe or to answer questions about the visual appearance of objects. Subjects with a deficit in the image generation process showed a consistent trend in lesion site.

Most of the subjects had most or all of their damage in the posterior left quadrant of the brain. This evidence argues against a right-hemisphere hypothesis for mental imagery. It also suggests that some properties of imagery may be mediated in the left hemisphere.

The possibility of image generation being mediated in the left hemisphere is further supported by Farah et al. in a study involving a split-brain subject [42]. The study included an imagery task as well as control tasks that required all of the same cognitive operations as the imagery task except the generation and inspection of the image itself. The task used was a letter detection classification presented laterally to each hemisphere. It was found that both the left and the right hemisphere performed well on the control tasks, but only the left hemisphere performed the imagery task.

In another study, Farah, Peronnet, Weisberg, and Monheit found that the generation of mental images from memory is accompanied by a characteristic pattern of electrophysiological activity [43]. The act of generating an image from memory caused changes in event-related potentials (ERPs) which were maximal on the scalp areas over the left visual cortex. This provides further evidence for the mediation of imagery in the left hemisphere.

Also, in an investigation of normal subjects by Farah, additional evidence was provided for the left hemisphere to generate mental images [44]. In a choice reaction time study, subjects determined whether a lateralized stimulus for 50 msec belonged to a target stimulus set. In the baseline condition, subjects performed the task without the use of imagery. In the imagery condition, before each trial, subjects were instructed to create an image of one of the target stimuli in the area of the visual field where the subsequent stimulus would appear. Farah hypothesized that the image could be used as a template to facilitate stimulus evaluation, especially when the image and the stimulus were the same. This was expected to produce faster reaction times than those in the baseline condition. Hemispheric specialization for the generation of images was inferred from a faster reaction time for an image generated in one visual hemifield than the other. Farah concluded that there existed a greater reduction in reaction time for right hemi-field images, suggesting a left-hemisphere locus for image generation.

Biggins, Turetsky, and Fein [45] discovered several methodological problems in Farah's [44] study. First, although subjects were instructed to focus on a central fixation point during each trial, eye position and eye movements were not monitored. Farah's findings may have resulted from preferential eye gaze or eye movement toward one hemi-field during the imagery condition. A second problem was that all of the subjects performed the task under the baseline condition followed by the imagery condition; order effects were confounded with the baseline-imagery comparison. The final problem described by Biggins et al. was that the Farah study was biased toward finding an effect of imagery because subjects who did not have a shortened reaction time in the imagery condition were excluded from the experiment.

After dealing with the aforementioned issues, Biggins et al. [45] failed to replicate Farah's finding of a preferentially left-hemispheric generation of images. They also failed to find support for a right-hemispheric locus for image generation. They interpreted their findings to be consistent with the hypothesis that both hemispheres are able to generate images.

This hypothesis has received support from Kosslyn [8]. He argued that some of the processes used to arrange parts of images are more effective in the left hemisphere, and some are more effective in the right. He found that the act of generating an image involves at least two classes of processes; ones that activate stored shapes and ones that arrange shapes into images. His discovered that the left hemisphere is better at arranging shapes when categorical information is appropriate, and the right hemisphere is better when coordinate information is necessary. Kosslyn argued that neither hemisphere can be called the seat of mental imagery; it is carried out by processes in different parts of the brain.

Farah has also concluded that different components of imagery processing appear to be differentially lateralized [46]. She maintains that the generation of mental images from memory primarily depend on structures in the left hemisphere and the rotation of mental images depends on structures in the right hemisphere.

One consequence resulting from the interest in hemispheric differences is that there is a tendency to classify human behavior as under the control of either the right hemisphere or the left hemisphere. The most widely cited characteristics can be divided into five groups. The left hemisphere is classified as 1) verbal, 2) sequential, temporal, digital, 3) gestalt, synthetic, 4) intuitive, and 5) Eastern thought [31].

Several years ago, Bradshaw and Nettleton claimed that the traditional verbal/ nonverbal dichotomy was inadequate for describing cerebral lateralization [47]. They maintained that musical functions were not necessarily mediated by the right hemisphere as traditionally believed. They believed that evidence for a specialist left-hemisphere mechanism dedicated to the encoded speech signal is weakening. They also believed that the right hemisphere possesses considerable comprehensional powers, an ability usually assumed to be reserved for only the left hemisphere. Bradshaw and Nettleton believe that there is a continuum of function between the hemispheres rather than a rigid dichotomy. They say that differences are quantitative, not qualitative.

Levy also argues against the "two-brain myth" [48, p. 20]. In her summary of scientific evidence, she outlines five points against the inferences derived from the myth. First, she believes that the hemispheres are so similar that when they are disconnected in a surgical procedure, each functions very well, although imperfectly. Second, the differences seen in the abilities of each hemisphere are seen in the contrasting contributions each side makes to all cognitive activities. Third, logic is not confined to the left hemisphere. Fourth, she believes there is no evidence that creativity and intuition are the exclusive property of the right hemisphere. Last, since the two hemispheres do not function independently, and since each hemisphere contributes its special capacities to all cognitive activities, it is impossible to educate one hemisphere at a time. Levy believes that there are individual differences; people vary in the relative balance of activation in the hemispheres. She maintains that the balance of activation is a continuum, and that these differences are only one of many factors that affect the way people think. Levy says that the myths are merely interpretations and wishes, not scientific observations. Normal people use one "gloriously differentiated brain" [48, p. 20], with each hemisphere contributing specialized abilities.

A further examination of hemispheric activity during the performance of various mental tasks was conducted by Erlichman and Weiner [49]. They conducted a study where subjects performed eighteen different covert mental tasks while EEGs were recorded from right and left tempoparietal leads. Some of the tasks were chosen with the intent of engaging either verbal or visuospatial processes; some of the tasks were unstructured and could have elicited any EEG pattern. The tasks resembled natural thinking with no external stimuli or overt responses. For this reason, the relationship between EEG asymmetry and cognitive task differences would be strong evidence that the EEG measurement reflected lateralized activity.

During the experiment, subjects were instructed to engage in each of the tasks (covert, self-generated types of mental activities) while lying quietly on a cot with eyes closed. Subjects were asked to perform tasks in this position because Gevins et al. have argued that differences in EEG asymmetries between verbal and visuospatial tasks are artifacts of differences in stimulus conditions or motor requirements, and therefore do not indicate lateralized cognitive functioning [50]. Since the procedure used by Erlichman and Weiner involved no overt movement or presentation of external stimuli, the relationship between EEG asymmetry and cognitive task differences would be evidence that EEG measurements do reflect lateralized cognitive activity [49].

In the Erlichman and Weiner study, each subject received the tasks in a different random order. After each task, subjects used a 7-point scale to orally rate the degree of covert verbalization, affect, visual imagery, and concentration that was required. It was found that higher verbal and concentration ratings were associated with relatively greater left hemisphere activation; stronger imagery and affect were associated with greater right hemisphere activation. After further analyses, an interesting pattern was observed for the verbal scale. Comparing the hemispheres, data suggested that verbal thinking may have affected EEG activity in the left hemisphere more than in the right hemisphere, but no such trend was found for the imagery scale. Also, verbalization ratings were significantly related to EEG asymmetry, accounting for 34.3 percent of the total between-task variance. For the left hemisphere, verbal and concentration ratings accounted for 17.6 percent and 15.5 percent, respectively, of the variance in the integrated amplitude and time within a specified bandpass (subjects were run either with a 2-12 Hz or a 8-12 Hz bandwidth). For the right hemisphere, neither of the scales (verbal and concentration) accounted for more than 1 percent of the variance. In contrast, the affect and imagery scales were related to integrated amplitude in both hemispheres.

It was concluded that covert mental tasks which could be classified as primarily involving left or right hemisphere cognitive processes showed clear differences in EEG asymmetry. The investigators maintained that if any generalization can be drawn from their findings, it is that EEG asymmetry is very responsive to the presence or absence of verbal processes, but may be indifferent to the presence or absence of visuospatial processes, at least the process of visual imagery. Erlichman and Weiner suggested that the reason EEG asymmetry is more sensitive to variation in verbal as opposed to visuospatial is that verbal processes may be more lateralized than visuospatial processes. The single hemisphere correlations support this hypothesis; verbal ratings were more strongly correlated with left integrated amplitude in contrast to the imagery ratings which were about equally correlated with integrated amplitudes in both hemispheres. Thus, imaging may be a function of both hemispheres, and which hemisphere is dominant may often be a function of the type of task the subject is asked to perform or mediate with imagery.

Erlichman and Weiner included among their covert tasks five which seemed to involve processes typically associated with the left hemisphere: 1) *multiplication,* where subjects were instructed to take the number 2 and subvocally raise it to the highest power before being asked to stop, 2) *letter/speech,* where subjects were asked to compose a letter or speech subvocally about some topic of interest, 3) *foreign counting* or counting in a foreign language, 4) *verbal counting in English,* where subjects were asked to count subvocally starting from one to whatever number they reached when asked to stop, and 5) *verbal long-term memory,* where subjects were asked if there was any poem, speech, or any other verbal composition that could be recalled from memory, and then to subvocally repeat the composition.

Five tasks which seemed to involve the right hemisphere were also chosen: 1) *music without words,* where subjects were asked if there was any nonvocal or orchestral melody with which they were familiar and that they could mentally produce; subjects were then asked to concentrate on hearing that melody in their minds for two minutes, not humming it, but rather hearing it, 2) *visual kinesthetic imagery,* where subjects were asked to visualize themselves doing some form of bodily action, either dancing or playing a sport, not as a spectator, but rather from the vantage point of a participant, 3) *visual long-term memory,* where subjects were asked to recall from memory pictures, places, faces, visual scenes from a movie, or rooms in their house or apartment, 4) *body feelings,* where subjects were asked to relax and concentrate on bodily feelings; for example, concentrating on internal organs, blood flowing through veins and arteries, then on the limbs, and 5) *visual counting,* where subjects were asked to visually count as high as possible by imagining a blackboard and writing the numbers on the board. After each number, subjects were to visualize the number being erased before the next number was written on the board.

IMAGERY UTILIZATION, IMAGING ABILITY, AND HYPNOSIS

Based on the findings reported by Erlichman and Weiner concerned with hemispheric laterality and imaging abilities, Wallace and Turosky [51] attempted to determine if visual imagery utilization depends on the specificity of the task and the hemisphere in which a given task is theoretically mediated. To determine if this was the case, left-hemisphere tasks as well as right-hemisphere tasks as defined by Erlichman and Weiner were used. Based on the assumption that right-hemisphere imagery is more visually mediated and vivid compared to left-hemisphere imagery [34, 52], they predicted that left-hemisphere imagery tasks should result in lower scores on a questionnaire designed to assess visual imagery utilization (the Sensory Imagery Utilization Questionnaire or SIUQ). Right-hemisphere imagery tasks were expected to produce higher questionnaire scores because of their greater reliance on visual imagery.

In addition to examining task type and hemispheric laterality involvement as a function of imagery ability, Wallace and Turosky also considered hypnotic susceptibility as it related to the aforementioned. This was the case since Wallace reported a relationship between imaging ability and hypnotic susceptibility in a gestalt closure task [53]. Specifically, when subjects were required to identify fragmented stimuli in the Closure Speed Test [54], in the Street [55] Test, or as afterimages, the greatest number of correct closures was reported by those who were both high in hypnotic susceptibility and vivid in imaging ability. Given that subjects who are both vivid imagers and high in hypnotic susceptibility seem to perform best, at least in a gestalt closure task, Wallace and Turosky examined the possibility that hypnotic susceptibility interacts with imaging ability in the performance of various right- and left-hemisphere tasks.

Results from the Wallace and Turosky study showed that right-hemisphere tasks did indeed produce higher SIUQ scores when contrasted to left-hemisphere tasks. In addition, vivid imagers performed in a superior fashion compared to poor imagers. Also, when hypnotic susceptibility was considered, imagery utilization was superior for those judged to be both vivid imagers and high in hypnotic susceptibility. This was true for both right- and left-hemisphere tasks.

In addition, some evidence has been produced to indicate that hypnosis may be associated with hemispheric shifts in EEG activity. MacLeod-Morgan and Lack reported an apparent shift in cortical activation, as measured by alpha EEG activity, from the left to the right hemisphere when individuals were hypnotized [56]. Also, London, Hart, and Leibovitz found that subjects, judged to be highly responsive to hypnotic suggestions, tended to show more alpha-wave activity during the waking state than subjects with low responsiveness to hypnotic suggestions [57]. However, London et al.'s study has not been replicated [58], nor has the one by MacLeod-Morgan and Lack [59]. Interestingly, DePascalis et al. who failed to replicate MacLeod-Morgan and Lack did report that highly hypnotizable subjects exhibited significantly higher alpha brain wave amplitude compared to low hypnotizable subjects.

Bakan has suggested a relationship between hypnosis or hypnotizability and information processing in the right hemisphere [60]. He found that subjects who were highly hypnotizable would, in response to a question, move their eyes to the left more often than to the right; for low hypnotizables, a movement produced to the right was most common. He interpreted this as indicating that high hypnotizability was associated with activity mediated by the right hemisphere. This hypothesis has received some empirical support [61-63].

CONCLUSIONS

It appears that mental imagery, both its control and utilization, is mediated by both cerebral hemispheres. This conclusion is supported by the results reported by Wallace and Turosky as well as by other studies cited in this chapter. Thus, the belief that imagery is predominantly a right-hemisphere process appears to be an oversimplification.

In their review of the literature concerned with right hemispheric specialization for mental imagery, Erlichman and Barrett concluded that the evidence supporting the right-hemisphere hypothesis was insufficient [49]. Most of the studies they examined contained results consistent with the hypothesis that imagery is a bilateral process. In addition, a number of studies have emphasized a left-hemisphere dominance in the ability to generate images [42, 43]. In essence, then, imagery production appears bilateral.

Also, while there has been tentative information provided to indicate that shifts in alpha EEG occur during hypnosis, this shift activity has not been replicated beyond the laboratory of MacLeod-Morgan and Lack. Because of this inability to replicate their findings, studies that would examine the relationship between shifts in EEG during hypnosis with hemispheric mediation of specific imagery tasks [49] have not been forthcoming. While there appears to be sufficient evidence to show that hemispheric specificity exists with regard to performing tasks involving the use of imagery and that hypnotizability may be mediated by the right hemisphere, it is unclear if a relationship exists between these observations. Hopefully, future research will address this possibility.

REFERENCES

1. R. G. Kunzendorf (ed.), *Mental Imagery,* Plenum, New York, 1991.
2. Z. Pylyshin, What the Mind's Eye Tells the Mind's Brain: A Critique of Mental Imagery, *Psychological Bulletin, 80,* pp. 1-24, 1973.

3. R. N. Shepard, The Mental Image, *American Psychologist, 33,* pp. 125-137, 1978.
4. M. Wertheimer, *Productive Thinking,* Harper, New York, 1945.
5. G. Holton, On Trying to Understand Scientific Genius, *American Scholar, 41,* pp. 95-110, 1972.
6. D. O. Hebb, Concerning Imagery, *Psychological Review, 75,* pp. 466-477, 1968.
7. J. C. Eccles, The Physiology of Imagination, *Scientific American, 199,* pp. 135-149, 1958.
8. S. M. Kosslyn, *Image and Mind,* Harvard University Press, Cambridge, Massachusetts, 1980.
9. B. Wallace and B. G. Hofelich, Process Generalization and the Prediction of Performance on Mental Imagery Tasks, *Memory and Cognition, 20,* pp. 695-704, 1992.
10. P. W. Sheehan, A Shortened Form of Betts' Questionnaire upon Mental Imagery, *Journal of Clinical Psychology, 23,* pp. 386-389, 1967.
11. D. F. Marks, Visual Imagery Differences in the Recall of Pictures, *British Journal of Psychology, 64,* pp. 17-24, 1973.
12. R. Gordon, An Investigation into Some of the Factors that Favor the Formation of Stereotyped Images, *British Journal of Psychology, 39,* pp. 156-167, 1949.
13. R. C. Gur and E. R. Hilgard, Visual Imagery and the Discrimination of Differences between Altered Pictures Simultaneously and Successively Presented, *British Journal of Psychology, 66,* pp. 341-345, 1975.
14. D. F. Marks, Construct Validity of the Vividness of Visual Imagery Questionnaire, *Perceptual and Motor Skills, 69,* pp. 459-465, 1989.
15. A. Ahsen, Unvividness Paradox, *Journal of Mental Imagery, 9,* pp. 1-13, 1985.
16. A. Ahsen, Prologue to Unvividness Paradox, *Journal of Mental Imagery, 10,* pp. 1-8, 1986.
17. A. Ahsen, Epilogue to Unvividness Paradox, *Journal of Mental Imagery, 11,* pp. 13-60, 1987.
18. B. Wallace, Imaging Ability, Visual Search Strategies, and the Unvividness Paradox, *Journal of Mental Imagery, 12,* pp. 173-184, 1988.
19. R. A. Finke, Levels of Equivalence in Imagery and Perception, *Psychological Review, 87,* pp. 113-132, 1980.
20. K. Berbaum and C. P. Chung, Mueller-Lyer Illusion Induced by Imagination, *Journal of Mental Imagery, 5,* pp. 125-128, 1981.
21. B. Wallace, Apparent Equivalence between Perception and Imagery in the Production of Various Visual Illusions, *Memory and Cognition, 12,* pp. 156-162, 1984.
22. J. H. Jackson, On the Nature and Duality of the Brain, *Medical Press, 1,* p. 19, 1874.
23. R. G. Ley, Cerebral Laterality and Imagery, in *Imagery: Current Theory, Research, and Applications,* A. A. Sheikh (ed.), John Wiley & Sons, New York, pp. 252-287, 1983.
24. M. G. McGee, Human Spatial Abilities: Psychometric Studies and Environmental, Genetic, Hormonal, and Neurological Influences, *Psychological Bulletin, 86,* pp. 889-918, 1979.
25. F. Newcombe, *Missile Wounds to the Brain,* Oxford University Press, London, 1969.
26. M. D. Humphrey and O. L. Zangwill, Cessation of Dreaming after Brain Injury, *Journal of Neurology, Neurosurgery, and Psychiatry, 14,* pp. 322-325, 1951.
27. M. Jones-Gotman, and B. Milner, Right Temporal Lobe Contribution to Imagery-mediated Verbal Learning, *Neuropsychologia, 16,* pp. 61-71, 1978.
28. P. L. Short, The Objective Study of Mental Imagery, *British Journal of Psychology, 44,* pp. 38-51, 1953.

29. A. H. Morgan, P. J. McDonald, and H. MacDonald, Difference in Bilateral Alpha Activity as a Function of Experimental Task with a Note on Lateral Eye Movements and Hypnotizability, *Neuropsychologia, 9,* pp. 459-469, 1971.
30. M. S. Myslobodsky and J. Rattok, Bilateral Electrodermal Activity in Working Man, *Acta Psychologica, 14,* pp. 273-282, 1977.
31. S. P. Springer and G. Deutsch, *Left Brain, Right Brain* (3rd Edition), Freeman, New York, 1989.
32. H. Erlichman and J. Barrett, Right Hemispheric Specialization for Mental Imagery: A Review of the Evidence, *Brain and Cognition, 2,* pp. 55-76, 1983.
33. P. Greenwood, D. H. Wilson, and M. S. Gazzaniga, Dream Report following Commissurotomy, *Cortex, 13,* pp. 311-316, 1977.
34. J. G. Seamon and M. S. Gazzaniga, Coding Strategies and Cerebral Laterality Effects, *Cognitive Psychology, 5,* pp. 249-256, 1973.
35. M. Kinsbourne, Eye and Head Turning Indicates Cerebral Lateralization, *Science, 176,* pp. 539-541, 1972.
36. J. G. Beaumont, A. W. Young, and I. C. McManus, Hemisphericity: A Critical Review, *Cognitive Neuropsychology, 1,* pp. 191-212, 1984.
37. H. Erlichman and M. S. Weinberger, Lateral Eye Movements and Hemispheric Asymmetry: A Critical Review, *Psychological Bulletin, 85,* pp. 1080-1101, 1978.
38. W. Owens and J. Limber, Lateral Eye Movements as a Measure of Cognitive Ability and Style, *Perceptual and Motor Skills, 56,* pp. 711-719, 1983.
39. K. I. Robbins and D. W. McAdam, Interhemispheric Alpha Asymmetry and Imagery Mode, *Brain and Language, 1,* pp. 189-193, 1974.
40. M. C. Corballis and J. Sergent, Imagery in a Commissurotomized Patient, *Neuropsychologia, 26,* pp. 13-26, 1988.
41. M. J. Farah, The Neurological Basis of Mental Imagery: A Componential Analysis, *Cognition, 18,* pp. 228-235, 1984.
42. M. J. Farah, M. S. Gazzaniga, J. D. Holtzman, and S. M. Kosslyn, A Left Hemisphere Basis for Visual Mental Imagery?, *Neuropsychologia, 23,* pp. 115-118, 1985.
43. M. J. Farah, F. Peronnet, L. L. Weisberg, and M. A. Monheit, Brain Activity Underlying Mental Imagery: Event-related Potentials during Mental Image Generation, *Journal of Cognitive Neurosciences,* in press.
44. M. J. Farah, The Laterality of Mental Image Generation: A Test with Normal Subjects, *Neuropsychologia, 24,* pp. 541-551, 1986.
45. C. A. Biggins, B. Turetsky, and G. Fein, The Cerebral Laterality of Mental Image Generation in Normal Subjects, *Psychophysiology, 27,* pp. 57-67, 1990.
46. M. J. Farah, The Neural Basis of Mental Imagery, *Trends in Neurosciences, 12,* pp. 398-399, 1989.
47. J. L. Bradshaw and N. C. Nettleton, The Nature of Hemispheric Specialization in Man, *Behavioral and Brain Sciences, 4,* pp. 51-91, 1981.
48. J. Levy, Right Brain, Left Brain: Fact and Fiction, *Annual Editions 90/91: Psychology, 20,* pp. 18-21, 1990.
49. H. Erlichman and M. S. Weiner, EEG Asymmetry during Covert Mental Activity, *Psychophysiology, 17,* pp. 228-235, 1980.
50. A. S. Gevins, G. M. Zeitlin, J. C. Doyle, R. E. Shaffer, C. D. Yingling, E. Callaway, and C. L. Yeager, EEG Correlates of Higher Cortical Functions, *Science, 203,* pp. 665-668, 1979.
51. B. Wallace and D. D. Turosky, Hemispheric Laterality, Imaging Ability, and Hypnotic Susceptibility, *Journal of Mental Imagery, 18,* pp. 183-196, 1994.
52. K. Klein and R. Armitage, Rhythms in Human Performance: 1 1/2-hour Oscillations in Cognitive Style, *Science, 204,* pp. 1326-1328, 1979.

53. B. Wallace, Imagery Vividness, Hypnotic Susceptibility, and the Perception of Fragmented Stimuli, *Journal of Personality and Social Psychology, 58,* pp. 354-359, 1990.
54. L. L. Thurstone and T. E. Jeffrey, *Closure Speed Test Administration Manual,* Industrial Relations Center, University of Chicago, Chicago, 1966.
55. R. F. Street, *A Gestalt Completion Test* (Contributions to Education No. 481), Columbia University Teachers College, New York, 1933.
56. C. MacLeod-Morgan and L. Lack, Hemispheric Specificity: A Physiological Concomitant of Hypnotizability, *Psychophysiology, 19,* pp. 687-690, 1982.
57. P. London, J. T. Hart, and M. P. Leibovitz, EEG Alpha Rhythms and Susceptibility to Hypnosis, *Nature, 219,* pp. 71-72, 1968.
58. F. J. Evans, Hypnosis and Sleep: Techniques for Exploring Cognitive Activity during Sleep, in *Hypnosis: Developments in Research and New Perspectives,* E. Fromm and R. E. Shor (eds.), Aldine, New York, 1979.
59. V. DePascalis, A. Silveri, and G. Palumbo, EEG Asymmetry during Covert Mental Activity and Its Relationship with Hypnotizability, *International Journal of Clinical and Experimental Hypnosis, 36,* pp. 38-52, 1988.
60. P. Bakan, Hypnotizability, Laterality of Eye Movements, and Functional Brain Asymmetry, *Perceptual and Motor Skills, 28,* pp. 927-932, 1969.
61. H. J. Crawford, Hypnotic Susceptibility and Gestalt Closure, *Journal of Personality and Social Psychology, 40,* pp. 376-383, 1981.
62. L. R. Frumkin, H. S. Ripley, and G. B. Cox, Changes in Cerebral Hemispheric Lateralization with Hypnosis, *Australian Journal of Hypnosis, 13,* pp. 741-750, 1978.
63. J. Gruzelier, T. Brow, A. Perry, J. Rhonder, and M. Thomas, Hypnotic Susceptibility: A Lateral Predisposition and Altered Cerebral Asymmetry under Hypnosis, *International Journal of Psychophysiology, 2,* pp. 131-139, 1984.

CHAPTER 13

Cerebral Brain Dynamics of Mental Imagery: Evidence and Issues for Hypnosis

HELEN J. CRAWFORD

There is good evidence for the age-old belief that the brain has something to do with . . . mind. Or, to use less dualistic terms, when behavioral phenomena are carved at their joints, there will be some sense in which the analysis will correspond to the way the brain is put together. . . . In any case each time there is a new idea in psychology, it suggests a corresponding insight in neurophysiology, and vice versa. The procedure of looking back and forth between the two fields is not only ancient and honorable—it is always fun and occasionally useful [1, p. 196], as quoted in Pribram [2, p. 1].

INTRODUCTION

Perceptual alterations and suggested hallucinations are the core phenomena of hypnosis [3]. Commonly given hypnotic suggestions ask persons to "image" or "imagine" an arm getting stiff, regressing to an earlier age, seeing something that is not present (e.g., hallucinating a person not present), or not seeing or feeling or smelling something that is actually present (e.g., not experiencing pain, hypnotic analgesia). These imaginal processes, whose roots are found in the Latin word *imitari,* to imitate, refer to the development of a mental representation of anything not actually in the senses. These mental images may or may not occur in conjunction with incoming sensory stimuli (e.g., hypnotic analgesia). Such complex, higher order cognitive processes involve various neurophysiological systems (e.g., [4, 5]) yet little attention has been given to integrating hypnosis findings into more recent neurophysiological studies of perceptually- and mentally-based imaging (e.g., [2, 6-10]).

Within the domain of hypnosis, these imaginal processes are variously hypothesized to draw on abilities such as imagery (e.g., [11-14]), imaginative involvement [15], absorption (e.g., [16, 17]), sustained attention [18], giving up reality testing

253

[19], and topographic regression [20]. A massive literature has examined the relationships between these individual cognitive abilities and hypnotizability, reporting at most moderate correlations in the .40s. Enhancements in imaginal processing during hypnosis for highly hypnotizable persons (subsequently referred to as highs) but not low hypnotizable persons (lows) have also been reported (e.g., [21, 22]; for review, see [11]).

No longer can one hypothesize hypnosis to be a right-hemisphere task, a commonly espoused theory (e.g., [23, 24]) popular since the 1970s, or that highly hypnotizable individuals exhibit greater right hemisphericity [25]. Rather, there is growing evidence (for reviews, see [4, 26-28]) that hypnotic phenomena selectively involve cortical and subcortical processes of either hemisphere, dependent upon the nature of the task, as well as shifts in attention and "disattention" processes. Highs apparently exhibit greater cognitive flexibility [21, 29], physiological hemispheric specificity [29, 30], and sustained attentional and disattentional processing [18] possibly due to differences in the prefronto-limbic attentional system [18, 26, 27, 31]. Thus, hypnosis instructions "can be seen to trigger a process that alters brain functional organization—a process that at the same time is dependent on individual differences in existing functional dynamics of the central nervous system" [4, p. 265]. The lack of "self-consciousness" so that hypnotic hallucinations become "unmonitored" images (e.g., [32, 33]) or disassociated (e.g., [34]) suggests possible greater involvement of prefrontal, dissattentional brain systems. Thus, hypnotic phenomena may differentially involve left and right hemispheres, anteriorly and posteriorly, in different cortical and subcortical subsystems. Such differences may depend upon the type of imagery generated, the strategies employed, the accompanying emotional affect, the degree of effortful or willful attention involved, and the imagery or attentional skills of the individual. This chapter is directed toward reevaluating psychophysiological studies of imaginal processing during waking and hypnosis, as moderated by hypnotic level, in light of recent shifts in theoretical thinking about the neuropsychophysiological substrates of mental imagery.

IMAGINAL PROCESSING AND HYPNOSIS

Correlates of Hypnotic Susceptibility

Relationships between hypnotic susceptibility level and self reports of imaginal processing or performance on perceptual and cognitive tasks involving imagery have been reported, albeit not consistently, by a number of researchers (e.g., for reviews, see [11-14, 35-37]). While imagery is most commonly assessed by Marks' [38] Vividness of Visual Imagery Questionnaire or Sheehan's [39] imagery questionnaire, such self-report questionnaires may be affected by potential demand characteristics, subject expectations and social desirability [40, 41]. Work by Barrett suggests that there are two subgroups of highs: those who are high on absorption and describe their hypnotic experiences as being much like their waking fantasy life; and the others who are lower in absorption and more likely to exhibit dissociative-like experiences in waking and hypnosis [42]. Kunzendorf and Boisvert provided some fascinating auditory brainstem evoked potential data that discriminates between these two groups of highs [43]. Hypnotic responsiveness is typically seen as being multidimensional, involving both multiple enduring abilities and situational influences (e.g., [37]. Thus, multivariate studies potentially provide more understanding about attentional [18] and imaginal [44] ability correlates. As seen below, a preference for and ease with imaginal-associated processing strategies may be more important than vividness per se in the imagery/ hypnotizability relationship.

Gestalt closure tasks require subjects to organize fragmented stimuli into identifiable objects or scenes via gestalt processes of closure. Crawford found highs performed better, possibly because of their greater ability to be imaginal, holistic, and associational in strategies [45]. Wallace (Experiment 1) replicated these findings and additionally found that "the greatest number of correct closures was reported by those who were both high in hypnotic susceptibility and vivid in imaging ability" [46, p. 354].

Hypnotic susceptibility has been found to be associated with superior performance on visual search tasks [47, 48], and searches for an object embedded within a pictorial scene [49, 50]. It is thought that perceptual judgments of visual figural reversals require sustained concentration without distraction. Thus, hypnotizability has been shown to correlate with frequency of reversals of the Necker Cube as well as other visual illusions [18, 51-53]. Highs also report significantly more autokinetic movement in a dark environment [54, 55]. Consistently, these researchers have proposed that such relationships, as well as findings that highs perform better on sustained attentional tasks, are due to highs possessing greater sustained attentional and disattentional abilities [27]. Like research previously discussed, Wallace (Experiment 2) found that highs who also are vivid imagers report significantly longer after-images than either highs who are poor imagers or lows who are either vivid or poor imagers [46]. Thus, Wallace's innovative work provides new evidence of the importance of vivid imagery abilities moderating cognitive performance.

Shifts in Imaginal Processing during Hypnosis

Phenomenologically, imagery is often experienced as being more intense and hallucinatory during hypnosis [32]. Whether this is due to increased activation of imaging systems, shifts in thinking strategies, enhanced focused attention, expectations, or other cognitive factors is open to debate. From a clinical perspective, imagery

> constitutes a very powerful uncovering technique because it is a symbolic representation of the activity of the patient's internal world, of unconscious

feelings, thoughts, and conflict [56, 57]. Imagery reveals these undercurrents more clearly than logical, reality-oriented, rational thinking . . . hypnotic imagery has often been found to represent problem-solving activity . . . [58, pp. 216-217].

In addition, imagery has been used within hypnotic and nonhypnotic contexts to influence bodily (e.g., psychoneuroimmunological) functioning with quite mixed results (for reviews, see [59-63]). The employment of imagery during hypnotically suggested analgesia is quite useful for pain control (for review, see [64]).

The enhancing effects of hypnosis upon self-reports of imagery vividness and/or controllability have been found in some studies but not others (e.g., [21, 65-67]). Bizarreness of imagery may also be increased (e.g., [68]). Encouraging, but mixed results have been reported on the facilitative effect of hypnosis upon creative task performance (for reviews, see [69, 70]).

Enhanced imaginal processing of information, particularly when the information to be remembered is literal or untransformed representations, has been shown to occur more consistently during hypnosis among hypnotically responsive individuals. Crawford and Allen examined performance on a sequential visual discrimination task that required detecting differences between successively presented picture pairs during waking and hypnosis [21]. While lows and highs did not differ significantly from one another in waking, highs showed enhanced performance in number correct during hypnosis but lows did not. Subjects reported two major strategies: 1) detail strategy, which involves the examination and rehearsal of individual details for memory, and 2) holistic strategy, which involves the examination and remembrance imaginally of whole pictures. Highs reported shifting to a more holistic, imagery-oriented strategy during hypnosis, while lows reported a preponderance of detail-oriented strategies in both conditions. In another study, Crawford, Nomura, and Slater found that subjects (both lows and highs) who reported during hypnosis experiencing significant shifts from a more detail-oriented strategy to a more holistic-oriented strategy, with reports of accompanying enhanced imagery, performed significantly better on a spatial memory for abstract forms test [71]. An alternative hypothesis to be considered is that hypnosis instructions facilitated a more focused and sustained attentional condition that led to enhanced performance.

A small percentage of high hypnotizables can produce eidetic-like visual memory imagery (remembering a random set of dots and superimposing this memory image upon a second set of dots in order to perceive a pattern of an object) during hypnosis [22, 72, 73] (for negative results, see [74]). Studies in the laboratories of Crawford and Wallace suggest that "this enhanced processing may be accompanied by reports of shifts in cognitive processing modes from a more verbal, detail-oriented style during waking to a more imaginal, holistic style during hypnosis" [29, p. 156]. In theoretically related research, longer sustaining of after-images during hypnosis by highs but not lows was reported by Atkinson [75].

Inspired by Paivio's dual-coding theory which proposes there are functionally separate but interactive imaginal and verbal processing systems, other research has examined the remembrance of more complex stimuli [76, 77]. The learning of high imagery, concrete words for subsequent recall is substantially easier than the learning of low imagery, abstract words. Traditionally, it is thought that imaginal processes are used for the processing of high imagery words (e.g., [76, 77]), although an alternate interpretation would suggest ease of verbal elaboration might also contribute. In light of this, several studies have examined paired-associate learning of high and low imagery words during hypnosis and waking with mixed results [78-81]. Positive relationships between hypnotizability and imagery-mediated learning was reported by 'T Hoen [81] but were not found by Sweeney, Lynn, and Bellezza [80]. By contrast, Crawford found lows recalled more low and high imagery words than did highs [78]. The facilitative effects of hypnosis on paired-associated learning was reported by Smith and Weene [79], but this study is limited by the lack of an assessment of the hypnotizability level of their subjects. Sweeney et al. reported no facilitative effect of hypnosis [80]. Crawford found highs recalled more words during hypnosis than waking, but the finding was not robust in all experimental orders [78].

Several studies by Friedman et al. found no hypnotizability-performance relationships for a speed of visual information processing, backward-masking task, but did find that subjects in the hypnosis condition performed significantly faster [82, 83]. Of interest to this chapter is that Friedman et al. found imagery suggestions had no influence on performance either in hypnotized or waking conditions [83].

Friedman, Taub, Sturr, and Monty suggested that imaginal differences between lows and highs after that favor highs may be more observable in more basic perceptual processes than in complex cognitive tasks [84]. The literature (for review, see [60]) reports enhanced performance during hypnosis more consistently for information to be remembered that is literal or untransformed representations. As Holroyd concluded, "The associated changes in imagery processing are more complex than simply changes in vividness, which heretofore was the principal attribute of interest" [60, p. 207]. Most certainly the observation of Friedman et al. [84] is an intriguing one that needs further systematic investigation in conjunction with the simultaneous evaluation of attentional and disattentional processes (e.g., [4, 26, 27]). Consideration of the rich literature on the neurophysiological correlates of imagery and hypnosis (discussed in subsequent sections) will also help guide future studies.

IMAGERY AND NEUROPHYSIOLOGICAL PROCESSING: GENERAL OVERVIEW

When the neurophysiology of perception is considered, a set of processes emerges, each served by a separate neural system. These systems are shown

to act in concert with other neural systems anatomically and/or biochemically
related to them [2, p. 2].

... neither hemisphere can be said to be the seat of mental imagery; imagery
is carried out by multiple processes, not all of which are implemented equally
effectively in the same part of the brain [85, p. 1626].

Any mental thought is not an island unto itself. Rather, it is involved in a
complexly orchestrated interplay—a reciprocal connectivity of top-down and
bottom-up processing both within and between brain systems. Imagery involves
an accessing of long-term memories about sensory experiences—visual as well as
auditory and kinesthetic—so that at a phenomenological level it is experienced as
if it were a perception. Whether imagery is a quasi-perceptual experience which
shares some of its generational processes with perception has been the subject of
a long-standing debate. There are two major sides with different models: top-
down activation of perceptual representations models (e.g., [9, 86, 87]) and
models maintaining that the representations imagery uses are distinct from actual
perceptual representations (e.g., [88]). It is my working thesis that the creation of
a mental image requires cognition, "an input independent of direct, current sensory stimulation" [2, p. 165] that reactivates downstream stored memory and
perceptual systems—previously laden associative schemata—that then act in a
similar manner to the percept imaging of external stimuli. If so, one may see
certain similar brain systems activated during mental imagery and actual perception within the same sensory modality, if they have been equated in (among other
additional dimensions) three distinguishable brain systems: the image, the object
and the category [2].

Traditionally, mental imagery processing has often been assumed to be associated with the right hemisphere in the cerebral laterality literature. This was
largely based upon a false formulation of a verbal/non-verbal split between the
two hemispheres. One of the first challenges was a review of the neuropsychological literature by Paivio and te Linde [89]. They concluded that both hemispheres were involved with the right posterior hemisphere being more involved in
image generation and manipulation processes. After a massive review of studies
of lateral eye movement, EEG, and behavioral evaluations of brain damaged,
commissurotomized, and normal subjects, Ehrlichman and Barrett concluded that
there was insufficient empirical data for considering imagery as a right hemisphere function [90]. These challenging reviews subsequently led researchers
to evaluate further how the various brain systems orchestrate together mental
imagery.

There is growing evidence that specific components of imagery tasks can
involve the left hemisphere, the right hemisphere, or bilaterally shared functioning
of both hemispheres (e.g., [6-9, 91-93]). Not only is there differential hemispheric
organization, but also there are important distinctions between the frontal and
more posterior systems, with intimate interconnections, evident in both primates
and humans [94]; (for review, see [2]). Thus, imagery processing can, like any

other mental process, be "decomposed into multicomponent information-processing systems" [85, p. 1621]. In addition, individual differences in mental imagery and other cognitive abilities may modulate how the brain processes mental imagery (e.g., [29, 38, 94, 95]). Hypotheses about the multicomponent imaginal systems, and the degree to which higher thought processes involved in mental imagery activate direct perceptual systems, in reciprocal connections between brain systems, can be tested by an increased availability of physiological neuroimaging methods such as computerized electroencephalographic (EEG) frequency analysis, EEG topographic brain mapping, evoked potential (EP) analysis, regional cerebral blood flow (rCBF), positron emission tomography (PET), and single photon emission computer tomography (SPECT).

In a landmark review, Farah [7] demonstrated how neurophysiological evidence on the relation between imagery and perception may eventually answer the long-debated question among cognitive psychologists: "Does visual imagery engage some of the same representations used in visual perception?" Earlier, Farah [6, 8] had demonstrated that for brain-damaged patients with a loss of imagery the posterior left hemisphere is critical for the imagery generation process, while right posterior damaged patients may demonstrate hemi-inattention to the left visual fields of actual and imagined perceptions [96]. The left hemisphere of split-brain patients is better than the right hemisphere in generating mental images [97, 98], apparently when multipart images are involved [98]. Whereas Farah [99] found the left hemisphere to be better at using imagery to prime perceptual recognition in a visual-field paradigm, a methodologically improved replication [100] found no evidence for a preferential locus of simple mental image generation in either hemisphere. A left hemisphere advantage was found for an imaginal scanning strategy with simple dot patterns [101]. By contrast, during more complex mental imaging of the spatial rotation, utilizing Shepard and Metzler's [102] paradigm, right hemispheric specialization was found in both normal and brain-damaged (left vs. right parietal) subjects [103]. Sergent's scathing review of research advocating the exclusive left hemisphere involvement in image generation makes us pause and reevaluate even further the contribution of the two hemispheres to the generation of mental images [104]. Sergent's conclusion is that both hemispheres house processing structures involved in generating multipart images. Deficit object or part-object imagery appears to be usually a consequence of left posterior damage [6, 8], whereas loss of spatial imagery (topographical memory) is a result of right posterior damage (e.g., [105]).

The contributions of the two hemispheres during imagery have emerged not only in Farah's work but also in Kosslyn's [9, 10, 85] multicomponent model that involves low-level and high-level processing by an image analysis system, and Marks' [106] model that views imagery as resulting from the "triggering of the relevant associative schemata" similar to Hebb's [107, 108] cell assemblies. Recently, Tippett [109] provided a comparative review of the theoretical "houses" of Farah, Kosslyn, Goldenberg, and Corballis. Pribram's seminal works on holonomy and structure in figural processing [2] and the languages of the brain [110] have yet to be integrated into mental imagery research.

Pribram has provided an eloquent theory of brain and perception that should resonate to mental imagery researchers [2]. Unlike many neurophysiological theories of perception that only emphasize bottom-up, forward propagation of stimuli from the sensory organs to higher order "associative" cortex areas, Pribram reviews additional evidence for the likewise important top-down, higher-order influences on sensory cortex and demonstrates there are corticofugal connections even to the spinal reflex level (e.g., [1]) and the retinal processing stages [111, 112]. Dependent upon the imagery mode called upon, activation differences could be evident in the posterior convexity of the cerebrum if the mode is visual or auditory, the frontolimbic forebrain if olfactory/gustatory or pain/temperature, or the midarea around the central (Rolandic) fissure if tactile. Additional "computational spaces" may be activated within reciprocal brain systems when object-form or categorization is involved, or when there are multisensory mental images.

Kosslyn's still evolving theory of visual perception, drawn from a rich neurophysiological literature (e.g., [2]), has been applied more recently to mental imagery [10] with a rather successful attempt to explain individual differences in imaging visuospatial and imaginal information. Kosslyn [9, 85] proposed that low-level processing involves two cortical visual systems: the shape pathway, leading from the occipital lobe down to the inferior temporal lobe, and the location pathway, leading from the occipital lobe up to the parietal lobe [9, 85]. They connect via fibers to the frontal lobe. The subsystems of the high-level visual system are a visual buffer and an attention window that routes to the ventral system for shapes and the dorsal system for locations. The ventral system is involved in preprocessing or extracting "stable features of the stimulus that do not change when viewpoint or visual angle change" [10, p. 46], pattern activation and matching of shapes, and feature detection of properties (e.g., texture, color, location, simple shape features) that do require focal attention. The dorsal, location-encoding system involves spatiotopic mapping, encoding of categorical relations, and encoding of coordinate relations. In the hypnothesis-testing system, subsystems of coordinate lookup, categorical lookup, categorical-coordinate conversion, attentional shifting, and transformation shifts are described. Kosslyn et al. [10] assumed "that the connections between the frontal lobe and the parietal lobe are involved" in the hypothesis-testing system, but have yet to elaborate upon these processes (see below).

Thus, Kosslyn has demonstrated that

> the act of generating a visual mental image involves at least two classes of processes—ones that activate stored shapes and ones that use stored spatial relations to arrange shapes into an image. The discovery that the left hemisphere is better at arranging shapes when categorical information is appropriate, whereas the right hemisphere is better when coordinate information is

necessary, suggests that the processes that arrange parts can be further decomposed into two classes that operate on different sorts of information [85, p. 1626].

The left hemisphere is the "speech output controller," whereas the right hemisphere is the "search controller across the entire visual field" [9]. Similarly, the right hemisphere focuses more on the entire auditory field [113]. Thus, attention is also lateralized: the right hemisphere apparently is more dominant in the maintenance of attention over time and in vigilant, "preattentive focusing" (e.g., [114]), whereas the left hemisphere is superior at focusing on specific aspects of something (for review, see [92]).

Negative and positive affective states often accompany mental imagery and affect psychophysiological organization (for a review, see [115]). Langhinrichsen and Tucker's suggestion of an additional potential factor is worthy of noting:

> Perhaps the right hemisphere and the left hemisphere have qualitatively different modes of experiencing and elaborating imagery. For example, consistent with notions of left hemisphere function, left hemisphere imagery might be detail-oriented, subvocally or verbally mediated, and connect to motor systems. Perhaps this left hemisphere imagery is related to the anxiety-relaxation dimension. In contrast, right hemisphere imagery may appear as a holistic or global display. It may well be past-oriented and unconnected to any perception of threat or anxiety. Right hemisphere imagery may be aligned with the mood dimension ranging from elation to depression. The right hemisphere may use imagery to facilitate access to affectively valanced long term memory [91, pp. 171-172].

Finally, the importance of the prefrontal executive control system [2, 34] or supervisory attentional system [116, 117] that directs and allocates the resources of the rest of the brain is deemphasized or often missing from mental imagery models. Petsche, Lacroix, Lindner, Rappelsberger, and Schmidt-Henrich suggest that sustained and elaborated verbal or imaginal thinking involves strongly the frontal regions as well as other neuroanatomical regions [93]. The three prefrontal subsystems direct the what, when, and how of processing:

> The orbital cortex becomes involved when the question is what to do; the lateral frontal cortex becomes active when the question is how something is to be done and the dorsal portions of the lobe mediate when to do it. With regard to perceptual processing . . . "what" translates into propriety; "how" into practicality and "when" into priority. But . . . envisioning what to do when also involves where" [2, p. 242].

Thus, the type of mental thought processes involved may well activate different divisions of the prefrontal system.

These three major prefrontal subsystems have both cortical and subcortical connections, yet the probable additional involvement of the limbic system (e.g., amygdala, hippocampus, thalamus (see [2]) in imagery processes is not addressed adequately by mental imagery theories. Specifically, neuroanatomical evidence (for reviews, see [2, 118, 119]) shows the orbital system to be reciprocally connected with the amygdala and other parts of the basal ganglia, augmenting and enhancing sensitivities based on episodic processing (and thus involved in deja and jamais vu phenomena). The dorsolateral system connects with the hippocampal system (including the limbic medial fronto-cingulate cortex), augmenting and enhancing both efficiency (hippocampus) and "the ordering of priorities to ensure effective action" [2, p. 242]. The third system, a ventrolaterally located system, has "strong reciprocal connections with the posterior cerebral convexity . . . [and] involves the far frontal cortex in a variety of sensory-motor modalities when sensory input from the consequences of action incompletely specifies the situation. In such situations practical inference becomes necessary" [2, p. 243].

With this as a background, mental imagery and hypnosis researchers need to be more cognizant of cortical and subcortical involvement in the what, when, and how of perceptual, cognitive, and neurophysiological processing underlying their various experimental manipulations and tasks. Such neurophysiological knowledge will assist in the development of hypotheses about the activation of specific brain systems dependent upon the type of imagery task. The imaging of simple and complex perceptual stimuli may call upon different processes. The imaging of concrete words may call upon verbal processing, while spontaneous daydreaming or imaging a walk in the woods may call upon other processes. Imaging animals may call upon the object system, while imaging the locations of things ("imagine your living room") may call upon the location and object systems. When effortful strategies are imposed or stimuli are still novel and unhabituated, frontal lobe activation is likely (e.g., [117]). Individual differences in imagery and other cognitive abilities and the experienced state of consciousness may well be additional moderators.

Preliminary experimental research supporting such differentiations accompanying imaginal processing in nonhypnosis and hypnosis studies are discussed in the next section. Past psychophysiological reviews have explored possible relationships between imagery and electrocortical activity, eye movements, pupillary reactions, electrodermal activity, and visceral activity. The reader is referred to Crawford and Gruzelier's in-depth review of the hypnosis literature and their neuropsychophysiological model of hypnosis [4]. Other, more specialized reviews address evoked potentials [5] and EEG alpha band production [120]. Because of the newness of the field and the exciting implications of such research, as well as imposed page limitations, this review limits itself mainly to "neuroimaging" studies of cerebral blood flow.

NEUROIMAGING STUDIES OF IMAGINAL PROCESSING: NONHYPNOTIC STUDIES

Not very long ago, the feasibility of mapping the distinguishable regions of the human brain in relation to their functional roles seemed remote. With the tremendous advances in neurosciences in the past two decades, however, the opportunity now exists to approach the integrated understanding of brain structure and functioning necessary to clarify the neurobiological basis of human thought and emotion and to discern the mechanisms that underlie sensory perception and locomotor functions [121, p. 25].

Recent neuroimaging techniques (fMRI, PET, SPECT, rCBF) that assess regional brain metabolism offer a sensitive and reliable evaluation of brain function and cerebral organization during cognitive task activity. Changes in regional CBF accompany local changes in neuronal activity in the brain and been shown to be a valid marker of cerebral activation (e.g., for a review, see [122]). There are consistent increases in metabolic activity, with regional specificity often present, during cognitive tasks compared to resting baseline (e.g., [123-125]). The research provides us now with partial localization of language (e.g., [126]), memory (e.g., [127]), and attentional (e.g., [128, 129]) processing.

The prefrontal lobe that subserves the "executive processor" [2, 34] or the "supervisory attentional system" [SAS; 116, 117] becomes activated particularly when cognitive tasks are not routine but rather involved with novelty and attentional effort. Certainly, it does not act alone but in concert with other parts of the brain. As Frith summarized:

> It is not that frontal cortex solves difficult problems, while temporal cortex solves easy ones. The frontal cortex solves difficult problems by interacting with other parts of the brain. Thus Goldman-Rakic proposes that visuo-spatial problems involve parietal-prefrontal connections, while problems that entail use of memory involve limbic-prefrontal connections [131]. Shallice proposes that the SAS (frontal cortex) modulates lower-level systems (other parts of the brain) by activating or inhibiting particular schemata [117]. PET scanning techniques are particularly suitable for studying interactions between prefrontal cortex and other parts of the brain [130, pp. 185-186].

As we turn our attention now to the activation of brain structures and processes after imagery instructions and during imaginal processing during nonhypnotic and hypnotic conditions, it is important to separate spontaneous imagining (e.g., daydreams or visualizations without an external source) from imagining that accompanies external stimuli (e.g., paired associate words), as well as object-form imagery from spatial imagery, as they may activate different associate schemas or memory systems.

Spontaneous Imagining

Roland and Friberg showed that visualizing a walk through one's neighborhood increased cerebral metabolism in the occipital lobe, the posterior superior parietal area and the posterior inferior temporal area; mental arithmetic and recalling sequential verbal aspects of a musical piece did not [132]. When asked to imagine their living room and describe all the furniture in it, subjects showed the greatest prefrontal activation of all the purely mental tasks studied. In a

SPECT study those subjects reporting spontaneous imagery during the rest condition had significantly higher flow indices in both orbitofrontal regions and lower flow indices in the left middle frontal and left inferior parietal regions [133]. Effortful organizing and controlling of cognitive processing is a function of the far frontal cortex, as demonstrated in other CBF studies (e.g., [134, 135]).

Finally, Goldenberg found that when he himself was experiencing spontaneous visual daydreaming there was an activation of the whole occipital lobe, the hippocampus, the left lateral inferior temporal region, and most strongly the left inferior occipital region [136].

Imaginal Processing Accompanying External Stimuli

Paivio's [76, 77] conceptual framework of a dual-coding theory has led him to argue that the two symbolic systems, verbal and nonverbal, are dependent on different brain systems (e.g., [137]). When referential processing activates an interconnectiveness between the two systems, Paivio hypothesized that the left hemisphere "dominates" [137, p. 210], such as during the imaginal processing of words and sentences. Goldenberg et al., in a series of studies reviewed below, have found somewhat consistent evidence that the left occipital brain region plays a prominent role in visual imagery, with interindividual variance having an effect on such cerebral activation patterns.

Goldenberg, Podreka, Steiner, and Willmes found that only in the resting condition and when subjects were asked to memorize concrete words without imagery were there large hemispheric asymmetries in favor of the right hemisphere [138]. Instructions to image concrete words led to leftward shifts of blood flow in the inferior occipital region, as well as in both superior frontal lobes and the left middle frontal lobe. Goldenberg, Podreka, Steiner, Willems, Suess, and Deecke (Experiment 1) found that imagery questions were accompanied by greater left inferior occipital blood flow than were low imagery questions when given to different groups of subjects [139]. In addition, the posterior temporal and posterior parietal visual processing areas were implicated only during imagery questions. Right anterior frontal flow rate was higher during low imagery conditions than during visual imagery, suggesting greater effort was expended (a confound was that more errors occurred with low imagery sentences). More recently, Goldberg et al. replicated the association of verifying high imagery sentences with higher flow rates in the left inferior occipital region and lower flow rates in the right anterior frontal region [140]. The decrease in right anterior frontal flow during imagery was replicated. When asked to use mental imagery strategies to memorize word lists, an increase of left middle frontal CBF was observed in another study [141]. Thus, differential involvement of the frontal lobes may occur with strategy differences. While Goldberg et al. [139] reported an unexplained bilateral increase of thalamic flow rates with imagery, another study [140] did not replicate it.

Spatial and topographical imagery is thought to involve the right hemisphere to a greater extent. In another SPECT study, three kinds of images—colors, faces, and a spatial map—were investigated in a between-subjects design [133]. In comparison to rest, color imaging led to a decrease in the left inferior occipital region. Face imaging led to increases in the left hippocampus and right inferior temporal region, as well as decreases in the left central region. Map imaging led to a decrease of the left superior medial frontal region. Like other neuropsychological research, this study suggests neuroanatomical differences for the activation of color, face, and map image processing. The amount of willful effort required for each may also have contributed to CBf differences.

Goldenberg et al. (Experiment 2) examined changes in CBF during the solution of a visuospatial task [133]. Subjects had to maintain an image of a capital letter for periods of eight to fifteen seconds before indicating the number of corners of the letter by flashing a light for each corner. For the control they had to count the number of letters between two earlier presented letters of the alphabet. Strategies were subsequently assessed. Significant increases in both inferior frontal regions were observed during the alphabet condition. Of most interest was the finding that as vividness of imagery increased in the corners condition, there were accompanying "decreasing flow-rates in regions of the frontal convexity and with increasing flow rates in the inferior temporal regions."

Different patterns of CBF may be associated with different strategies used in processing information. This is evident in activation studies of patients with specific strategy deficits, as well as normals (for reviews, see [125, 142]). In a PET study, Reivich, Alavi, Gur et al. (1985, as cited by [142]) reported that subjects who recalled tones during a tonal memory test by employing an analytical strategy activated the left hemisphere, whereas those employing a nonanalytical, holistic strategy activated the right hemisphere. Gender may also moderate CBF. For instance, Erwin, Mawhinney-Hee, Gur, and Gur reported that women, for unknown reasons (possibly strategy differences?), had greater hemispheric asymmetry of activation for verbal and spatial tasks [143].

Different patterns of CBF are also found in individuals differing in cognitive abilities. Gur and Reivich found increased CBF with the Xenon-133 technique in the left hemisphere with a verbal analogies task in comparison to rest [123]. Of particular interest to us is the finding that greater right hemispheric CBF increases correlated with better performance on a gestalt closure task, although for the whole sample it showed bilateral activation. Crawford found that highly hypnotizable persons perceived correctly more gestalt closure figures than did lows [45]. Thus, the blood flow research supports Crawford's earlier conclusion that highs may possess skills that permit greater right hemisphere involvement or preference for holistic processing.

High and low imagers while performing silent verb conjugation and mental imagery tasks, as well as rest, were studied by Charlot, Tzourio, Zilbovicius, Mazoyer, and Denis [144]. The left visual association and left frontal cortices showed increased CBF during the imagery task in both groups. Low imagers showed CBF increases over the whole cortex in both tasks, while high imagers were more region specific in their activation. Specifically, high imagers showed a right dominance in the visual association cortex in all conditions, and in the parietal association cortex at rest.

NEUROIMAGING STUDIES OF IMAGINAL PROCESSING: HYPNOSIS STUDIES

The importance of individual differences in cognitive abilities and strategies as moderators of cerebral blood flow during tasks has been documented in a few of the above reviewed studies. We may now turn to hypnosis studies which have used rCBF, PET, and SPECT techniques to ask whether 1) hypnosis has an effect upon CBF, and 2) individuals differing in hypnotic level have differing CBF patterns either in waking or hypnosis. Will the hypothesized focused state of hypnosis be accompanied by increased cerebral metabolism? Will lows and highs exhibit different cerebral activation patterns due to possible underlying cognitive strategy, ability, and/or neurophysiological differences in nonhypnotic conditions as well as hypnosis?

Substantial global increases in cerebral blood flow during hypnosis among hypnotically responsive subjects, both normally healthy [31, 145-148] and psychiatric [148-150], have been consistently reported. When included, lows do not demonstrate such global increases during hypnosis [31, 145, 148]. In light of consistent demonstrations of increased CBF during mental effort, these results support a growing belief (e.g., [14, 26, 27, 31, 34]) that hypnosis takes cognitive effort. Thus, there may be increased cortical involvement in the focusing of attention and disattention during hypnosis among hypnotically responsive individuals.

Regional CBF pattern differences between eyes closed waking and hypnotic rest (no specific instructions indicated) have been reported by Walter [148]. She examined SPECTs during counterbalanced waking and hypnosis rest, eyes closed conditions, in low and high hypnotic groups, as screened by the Stanford Hypnotic Susceptibility Scale, Form C [151]. Analyses were limited to men and women separately within the hypnotic groups. During hypnosis, highly hypnotizable women showed significant increases in the left superior frontal region as well as both left and right inferior frontal regions. They also showed significant decreases in the central region and both the left and right thalamus, possibly suggestive of less involvement in the screening of external stimuli. Male highs showed a significant CBF increase in the left basal ganglia and a decrease in the left inferior occipital region. Low women showed a CBF increase in the right inferior temporal region, whereas low men showed a CBF increase in the right superior parietal region and a decrease in the left superior occipital. This well conducted study documents excellently the increased involvement of the frontal cortex during hypnosis (see also [31]). Gender differences have once again cropped up, like in some other CBF studies (e.g., [143]). Whether the men and women were equally hypnotizable was not ascertainable, but remains a possible confound.

Halama used SPECT to study changes before and during hypnosis in seventeen patients (16 neurotic depression, 1 epileptic) [149]. Both before and during hypnosis there was a greater right than left CBF. There was a global blood flow increase during hypnosis. Of the seventeen patients, the eleven more deeply hypnotized patients showed greater CBF increases than those six patients who reported being distracted by noises and showed less hypnotic responsiveness. In hypnosis ten minutes after the induction, he found (in comparison to a rest waking control) "a cortical 'frontalization,' takes place particularly in the right hemisphere and in higher areas (7 cm above the meato-orbital-level) more than in the deeper ones (4 cm above the meato-orbital-level)" [149, p. 19]. These frontal regional increases included the gyrus frontal, medial and inferior, as well as the superior and precentral gyrus regions. By contrast, there was a significant decrease in brain metabolism in the left hemisphere in the gyrus temporalis and inferior region, as well as in areas 39 and 40.

Crawford, Gur, Skolnick, Gur, and Benson found substantial increases in CBF, as measured by the xenon inhalation method, during hypnosis in highs but not lows [31]. CBF increases for highs during hypnotic conditions of rest, and ischemic pain with and without suggested analgesia are evident in Figure 1. In this study healthy male subjects had been screened on three well known hypnotic scales [151-153] to ensure they represented the extremes of hypnotic susceptibility: lows ($N = 6$) who could not eliminate pain perception, and "virtuoso" highs ($N = 5$) who could eliminate all perception of cold pressor and ischemic pain. Lows and highs did not differ significantly on the Mark's [38] Vividness of Visual Imagery Questionnaire, but highs reported more absorption on the Tellegen Absorption Scale [154].

During eyes closed rest conditions in waking and hypnosis their subjects were asked to let their thoughts come and go, thinking of a past trip they had taken. No CBF differences between lows and highs were noted during waking. During hypnosis, only the highs showed significant regional enhancements (left and right hemispheres collapsed due to the lack of regional hemispheric differences), ranging from 13 percent to 28 percent, with the largest being in the temporal region, an area associated with long-term memory processing [unpublished data]. For the resting imagery conditions CBF values in waking and hypnosis, there was a significant State X Hemisphere interaction ($p < .05$), but no further interaction with hypnotic level. This interaction reflected higher left hemispheric values during hypnosis than waking for both low and highs. Attention paid to external stimuli results in a right hemisphere CBF increase [155]. It may have been that

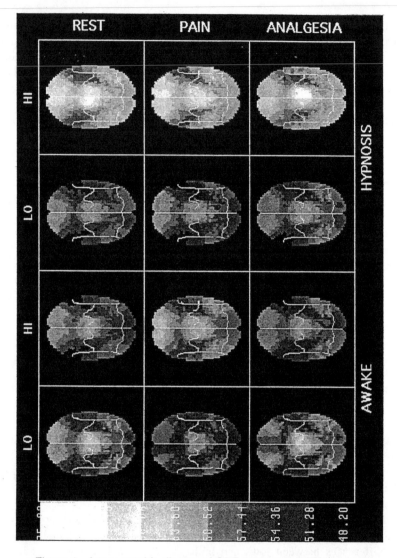

Figure 1. A topographic display of CBF gray-matter (IS) values in
three conditions: Rest (top row), pain (middle row), and Pain with Suggested
Analgesia (bottom row). The waking, nonhypnosis state is the first two
columns: low (column one) and high (column two) hypnotizable healthy
male subjects. The hypnosis state is the last two columns: low (column three)
and highly (column four) hypnotizable subjects. The lighter the shading the
greater the values. From "effects of hypnosis on regional cerebral blood flow
during ischemic pain with and without suggested hypnotic analgesia" (p. 189)
by H. J. Crawford, R. C. Gur, B. Skolnick, R. E. Gur, and D. M. Benson,
International Journal of Psychophysiology, 15, pp. 181-195, 1993.
Copyright 1993 by Elsevier Science Publishers. Reprinted by permission.

more attention was allocated to external activities in the room (sounds, although no talking occurring during the measurements) during waking while more attention was allocated to internal imaginal processing during hypnosis. Of further interest was a significant Hemisphere X Region X State interaction ($p < .0001$). In the temporal region there was a striking left greater than right CBF during waking, but this disappeared during hypnosis.

Crawford, Gur et al. examined CBF while experiencing ischemic pain to both arms under two counterbalanced conditions in waking and hypnosis: attend to pain and suggested analgesia [31] (Figure 1). Both lows and highs reported using similar imagery techniques to control pain, but only the highs were successful in eliminating all perception of pain. As anticipated, ischemic pain produced CBF increases in the somatosensory region. Of major theoretical interest was the finding that only the highs during hypnotic analgesia showed even further CBF increases: first, in the somatosensory region, and second, a bilateral CBF activation of the orbito-frontal cortex (Figure 2). Since PET studies (for a review, see [130]) show increased activity in the frontal cortex during the performance of willed actions, we [31] hypothesized that the mental effort involved in inhibiting painful stimuli was accompanied by increased cerebral blood flow in the frontal cortex. The increased CBF of the somatosensory cortex may be reflective of this inhibitory process since fibers do lead from the frontal lobes to more posterior regions, both cortico-cortical and cortico-subcortico-cortical [2].

Further support that changes in brain dynamics accompany hypnotically suggested analgesia is provided by recent somatosensory evoked potential [SEP; 26, 156, 157] and EEG Hz band [26, 158, 159] research conducted in my laboratory with collaborators. The SEP research demonstrated dramatic decreases in SEP in the prefrontal region during hypnotic analgesia, accompanied by decreases in SEPs in the more posterior regions of a different pattern [156, 157]. We have suggested that hypnotic analgesia involves the executive control system of the prefrontal cortex in a topographically specific inhibitory feedback circuit that cooperates in the regulation of thalamocortical activities, such as that discussed by Birbaumer, Elbert, Canavan, and Rockstroh [160].

Additional support for attentional shifts during hypnotic analgesia is found in Crawford's [26, 27, 158, 159] EEG research. Like Sabourin, Cutcomb, Crawford, and Pribram [161] and others ([62], for reviews, see [4, 163]), highs were found to generate more EEG theta power, hypothesized to be associated with focused attention, than lows. In addition, Crawford reported that highs showed asymmetrical EEG theta shifts during cold pressor pain focusing and disattention conditions, whereas lows did not [26, 158, 159]. Specifically, highs showed a left hemisphere (more anterior than posterior) dominance while focusing upon pain and a right hemisphere dominance while disattending the pain. In concert, these CBF, SEP, and EEG studies support the hypothesis that highly hypnotizable individuals have a more efficient and flexible fronto-limbic attentional-disattentional system [4, 26, 27, 164].

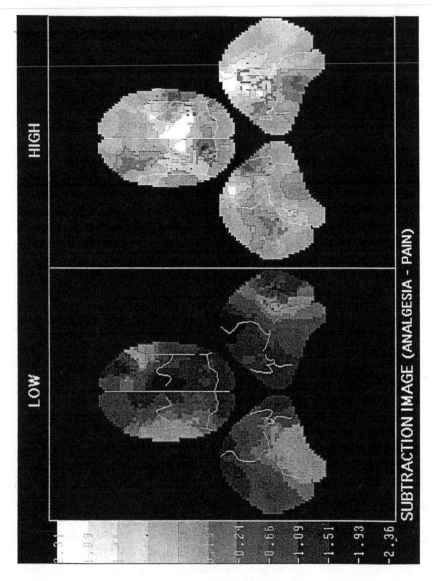

Figure 2. Blood flow activity unique to hypnotic analgesia: A topographic display reflection hypnosis analgesia after subtraction of pain condition during hypnosis. Low hypnotizables are on the left and high hypnotizables are on the right. The lighter the shading the greater the difference is.
From "effects of hypnosis on regional cerebral blood flow during ischemic pain with and without suggested hypnotic analgesia" (p. 190)
by H. J. Crawford, R. C. Gur, B. Skolnick, R. E. Gur, and D. M. Benson,
International Journal of Psychophysiology, 15, pp. 181-195, 1993.
Copyright 1993 by Elsevier Science Publishers. Reprinted by permission.

A SPECT comparison of seventeen psychotic patients who experienced auditory hallucinations was made with ten healthy, hypnotically responsive subjects experiencing music hallucinations by hypnotic suggestion by Walter et al. [148, 165]. In comparison to rest, during hallucinated music the healthy subjects experienced increased CBF in the left superior and mesio-frontal regions, whereas in the right superior occipital and superior temporal regions they demonstrated significant CBF decreases. The comparisons between the patients and healthy subjects is methodologically problematic for this reviewer because of their non-equivalence of phenomenological experiences and other potentially important dimensions.

In summary, this blood flow research is encouraging although it is still in its early infancy. Unlike EEG studies (e.g., [156-159]) which have reported greater theta power during waking among highs than lows, the CBF studies did not report differences in cerebral activation patterns between lows and highs in waking. The results of these CBF studies provide evidence that there are significant shifts in brain dynamics during hypnosis that varies dependent upon the task imposed. A rather consistent finding is an increase in CBF during hypnosis only among highly hypnotically responsive individuals. In view of the consistent findings of increased CBF during mental effort (reviewed previously), this research suggests that although a hypnotized person is often extremely relaxed at the physical level, at a cognitive level there is effort occurring that demands attentional and disattentional allocations. Thus, "dissociated" hypnotic phenomena may only be effortless and lack self-consciousness at a phenomenological level, yet they may still require directed, willful attention out of self-conscious awareness [27].

The differential involvement of the frontal and posterior regions of the brain during hypnosis was evident in several studies. Rather consistently there is increased involvement of regions within the frontal cortex during hypnotic suggestions [31, 147, 163]. This suggests the greater activation of the executive control system during imaginal activities, be they hypnotic or nonhypnotic. Alternate shifts in the posterior regions of the brain point out the importance of not only considering left and right hemisphere dynamics, but also anterior/posterior dynamics (e.g., [4]). Unexplained decreased activations found in the temporal regions during acoustic focused attention [146], music hallucinations [163], and sometimes hypnotic rest [148], need replication in order to verify their presence.

SUMMARY

It is now fairly well established that both hemispheres have the capacity for imagery, but they differ in the way they approach the material. The left hemisphere is more involved in object perception and the ordering of cognitive operations sequentially, whereas the right hemisphere is more involved in spatial perception and parallel, global processing. This chapter reviewed several theories of visual perception [2, 10] and their applicability to the understanding of mental imagery. Evidence for the neural basis of the generation and maintenance of mental imagery, with an emphasis upon cerebral blood flow studies, was evaluated. There is no single substrate of imagery, even within sensory modalities. Rather, dependent upon what kind of information is being depicted by the mental image (e.g., verbal vs. spatial) and the cognitive strategies employed, different brain systems are activated in a reciprocal interplay between cortical and sub-cortical systems. The occipital and temporal-parietal cortices were differentially activated during visual imagery, suggesting the reactivation of long-term memories and percept-like processes. The involvement of the far frontal cortex in the executive or attentional control of thought processes involving mental imagery was evident.

A review of the literature suggested that hypothesized enhanced imaginal processing during hypnosis occurs more consistently with information to be remembered or imaged that is more literal or untransformed representations: eidetic-like imagery [22, 72, 73]; sustaining of after-images [75]; remembrance of complex pictures for subsequent comparison to new ones that differ slightly [21]; and memory for spatial abstract forms [71]. By contrast, reports of enhanced memory performance during hypnosis may or may not be reported for more complex, verbally-mediated processing such as paired associate words [78-81].

Given the review of cerebral blood flow activation patterns accompanying mental processing, and differences in individuals differing in hypothesized mental imagery skills, one might expect CBF differences between lows and highs during waking. Not one reviewed hypnosis CBF study reported waking differences, although EEG differences for lows and highs have been reported (for review, see [41]). In addition, one might anticipate increases in CBF during hypnosis when there is more focused attention on suggestions and tasks. A robust finding is that highs do show increases in CBF during hypnosis [31, 146-150, 165]. Such increases may reflect greater focused attention and disattention involving the fronto-limbic attentional system during hypnosis among the highs [31]. The enhanced CBF involvement of the fronto-orbital region during hypnotic analgesia attests to the possible greater involvement of the executive processor "deciding" to dis-attend pain and attend to internally produced mental imagery instead. Open to subsequent research is the hypothesis that such inhibitory processes may also activate other cortical and subcortical regions, as in our CBF study of hypnotic analgesia [31], due to feedback inhibitory fibers from the frontal lobes to these regions [2].

As reviewed here and elsewhere [4, 26-28], there is growing evidence that hypnotic phenomena selectively involve cortical and subcortical processes of either hemisphere, dependent upon the nature of the task, as well as shifts in attention and dis-attention processes. To help refine hypotheses and theoretical thinking, hypnosis researchers interested in cognitive and/or neuropsychophysiological functioning can find guidance from general neurophysiological theories of visual functioning [2, 10] and hypnosis [4].

Future research using new neuroimaging techniques such as fMRI, rCBF, PET, and SPECT holds exciting opportunities to map the brain areas that constitute different types of cognitive and perceptual processing in individuals with varying cognitive abilities both in hypnotic and nonhypnotic conditions. rCBF with 133-xenon restricts one's view to cortical dynamics, whereas the use of three-dimensional physiological neuro-imaging techniques such as PET and SPECT provides much more detailed maps of cortical-subcortical brain dynamics. The much safer and less expensive SPECT should become more accessible to researchers desiring to pursue this exciting and challenging field of research.

As the "Decade of the Brain" progresses through the 1990s and we enter the twenty-first century, we shall learn more at a neurophysiological level how hypnosis, and other alternate states of awareness, lead to sometimes rather dramatic perceptual alterations and even hallucinations experienced at the phenomenological level. Perhaps we will discover, like Miller et al. [1], that there is much truth in the age-old belief that "the brain has something to do with . . . mind."

REFERENCES

1. G. A. Miller, E. H. Galanter, and K. H. Pribram, *Plans and the Structure of Behavior,* Holt, Rinehart & Winston, New York, 1960.
2. K. H. Pribram, *Brain and Perception: Holonomy and Structure in Figural Processing,* Erlbaum, Hillsdale, New Jersey, 1991.
3. E. R. Hilgard, *Hypnotic Susceptibility,* Harcourt, Brace, and World, New York, 1965.
4. H. J. Crawford and J. H. Gruzelier, A Midstream View of the Neuropsychophysiology of Hypnosis: Recent Research and Future Directions, in *Contemporary Hypnosis Research,* E. Fromm and M. R. Nash (eds.), Guilford Press, New York, pp. 227-266, 1992.
5. D. Spiegel and A. F. Barabasz, Psychophysiology of Hypnotic Hallucinations, in *The Psychophysiology of Mental Imagery: Theory, Research and Application,* R. G. Kunzendorf and A. A. Sheikh (eds.), Baywood Publishing Company, Amityville, New York, pp. 133-145, 1990.
6. M. J. Farah, The Neurological Basis of Mental Imagery: A Componential Analysis, *Cognition, 18,* pp. 245-269, 1984.
7. M. J. Farah, Is Visual Imagery Really Visual? Overlooked Evidence from Neuropsychology, *Psychological Review, 95,* pp. 307-317, 1988.
8. M. J. Farah, The Neuropsychology of Mental Imagery: Converging Evidence from Brain-damaged and Normal Subjects, in *Spatial Cognition: Brain Bases and Development,* J. Stiles-Davis, M. Kritchevsky, and U. Bellugi (eds.), Erlbaum, Hillsdale, New Jersey, pp. 33-56, 1988.
9. S. M. Kosslyn, Seeing and Imagery in the Cerebral Hemispheres: A Computational Approach, *Psychological Review, 94,* pp. 148-175, 1987.
10. S. M. Kosslyn, M. H. Van Kleeck, and K. N. Kirby, A Neurologically Plausible Model of Individual Differences in Visual Mental Imagery, in *Imagery: Current Developments,* P. J. Hampson, D. F. Marks, and J. T. E. Richardson (eds.), Routledge, London, pp. 39-77, 1990.
11. H. J. Crawford, Imagery Processing during Hypnosis: Relationships to Hypnotizability and Cognitive Strategies, in *Imagery: Recent Practice and Theory,* M. Wolpin, J. E. Shor, and L. Krueger (eds.), Plenum Press, New York, pp. 13-32, 1986.

12. H. J. Crawford and C. MacLeod-Morgan, Hypnotic Investigations of Imagery: A Critical Review of Relationships, in *International Review of Mental Imagery,* Vol. 2, A. A. Sheikh (ed.), Human Sciences Press, Inc., New York, pp. 32-56, 1986.
13. P. W. Sheehan, Hypnosis and the Processes of Imagination, in *Hypnosis: Developments in Research and New Perspectives,* E. Fromm and R. Shor (eds.), Aldine, New York, pp. 381-411, 1979.
14. P. W. Sheehan, Imagery and Hypnosis: Forging a Link, at Least in Part, *Research Communications in Psychology, Psychiatry, and Behavior, 7,* pp. 257-272, 1982.
15. J. R. Hilgard, *Personality and Hypnosis: A Study of Imaginative Involvement* (2nd Edition), University of Chicago Press, Chicago, 1979.
16. S. M. Roche and K. M. McConkey, Absorption: Nature, Assessment, and Correlates, *Journal of Personality and Social Psychology, 59,* pp. 91-101, 1990.
17. A. Tellegen and C. Atkinson, Openness to Absorbing and Self-altering Experiences ("Absorption"), a Trait Related to Hypnotic Susceptibility, *Journal of Abnormal Psychology, 83,* pp. 268-277, 1974.
18. H. J. Crawford, A. M. Brown, and C. E. Moon, Sustained Attentional and Disattentional Abilities: Differences between Low and Highly Hypnotizable Persons, *Journal of Abnormal Psychology, 102,* pp. 534-543, 1993.
19. R. E. Shor, Hypnosis and the Concept of the Generalized Reality Orientation, *American Journal of Psychotherapy, 13,* pp. 582-602, 1959.
20. M. R. Nash, Hypnosis as a Special Case of Psychological Regression, in *Theories of Hypnosis: Current Models and Perspectives,* S. J. Lynn and J. W. Rhue (eds.), Guilford Press, New York, pp. 171-194, 1991.
21. H. J. Crawford and S. N. Allen, Enhanced Visual Memory during Hypnosis as Mediated by Hypnotic Responsiveness and Cognitive Strategies, *Journal of Experimental Psychology: General, 112,* pp. 662-685, 1983.
22. H. J. Crawford, B. Wallace, K. Nomura, and H. Slater, Eidetic-like Imagery in Hypnosis: Rare But There, *American Journal of Psychology, 99,* pp. 527-546, 1986.
23. K. R. Graham, Perceptual Processes and Hypnosis: Support for a Cognitive-state Theory Based on Laterality, in *Conceptual and Investigative Approaches to Hypnosis and Hypnotic Phenomena,* W. E. Edmonston, Jr. (ed.), *Annals of the New York Academy of Sciences, 296,* pp. 274-283, 1977.
24. C. MacLeod-Morgan, EEG Lateralization in Hypnosis: A Preliminary Report, *Australian Journal of Clinical and Experimental Hypnosis, 10,* pp. 99-102, 1982.
25. R. C. Gur and R. E. Gur, Handedness, Sex and Eyedness as Moderating Variables in the Relation between Hypnotic Susceptibility and Functional Brain Asymmetry, *Journal of Abnormal Psychology, 83,* pp. 635-643, 1974.
26. H. J. Crawford, Brain Systems Involved in Attention and Disattention (Hypnotic Analgesia) to Pain, in *Origins: Brain and Self Organization,* K. Pribram (ed.), Erlbaum, New Jersey, pp. 661-679, 1994.
27. H. J. Crawford, Brain Dynamics and Hypnosis: Attentional and Disattentional Processes, *International Journal of Clinical and Experimental Hypnosis, 52,* pp. 204-232, 1994.
28. J. H. Gruzelier, The Neuropsychology of Hypnosis, in *Hypnosis: Current Clinical, Experimental and Forensic Practices,* M. Heap (ed.), Croom Helm, London, pp. 68-76, 1988.
29. H. J. Crawford, Cognitive and Physiological Flexibility: Multiple Pathways to Hypnotic Responsiveness, in *Suggestion and Suggestibility: Theory and Research,* V. Ghorghui, P. Netter, H. Eysenck, and R. Rosenthal (eds.), Plenum Press, New York, pp. 155-168, 1989.

30. C. MacLeod-Morgan and L. Lack, Hemispheric Specificity: A Physiological Concomitant of Hypnotizability, *Psychophysiology, 19,* pp. 687-690, 1982.
31. H. J. Crawford, R. C. Gur, B. Skolnick, R. E. Gur, and D. M. Benson, Effects of Hypnosis on Regional Cerebral Blood Flow during Ischemic Pain With and Without Suggested Hypnotic Analgesia, *International Journal of Psychophysiology, 15,* pp. 181-195, 1993.
32. R. G. Kunzendorf, Hypnotic Hallucinations as "Unmonitored" Images: An Empirical Study, *Imagination, Cognition and Personality, 5,* pp. 255-270, 1985-86.
33. R. G. Kunzendorf, Self-consciousness as the Monitoring of Cognitive States: A Theoretical Perspective, *Imagination, Cognition and Personality, 7,* pp. 3-22, 1987-88.
34. E. R. Hilgard, *Divided Consciousness: Multiple Controls in Human Thought and Action,* Wiley, New York, 1986.
35. H. J. Crawford, Hypnotizability, Daydreaming Styles, Imagery Vividness, and Absorption: A Multidimensional Study, *Journal of Personality and Social Psychology, 42,* pp. 915-926, 1982.
36. N. E. Heyneman, The Role of Imagery in Hypnosis: An Information Processing Approach, *International Journal of Clinical and Experimental Hypnosis, 38,* pp. 39-59, 1990.
37. I. Kirsch and J. R. Council, Situational and Personality Correlates of Hypnotic Responsiveness, in *Contemporary Hypnosis Research,* E. Fromm and M. R. Nash (eds.), Guilford Press, New York, pp. 267-291, 1992.
38. D. F. Marks, Visual Imagery Differences in the Recall of Pictures, *British Journal of Psychology, 64,* pp. 17-24, 1973.
39. P. W. Sheehan, A Shortened Form of Betts's Questionnaire upon Mental Imagery, *Journal of Clinical and Experimental Hypnosis, 23,* pp. 386-389, 1967.
40. F. J. DiVesta, G. Ingersoll, and P. Sunshine, A Factor Analysis of Imagery Tests, *Journal of Verbal Learning and Verbal Behavior, 10,* pp. 461-470, 1971.
41. A. H. Perlini, A. Lee, and N. P. Spanos, The Relationship between Imaginability and Hypnotic Susceptibility: Does Context Matter?, *Contemporary Hypnosis, 9,* pp. 35-41, 1992.
42. D. Barrett, Fantasizers and Dissociaters: Data on Two Distinct Subgroups of Deep Trance Subjects, *Psychological reports, 71,* pp. 1011-1014, 1992.
43. R. G. Kunzendorf and P. Boisvert, Presence vs. Absence of a 'Hidden Observer' during Total Deafness: The Hypnotic Illusion of Subconsciousness vs. the Imaginal Attenuation of Brainstem Evoked Potentials, in *Hypnosis and Imagination,* R. G. Kunzendorf, N. Spanos, and B. Wallace (eds.), Baywood Publishing Company, Amityville, New York, pp. 223-234, 1996.
44. R. Nadon, J.-R. Laurence, and C. Perry, Multiple Predictors of Hypnotic Susceptibility, *Journal of Personality and Social Psychology, 53,* pp. 948-960, 1987.
45. H. J. Crawford, Hypnotic Susceptibility as Related to Gestalt Closure Tasks, *Journal of Personality and Social Psychology, 40,* pp. 376-383, 1981.
46. B. Wallace, Imagery Vividness, Hypnotic Susceptibility, and the Perception of Fragmented Stimuli, *Journal of Personality and Social Psychology, 58,* pp. 354-359, 1990.
47. B. Wallace, Imaging Ability and Performance in a Proofreading Task, *Journal of Mental Imagery, 15,* pp. 177-188, 1991.
48. B. Wallace and S. L. Patterson, Hypnotic Susceptibility and Performance on Various Attention-specific Cognitive Tasks, *Journal of Personality and Social Psychology, 47,* pp. 175-181, 1984.

276 / HYPNOSIS AND IMAGINATION

49. F. A. Priebe and B. Wallace, Hypnotic Susceptibility, Imaging Ability and the Detection of Embedded Objects, *International Journal of Clinical and Experimental Hypnosis, 34,* pp. 320-329, 1986.
50. B. Wallace, Imaging Ability, Visual Search Strategies, and the Unvividness Paradox, *Journal of Mental Imagery, 12,* pp. 173-184, 1988.
51. R. J. Miller, Response to the Ponzo Illusion as Reflection of Hypnotic Susceptibility, *International Journal of Clinical and Experimental Hypnosis, 23,* pp. 148-157, 1975.
52. B. Wallace, Latency and Frequency Reports to the Necker Cube Illusion: Effects of Hypnotic Susceptibility and Mental Arithmetic, *Journal of General Psychology, 113,* pp. 187-194, 1986.
53. B. Wallace, T. A. Knight, and J. F. Garrett, Hypnotic Susceptibility and Frequency Reports to Illusory Stimuli, *Journal of Abnormal Psychology, 85,* pp. 558-563, 1976.
54. R. P. Atkinson and H. J. Crawford, Individual Differences in Afterimage Persistence: Relationships to Hypnotic Responsiveness and Visuospatial Skills, *American Journal of Psychology, 105,* pp. 527-539, 1992.
55. B. Wallace, J. B. Garrett, and S. P. Anstadt, Hypnotic Susceptibility, Suggestion, and Reports of Autokinetic Movement, *American Journal of Psychology, 87,* pp. 117-123, 1974.
56. J. Reyher, Free Imagery: An Uncovering Procedure, *Journal of Clinical Psychology, 19,* pp. 454-459, 1963.
57. J. E. Shor, *Psycho-Imagination Therapy,* Intercontinental Medical Book, New York, 1972.
58. E. Fromm, Significant Developments in Clinical Hypnosis during the Past 25 Years, *International Journal of Clinical and Experimental Hypnosis, 35,* pp. 215-230, 1987.
59. H. Hall, Imagery, Psychoneuroimmunology, and the Psychology of Healing, in *The Psychophysiology of Mental Imagery: Theory, Research and Application,* R. G. Kunzendorf and A. A. Sheikh (eds.), Baywood Publishing Company, Amityville, New York, pp. 203-227, 1990.
60. J. Holroyd, Hypnosis as a Methodology in Psychological Research, in *Contemporary Hypnosis Research,* E. Fromm and M. R. Nash (eds.), Guilford Press, New York, 1992.
61. R. G. Kunzendorf and A. A. Sheikh, Imagining, Imagery-monitoring, and Health, in *The Psychophysiology of Mental Imagery: Theory, Research and Application,* R. G. Kunzendorf and A. A. Sheikh (eds.), Baywood Publishing Company, Amityville, New York, pp. 185-202, 1990.
62. K. R. Pelletier and D. L. Herzing, Psychoneuroimmunology: Toward a Mindbody Model, *Advances, Institute for the Advancement of Health, 5,* pp. 27-56, 1988.
63. A. A. Sheikh and R. G. Kunzendorf, Imagery, Physiology, and Psychosomatic Illness, *International Review of Mental Imagery, 1,* pp. 95-138, 1984.
64. E. R. Hilgard and J. R. Hilgard, *Hypnosis in the Relief of Pain* (Rev. Edition), William Kaufmann, Los Altos, California, 1994.
65. T. X. Barber and S. C. Wilson, Hypnosis, Suggestions, and Altered States of Consciousness: Experimental Evaluation of the New Cognitive-behavioral Theory and the Traditional Trance-state Theory of "Hypnosis," in *Conceptual and Investigative Approaches to Hypnosis and Hypnotic Phenomena. Annals of the New York Academy of Sciences,* W. E. Edmonston, Jr. (ed.), *296,* pp. 34-47, 1977.
66. H. J. Crawford, Cognitive Processing during Hypnosis: Much Unfinished Business, *Research Communications in Psychology, Psychiatry, and Behavior, 7,* pp. 169-179, 1982.

67. K. M. Nilsson, The Effect of Subject Expectations of "Hypnosis" upon Vividness of Visual Imagery, *International Journal of Clinical and Experimental Hypnosis, 38,* pp. 17-24, 1990.
68. L. J. Shofield and K. Platoni, Manipulation of Visual Imagery under Various Hypnotic Conditions, *American Journal of Clinical Hypnosis, 18,* pp. 191-199, 1976.
69. P. G. Bowers and K. S. Bowers, Hypnosis and Creativity: A Theoretical and Empirical Rapprochement, in *Hypnosis: Developments in Research and New Perspectives* (2nd Edition), E. Fromm and R. E. Shor (eds.), Aldine, New York, pp. 351-379, 1979.
70. V. A. Shames and P. G. Bowers, Hypnosis and Creativity, in *Contemporary Hypnosis Research,* E. Fromm and M. R. Nash (eds.), Guilford Press, New York, pp. 334-363, 1992.
71. H. J. Crawford, K. Nomura, and H. Slater, Spatial Memory Processing: Enhancement during Hypnosis, in *Imagery: Theoretical Aspects and Applications,* J. C. Shorr, J. Conella, G. Sobel, and T. Robin (eds.), Plenum Press, New York, pp. 209-216, 1983.
72. N. S. Walker, J. B. Garrett, and B. Wallace, Restoration of Eidetic Imagery via Hypnotic Age Regression: A Preliminary Report, *Journal of Abnormal Psychology, 85,* pp. 335-337, 1976.
73. B. Wallace, Restoration of Eidetic Imagery via Hypnotic Age Regression: More Evidence, *Journal of Abnormal Psychology, 87,* pp. 673-675, 1978.
74. N. P. Spanos, F. Ansari, and H. J. Stam, Hypnotic Age Regression and Eidetic Imagery: A Failure to Replicate, *Journal of Abnormal Psychology, 88,* pp. 88-91, 1979.
75. R. H. Atkinson, Enhanced Afterimage Persistence in Waking and Hypnosis: High Hypnotizables Report More Enduring Afterimages, *Imagination, Cognition and Personality, 14,* pp. 31-41, 1994.
76. A. Paivio, *Imagery and Verbal Processes,* Holt, Rinehart & Winston, 1971.
77. A. Paivio, *Mental Representations: A Dual Coding Approach,* Oxford University Press, New York, 1986.
78. H. J. Crawford, Paired Associate Learning and Recall of High and Low Imagery Words: Moderating Effects of Hypnosis, Hypnotic Susceptibility Level, and Visualization Abilities, *American Journal of Psychology,* in press.
79. R. T. Smith and K. A. Weene, The Effects of Hypnosis on Recall of High and Low Imagery Paired-Associated Words, *Journal of Mental Imagery, 15,* pp. 171-176, 1991.
80. C. A. Sweeney, S. J. Lynn, and F. S. Bellezza, Hypnosis, Hypnotizability, and Imagery-mediated Learning, *International Journal of Clinical and Experimental Hypnosis, 34,* pp. 29-40, 1986.
81. P. 'T Hoen, Effects of Hypnotizability and Visualizing Ability on Imagery-mediated Learning, *International Journal of Clinical and Experimental Hypnosis, 26,* pp. 45-54, 1978.
82. H. Friedman and H. A. Taub, Hypnotizability and Speed of Visual Information Processing, *International Journal of Clinical and Experimental Hypnosis, 36,* pp. 234-241, 1986.
83. H. Friedman, H. A. Taub, J. F. Sturr, and R. A. Monty, Hypnosis and Hypnotizability in Cognitive Task Performance, *British Journal of Experimental and Clinical Hypnosis, 7,* pp. 103-107, 1987.
84. H. Friedman, H. A. Taub, J. F. Sturr, and R. A. Monty, Hypnosis and Hypnotizability in Cognitive Task Performance, *British Journal of Experimental and Clinical Hypnosis, 7,* pp. 103-107, 1990.

85. S. M. Kosslyn, Aspects of a Cognitive Neuroscience of Mental Imagery, *Science, 240,* pp. 1621-1626, 1988.

86. R. A. Finke, Levels of Equivalence in Imagery and Perception, *Psychological Review, 87,* pp. 113-132, 1980.

87. R. N. Shepard, Form, Formation, and Transformation of Internal Representations, in *Information Processing and Cognition,* R. Solso (ed.), Erlbaum, Hillsdale, New Jersey, 1975.

88. Z. W. Pylyshyn, What the Mind's Eye Tells the Mind's Brain: A Critique of Mental Imagery, *Psychological Bulletin, 80,* pp. 1-24, 1973.

89. A. Paivio and J. te Linde, Imagery, Memory, and the Brain, *Canadian Journal of Psychology, 36,* pp. 243-272, 1982.

90. H. Ehrlichman and J. Barrett, Right Hemisphere Specialization for Mental Imagery: A Review of the Evidence, *Brain and Cognition, 2,* pp. 55-76, 1983.

91. J. Langhinrichsen and D. M. Tucker, Neuropsychological Concepts of Mood, Imagery, and Performance, in *The Psychophysiology of Mental Imagery,* R. G. Kunzendorf and A. A. Sheikh (eds.), Baywood Publishing Company, Amityville, New York, pp. 167-184, 1990.

92. D. M. Tucker and P. A. Williamson, Asymmetric Neural Control Systems in Human Self-regulation, *Psychological Review, 91,* pp. 185-215, 1984.

93. H. Petsche, D. Lacroix, K. Lindner, P. Rappelsberger, and E. Schmidt-Henrich, Thinking with Images of Thinking with Language: A Pilot EEG Probability Mapping Study, *International Journal of Psychophysiology, 12,* pp. 31-39, 1992.

94. K. L. Chow and K. H. Pribram, Cortical Projects of the Thalamic Ventrolateral Nuclear Group in Monkeys, *Journal of Comparative Neurology, 104,* pp. 37-75, 1956.

95. B. Wallace and D. Turosky, Imagination and Hemispheric Laterality: An Examination of Individual Differences, in *Hypnosis and Imagination,* R. G. Kunzendorf, N. Spanos, and B. Wallace (eds.), Baywood Publishing Company, Amityville, New York, pp. 235-252, 1996.

96. E. Bisiach and C. Luzzatti, Unilateral Neglect of Representational Space, *Cortex, 14,* pp. 101-114, 1978.

97. M. J. Farah, M. S. Gazzaniga, J. D. Holtzman, and S. M. Kosslyn, A Left Hemisphere Basis for Visual Mental Imagery?, *Neuropsychologia, 23,* pp. 115-118, 1985.

98. S. M. Kosslyn, J. D. Holtzman, M. S. Gazzaniga, and M. J. Farah, A Computational Analysis of Mental Image Generation: Evidence from Functional Dissociations in Split-brain Patients, *Journal of Experimental Psychology: General, 114,* pp. 311-341, 1985.

99. M. J. Farah, The Laterality of Mental Image Generation: A Test with Normal Subjects, *Neuropsychologia, 24,* pp. 541-551, 1986.

100. C. A. Biggins, B. Turetsky, and G. Fein, The Cerebral Laterality of Mental Image Generation in Normal Subjects, *Psychophysiology, 27,* pp. 57-67, 1990.

101. C. C. French and P. Brightwell, Spontaneous Imagery Scanning and Hemisphere Function, *Neuropsychologia, 27,* pp. 1105-1108, 1989.

102. R. E. Shepard and F. Metzler, Mental Rotation of Three-dimensional Objects, *Science, 171,* pp. 701-703, 1971.

103. P. L. Ditunno and V. A. Mann, Right Hemisphere Specialization for Mental Rotation in Normals and Brain Damaged Subjects, *Cortex, 26,* pp. 177-188, 1990.

104. J. Sergent, The Neuropsychology of Visual Image Generation: Data, Method and Theory, *Brain and Cognition, 13,* pp. 98-129, 1990.

105. A. L. Benton, H. S. Levin, and M. W. von Allen, Geographic Orientation in Patients with Unilateral Cerebral Disease, *Neurology, 25,* pp. 907-910, 1974.

106. D. F. Marks, On the Relationship between Imagery, Body, and Mind, in *Imagery: Current Developments*, P. J. Hampson, D. F. Marks, and J. T. E. Richardson (eds.), Routledge, London, pp. 1-38, 1990.

107. D. O. Hebb, *The Organization of Behavior*, Wiley, New York, 1949.

108. D. O. Hebb, *Essay on Mind*, Erlbaum, Hillsdale, New Jersey, 1980.

109. L. J. Tippett, The Generation of Visual Images: A Review of Neuropsychological Research and Theory, *Psychological Bulletin, 112*, pp. 415-432, 1992.

110. K. H. Pribram, *Languages of the Brain: Experimental Paradoxes and Principles in Neuropsychology*, Prentice-Hall, Englewood Cliffs, New Jersey, 1971.

111. D. N. Spinelli, K. H. Pribram, and M. Weingarten, Centrifugal Optic Nerve Responses Evoked by Auditory and Somatic Stimulation, *Experimental Neurology, 12*, pp. 303-319, 1965.

112. D. N. Spinelli and M. Weingarten, Afferent and Efferent Activity in Single Units of the Cat's Optic Nerve, *Experimental Neurology, 13*, pp. 347-361, 1966.

113. K. M. Heilman and E. Valenstein, Auditory Neglect in Man, *Archives of Neurology, 26*, pp. 32-35, 1972.

114. M. Kinsbourne, Mechanisms of Hemispheric Interaction in Man, in *Hemispheric Disconnection and Cerebral Function*, M. Kinsbourne and W. L. Smith (eds.), Charles C. Thomas, Springfield, Illinois, 1974.

115. G. E. Schwartz, Emotion and Psychophysiological Organization: A Systems Approach, in *Psychophysiology: Systems, Processes, and Applications*, M. G. H. Coles, E. Donchin, and S. W. Porges (eds.), Guilford Press, New York, pp. 354-377, 1986.

116. D. A. Norman and T. Shallice, Attention to Action: Willed and Automatic Control of Behavior, in *Consciousness and Self-Regulation. Advances in Research and Theory*, Vol. 4, R. J. Davidson, G. E. Schwartz, and D. Shapiro (eds.), Plenum Press, New York, pp. 1-18, 1986.

117. T. Shallice, *From Neuropsychology to Mental Structure*, Cambridge University Press, Cambridge, 1988.

118. K. H. Pribram, Subdivisions of the Frontal Cortex Revisited, in *The Frontal Lobes Revisited*, E. Brown and E. Perecman (eds.), NRBN Press, New York, pp. 11-39, 1987.

119. K. H. Pribram, The Frontal Cortex—A Luria/Pribram Rapprochement, in *Contemporary Neuropsychology and the Legacy of Luria*, E. Goldberg (ed.), Lawrence Erlbaum Associates, Hillsdale, New Jersey, pp. 77-97, 1990.

120. A. H. Perlini and N. P. Spanos, EEG Alpha Methodologies and Hypnotizability: A Critical Review, *Psychophysiology, 28*, pp. 511-530, 1991.

121. C. M. Pechura and J. B. Martin (eds.), *Mapping the Brain and its Functions: Integrating Enabling Technologies into Neuroscience Research*, National Academy Press, Washington, D.C., 1991.

122. M. E. Raichle, Circulatory and Metabolic Correlates of Brain Function in Normal Humans, in *Handbook of Physiology, Vol. 5: Higher Cortical Functions of the Brain*, F. Plum and V. B. Mountcastle (eds.), American Physiological Society, Washington, D.C., 1987.

123. R. C. Gur and M. Reivich, Cognitive Task Effects on Hemispheric Blood Flow in Humans: Evidence for Individual Differences in Hemispheric Activation, *Brain and Language, 9*, pp. 78-92, 1980.

124. J. Risberg, Regional Cerebral Blood Flow in Neuropsychology, Special Issue: Methods in Neuropsychology, *Neuropsychologia, 24*, pp. 35-140, 1986.

125. R. C. Gur and R. E. Gur, The Impact of Neuroimaging on Human Neuropsychology, in *Perspectives on Cognitive Neuroscience*, R. G. Lister and H. J. Weingartner (eds.), Oxford University Press, Oxford, pp. 417-435, 1991.

126. R. Wise, U. Hadar, D. Howard, and K. Patterson, Language Activation Studies with Positron Emission Tomography, in *Exploring Brain Functional Anatomy with Positron Emission Tomography* (Ciba Foundation Symposium 163), D. H. Chadwick and J. Whelan (eds.), Wiley, New York, pp. 198-217, 1991.
127. M. E. Raichle, Memory Mechanisms in the Processing of Words and Work-like Symbols, in *Exploring Brain Functional Anatomy with Positron Emission Tomography* (Ciba Foundation Symposium 163), D. H. Chadwick and J. Whelan (eds.), Wiley, New York, pp. 198-217, 1991.
128. M. Corbetta, F. J. Miezin, G. L. Shulman, and S. E. Petersen, Selective Attention Modulates Extrastriate Visual Regions in Humans during Visual Feature Discrimination and Recognition, in *Exploring Brain Functional Anatomy with Positron Tomography* (Ciba Foundation Symposium 163), D. J. Chadwick and J. Whelan (eds.), John Wiley & Sons, Chicester, England, pp. 165-175, 1991.
129. J. V. Pardo, P. T. Fox, and M. E. Raichle, Localization of a Human System for Sustained Attention by Positron Emission Tomography, *Nature, 349,* pp. 61-64, 1991.
130. C. Frith, Positron Emission Tomography Studies of Frontal Lobe Function: Relevance to Psychiatric Disease, in *Exploring Brain Functional Anatomy with Positron Emission Tomography* (Ciba Foundation Symposium 163), D. H. Chadwick and J. Whelan (eds.), Wiley, New York, pp. 181-197, 1991.
131. P. S. Goldman-Rakic, Circuitry of Primate Prefrontal Cortex and Regulation of Behavior by Representational Memory, in *Handbook of Physiology, Section a: The Nervous System, Vol. 5: Higher Functions of the Brain,* F. Plum (ed.), Oxford University Press (American Physiological Society, Bethesda), Oxford, England, 1987.
132. P. E. Roland and L. Friberg, Localization of Cortical Areas Activated by Thinking, *Journal of Neurophysiology, 53,* pp. 1219-1243, 1985.
133. G. Goldenberg, I. Podreka, F. Uhl, M. Steiner, K. Willmes, and L. Deecke, Cerebral Correlates of Imagining Colors, Faces and a Map—I. SPECT of Regional Cerebral Blood Flow, *Neuropsychologia, 27,* pp. 1315-1328, 1989.
134. D. H. Ingvar, Serial Aspects of Language and Speech Related to Prefrontal Cortical Activity. A Selective Review, *Human Neurobiology, 2,* pp. 177-190, 1983.
135. P. E. Roland, Metabolic Measurements of the Working Frontal Cortex in Man, *Trends in Neuroscience, 7,* pp. 430-435, 1984.
136. G. Goldenberg, I. Podreka, and M. Steiner, The Cerebral Localization of Visual Imagery: Evidence from Emission Computerized Tomography of Cerebral Blood Flow, in *Imagery: Current Developments,* P. J. Hampson, D. F. Marks, and J. T. E. Richardson (eds.), Routledge, London, pp. 307-332, 1990.
137. A. Paivio, A Dual Coding Perspective on Imagery and the Brain, in *Neuropsychology of Visual Perception,* J. W. Brown (ed.), Erlbaum, Hillsdale, New Jersey, 1989.
138. G. Goldenberg, I. Podreka, M. Steiner, and K. Willmes, Patterns of Regional Cerebral Blood Flow Related to Memorizing of High and Low Imagery Words—An Emission Computer Tomography Study, *Neuropsychologia, 25,* pp. 473-485, 1987.
139. G. Goldenberg, I. Podreka, M. Steiner, K. Willmes, E. Suess, and L. Deecke, Regional Cerebral Blood Flow Patterns in Visual Imagery, *Neuropsychologia, 25,* pp. 641-664, 1989.
140. G. Goldenberg, M. Steiner, I. Podreka, L. Deecke, Regional Cerebral Blood Flow Patterns Related to Verification of Low- and High-imagery Sentences, *Neuropsychologia, 30,* pp. 581-586, 1992.
141. G. Goldenberg, I. Podreka, M. Steiner, P. Franzen, and L. Deecke, Contributions of Occipital and Temporal Brain Regions to Visual and Acoustic Imagery—A SPECT Study, *Neuropsychologia, 29,* pp. 685-702, 1991.

142. N. D. Volkow and L. R. Tancredi, Biological Correlates of Mental Activity Studied with PET, *American Journal of Psychiatry, 148,* pp. 439-443, 1991.
143. R. J. Erwin, M. Mawhinney-Hee, R. C. Gur, and R. E. Gur, Effects of Task and Gender on EEG Indices of Hemispheric Activation: Similarities to Previous rCBF Findings, *Neuropsychiatry, Neuropsychology, and Behavioral Neurology, 2,* pp. 248-260, 1989.
144. V. Charlot, N. Tzourio, M. Ziblovicium, B. Mazoyer, and M. Denis, Different Mental Imagery Abilities Result in Different Regional Cerebral Blood Flow Activation Patterns during Cognitive Tasks, *Neuropsychologica, 30,* pp. 565-580, 1992.
145. G. De Benedittis and G. P. Longostreui, *Cerebral Blood Flow Changes in Hypnosis: A Single Photon Emission Computerized Tomography (SPECT) Study,* paper presented at the 4th International Congress of Psychophysiology, Prague, July 1988.
146. G. De Benedittis and G. Carli, Psineurobiologia dell'ipnosi, in *Seminari sul dolore,* M. Tiengo (ed.), Centro Studi sull'Analgesia Universitá degli Studi di Milano, Milan Italy, pp. 59-116, 1990.
147. H. K. Meyer, B. J. Diehl, P. T. Ulrich, and G. Meinig, Anderungen der regionalen kortikalen durchblutung unter hypnose, *Zeitschrift fur Psychosomatische Medizin und Psychoanalyse, 35,* pp. 48-58, 1989.
148. H. Walter, *Hypnose: Theorien, neurophysiologische Korrelate und praktische Hinweise zur Hypnosetherapie,* Georg Thieme Verlag, Stuttgart, 1992.
149. P. Halama, Die Veranderung der corticalen Durchblutung vor under in Hypnose, *Experimentelle und Klinkische Hypnose, 5,* pp. 19-26, 1989.
150. P. Halama, Neurophysiologische Untersuchungen vor und in Hypnose am menschlichen Cortex mittels SPECT—Unterschung—Pilotstudie, *Experimentelle und Klinische Hypnose, 6,* pp. 65-73, 1990.
151. A. M. Weitzenhoffer and E. R. Hilgard, *Stanford Hypnotic Susceptibility Scale, Form C,* Consulting Psychologists Press, Palo Alto, California, 1962.
152. R. E. Shor and M. T. Orne, *Harvard Group Scale of Hypnotic Susceptibility, Form A,* Consulting Psychologists Press, Palo Alto, California, 1962.
153. A. M. Weitzenhoffer and E. R. Hilgard, *Revised Stanford Profile Scales of Hypnotic Susceptibility, Forms I and II,* Consulting Psychologists Press, Palo Alto, California, 1967.
154. A. Tellegen, *Brief Manual for the Multidimensional Personality Questionnaire,* unpublished manuscript, Department of Psychology, University of Minnesota, Minneapolis, 1982.
155. J. Risberg and I. Prohovnik, Cortical Processing of Visual and Tactile Stimuli Studied by Non-invasive rCBF Measurements, *Human Neurobiology, 2,* pp. 5-10, 1983.
156. H. J. Crawford, K. Pribram, P. Kugler, M. Xiu, B. Zhang, and T. Knebel, *Somatosensory Evoked Potential Brain Topographical Changes during Suggestion Hypnotic Anesthesia,* paper presented at the 6th International Congress of Psychophysiology, Berlin, Germany, September 1992.
157. J. D. Kropotov, H. J. Crawford, and Y. I. Polyakov, Somatosensory Event-related Potential Changes to Painful Stimuli during Hypnotic Analgesia: Anterior Cingulate Cortex and Anterior Temporal Cortex Intracranial Recordings in Obsessive-Compulsives, *International Journal of Psychophysiology,* accepted.
158. H. J. Crawford, Cognitive and Psychophysiological Correlates of Hypnotic Responsiveness and Hypnosis, in *Creative Mastery in Hypnosis and Hypnoanalysis: A Festscrift for Erika Fromm,* M. L. Fass and D. P. Brown (eds.), Erlbaum, Hillsdale, New Jersey, pp. 47-54, 1990.

159. H. J. Crawford, *Cold Pressor Pain With and Without Suggested Analgesia: EEG Correlates as Moderated by Hypnotic Susceptibility Level,* paper presented at the 5th International Congress of Psychophysiology, Budapest, Hungary, July 1990.
160. N. Birbaumer, T. Elbert, A. G. M. Canavan, and B. Rockstroh, Slow Potentials of the Cerebral Cortex and Behavior, *Physiological Reviews, 70,* pp. 1-41, 1990.
161. M. E. Sabourin, S. D. Cutcomb, H. J. Crawford, and K. Pribram, EEG Correlates of Hypnotic Susceptibility and Hypnotic Trance: Spectral Analysis and Coherence, *International Journal of Psychophysiology, 10,* pp. 125-142, 1990.
162. H. J. Crawford and S. N. Clark, Self-generated Happy and Sad Emotions in Low and Highly Hypnotizable Persons during Waking and Hypnosis: Laterality and Regional EEG Activity Differences, *International Journal of Psychophysiology,* accepted.
163. D. L. Schacter, EEG Theta Waves and Psychological Phenomena: A Review and Analysis, *Biological Psychology, 5,* pp. 47-82, 1977.
164. J. H. Gruzelier and K. Warren, Neuropsychological Evidence of Reductions on Left Frontal Tests with Hypnosis, *Psychological Medicine, 23,* pp. 93-101, 1993.
165. H. Walter, I. Podreka, M. Steiner, E. Suess, N. Benda, M. Hajji, O. M. Lesch, M. Musalek, and V. Passweg, A Contribution to Classification of Hallucinations, *Psychopathology, 23,* pp. 97-105, 1990.

[The writing of this chapter was supported by a National Institutes of Health grant [1 R21 RR09598] to the author. Earlier research reported herein was supported by The Spencer Foundation, National Institute of Health Biomedical Research Support grants, and intramural grants from Virginia Polytechnic Institute and State University and the University of Wyoming to the author.]

CHAPTER 14

Hypnosis and the Brain: The Relationship between Subclinical Complex Partial Epileptic-Like Symptoms, Imagination, Suggestibility, and Changes in Self-Identity

MICHAEL A. PERSINGER

INTRODUCTION

The principles of modern neuroscience predict that all phenomenological and subjective experiences are determined by brain activity. At any given moment of psychological time, the content of the person's stream of consciousness is a function of the themes of those spatial regions that are most metabolically active [1, 2]. From this perspective the brain can be viewed as a matrix and subjective experiences correspond to the relative dominance of activity between the elements of this matrix. If we can isolate those portions of the brain that are most associated with a behavior, then it can be more effectively controlled and predicted.

The capacity to be hypnotized (suggestibility) is assumed to be a normal correlate of brain function. Because of the strong cognitive component that is involved with hypnotizability, the role of cerebral structures would be primary. If this assumption is valid then hypnotizability should be associated with specific differences in psychological function both within and between the cerebral hemispheres. These patterns must be evident qualitatively in clinical populations (or in extreme cases) but only discernible *quantitatively* (assuming the restricted range problem is accommodated) within the normal population.

This chapter reviews the recent work of the Laurentian University Neuroscience Research Group. We have pursued the hypothesis that overt displays of hypnotizability are derived from neurocognitive processes that are very similar to those associated with synchronous electrical activity within the deep structures of the ventral cerebrum. If this hypothesis is correct, then there should be convergence between classes of psychological phenomena (perhaps hereto considered not related) that share functional association with these regions of the brain.

BASIC BRAIN AND SUGGESTIBILITY CORRELATES

Hypnotizability or suggestibility is most frequently associated with the capacity: 1) to engage in vivid imagery, 2) to continue generating elaborate, (personally) meaningful fantasy once the instructions have terminated, 3) to dissociate (with brief amnesic intervals), 4) to incorporate instructional or incidental material into the amnesic intervals and 5) to display modifications of memory [3, 4] and its major process: the sense of self-identity. Combinations of these capacities, often weighted differentially, contribute to each person's potential hypnotizability [5].

These major dimensions of hypnotizability are strongly correlated with functions that have been attributed to the deep, mesiobasal structures of the temporal lobes [6]. One of these structures, the hippocampus, is associated with memory consolidation, access to long-term (cerebral cortical) storage and dreaming. The other major structure, the amygdala, facilitates attribution of meaningfulness to sensory information. Both of these structures are reciprocally connected to the orbital frontal regions that are intimately involved with allocating temporal order and context-dependence to memory and its experience.

Because of the microstructural organization and pattern of vascular supply of the hippocampal-amygdaloid complex, these structures display the *lowest* electrical ("depolarizing") threshold of the human brain. This electrical lability, manifested most frequently as rapid burst-firing of aggregates of neurons, is the precondition that allows the extraordinary representation of environmental stimuli within the brain. Extreme forms of this lability, such as electrical seizures (epilepsy), is the price the mammalian brain pays for this mechanism of memory.

The continuum of hypnotizability and its cognitive correlates can be considered a function of the electrical lability (or sensitivity) of these deep temporal lobe structures [7]. If this assumption is valid, then experimentally-induced lability (or extreme conditions of this state) should generate most of the major characteristics that define hypnosis. Complex partial epilepsy or limbic epilepsy is one classic manifestation. During ictal periods, when paroxysmal discharges are emitted from the deep structures within the temporal, cingulate or orbital frontal regions, a variety of altered states (often without loss of consciousness) can occur [8].

These altered states are not always associated with the distinct epileptiform electroencephalographic activity that is measured by scalp electrodes. It only infers changes in the outer 5 mm of the cerebrum and is only altered if the phasic electrical discharges (from subcortical structures) access the dorsal and lateral cortices (the ventral cortices, such as the parahippocampal gyrus, lie at the base of the skull and hence are less accessible by scalp electrodes). Instead, altered states of consciousness appear to be a function of the percentages of neurons within an amygdaloid or hippocampal region that are recruited into the depolarizing wave [9]. There is a clear continuum between normal consciousness and its cessation (with convulsions) that is associated with all of the phenomenon normally attributed to hypnosis.

Alterations of the human experience of consciousness are not the only phenomena that are modulated by deep mesiobasal structures within the temporal and limbic lobes. Because of the significant neuroanatomical input into regions around the third ventricle (primarily the hypothalamus), amygdaloid and hippocampal stimulation significantly affects the release of neuropeptides from hypothalamic neurons; they control subsequent hypophyseal activity. For example the duration (in the order of seconds) of after-discharges [10] following electrical stimulation of the amygdala induces either decreases or increases in the blood concentrations of adrenocorticotrophic hormone (ACTH). This non-monotonic relationship would allow relatively subtle neurocognitive (psychological) stimuli to exert significant influence at the interface between immuno-facilitation (reduced ACTH) and immunosuppression (enhanced ACTH) levels.

The powerful effects of these limbic structures upon the hormonal processes that influence sexual arousal and reproduction are commensurate with the observed or the suspected association between limbic lability, latency to orgasm and the development of subjective pseudocyesis [11]. Amygdaloid stimulation promotes gastric section [12], fluid retention, alterations in heart rate and blood pressure and peripheral vasoconstriction or vasodilation [13]. Because of the direct non-myelinated, biogenic amine-containing fibers between the hypothalamus and the thymus, spleen and related immunological and hematopoietic organs [14], modulatory influence upon cellular immunity is very likely.

DIRECT OR SURGICAL STIMULATION OF THE TEMPORAL LOBES

Despite the revisions and arguments by several contemporary neurosurgeons [15], the stimulation experiments that were first reported by Penfield and his colleagues [16] are still frequently misinterpreted. These researchers found that stimulation of the temporal lobes (especially the deep structures) of complex partial ("temporal lobe") epileptic patients were associated with vivid experiences that appeared to be "memories." This conclusion was only partially correct.

Vivification of Ongoing Cognition

Horowitz offered a more general formulation for these current-evoked phenomenological patterns [17]. He suggested that temporal lobe stimulation "induced a state of mind that was favorable for the experience and reporting of internal images, no matter what the source." It could involve memories, emotional concerns, ongoing sensory information, or wishes. In more contemporary language, direct electrical stimulation of the temporal lobes enhances the *relative magnitude* of *all ongoing* cognitive activity. If the person was listening to a verbal instruction, the imagery and meaningfulness of the linguistic string could approach that associated with normal perceptual processing.

As predicted by the concept of the brain matrix, direct (and gross) electrical stimulation of the deep temporal lobe structures by surgical techniques generates vivid phenomenology that reflects the functions of these structures. Apprehension, floating sensations, complex vivid visual imagery (because of the powerful projections of the visual association cortex to the hippocampal gyrus and amygdala), dream-like states, dissociative (partial amnesic) periods, psychical-like experiences (out-of-body experiences, "sudden knowing") and the perception of temporal juxtapositions (sometimes designated as premonitional experiences) have been common correlates [18, 19].

Interictal Behavior

During the last century, several serious researchers [20, 21] have strongly suggested that recurrent electrical seizures within the mesiobasal temporal lobes alter behavior. Depending upon the lateralization of the focus, these chronic alterations are displayed as an increased *quantitative* incidence of circumstantiality, a sense of the personal (events happen with special reference to the person), infusion of personal meaning into odd or infrequent events and an interest in nascent themes and mystical/religious experiences. Counterarguments for the existence of interictal profiles are weak and invariably confuse qualitative incidence versus quantitative occurrence (the continuum) of these behaviors. Quantitative phenomena require psychometric measurement rather than clinical impression or a review of a list of symptoms.

Within the context of hypnosis and complex partial epilepsy, these interictal behaviors are manifested as an exaggerated egocentric emphasis and a cognitive mode that involves affective more than conceptual or semantic dimensions. Discourse planning during cognition is considered to rely upon a "tree geometry" whereby topical propositions occupy specific nodal positions within the arbour [22]. The relationship between the nodes is based upon the linguistic or perceptual categories. If nodal positions also contain an affective component [22], then selective enhancement of this component would direct cognition according to the emotional similarities of the words in the tree geometry.

A more accurate metaphor would be a tensor whereby the relationships between elements are a function of the affective dimensions [pleasant-unpleasant; active-passive] that are defined by the specific context. Cognition would diffuse according to affective pathways rather than develop through discrete sequential nodes. The dominance of the former would allow the simultaneous acceptance of logical incongruities [5] as long as the aggregate of propositions shared the same affective domain. This cognitive pattern would be similar to that associated with normal dreaming; the ideational contents of a sequence are more related to their shared affective domains rather than to conceptual, perceptual, or linguistic similarities.

These interictal characteristics are manifested within the highly hypnotizable subject as: 1) suspension of critical judgment, 2) affiliation with new events (because of overreactive amygdaloid activation and attribution of meaning to new events), 3) trance (incongruous) logic, 4) excellent memory (enhanced hippocampal lability) and the capacity for concentration (an indirect consequence of the same proces that promotes circumstantiality and viscosity).

Phenomenological Similarity between Complex Partial Seizures and Affective-Dissociative Disorders

Spiegel and Spiegel proposed a psychological model for the continuum of hypnotizability [5]. A high capacity for hypnotic induction should be displayed by people prone to hysterical reactions, hysterical dissociative disorders, hysterical conversions, depression, and mania. These syndromes were classified as affective disorders. A low capacity for hypnotizability should be dominated by people who display cognitive disorders such as the schizophrenias or obsessive-compulsions.

If a similar source of brain variance contributes to hypnotizability and to affective disorders, then one should expect strong concordance between the symptoms of the temporal lobe epileptic and affective patients. Robert Post has shown a marked overlap in symptoms between these two traditionally distinct nosologies [23]. Both classes of patients are prone to experience illusions of significance (egocentricism), altered sound intensity, changes in odors, formed auditory hallucinations, altered color intensity, derealization, amnesic periods, epigastric (rising, floating) sensations, and hallucinations. The dynamic relationship between ictal (hypermetabolic) and interictal (hypometabolic) stages and the phases of hypomania and depression is conspicuous.

Integration into Ongoing Experience

A brief anomalous amplification of the neural substrate of any phase of cognition should be experienced as ego-alien (intrusive and not from the "self.") However this intrusion would be incorporated into the ongoing fabric of awareness and its content would be primarily a function of the specific setting. Thus, the labels that are available, from the subtle perceptual or verbal context, would be expected to strongly affect the content of the phenomenology. This property has been observed within both hypnosis and direct surgical stimulation.

The best known experimental study involved a young woman who displayed an epileptic focus within the left temporofrontal lobe [24]. During periods of spontaneous narratives and answers (in response to questions by staff members), the patient's left temporal lobe (without her knowledge) was stimulated. Careful analysis of the interview tape-recordings indicated that the content of the "intrusive" ideational experiences was a function of her prestimulation mental set. For example immediately before a stimulation the patient was discussing her daughter's desire for a baby sister. The stimulation occurred and the patient heard a female voice say "I got a baby . . . sister."

This relationship between experimental (social) context, transient stimulation of the deep structures within the temporal lobes and the specific content of the subsequent vivid experience may be a primary property of human cognition. Hypnosis as a phenomenon and the capacity to generate situation-specific fantasy would be normal consequences of this property.

Integration into Memory and Temporal Order

The origin of a contemporary experience is not discriminated by the hippocampal formation. Mundane perceptions, wishes, thoughts, fantasies, and dreams are consolidated as memories. If they were not, the average person would not be able to remember any of these cognitive processes. Once an experience, evoked by usual or exotic sources has been consolidated, it can be remembered as real.

The capacity to discriminate between dreams, fantasies, wishes, and normative memories involves the prefrontal cortices. Mild dysfunction in prefrontal (orbito-frontal) activity, especially at the time of consolidation, should interfere with: 1) the capacity to discriminate between fantasies and veridical experiences, and 2) temporal references, for example, when the memories occurred in auto-biographical time. Patients who exhibit anomalies of the (right) frontotemporal region, for example, frequently exhibit confabulation [whereas delusions without obvious thought disorder emphasize left temporofrontal electrical disruptions]. Images that were evoked by instructions, contexts or questions that occurred after an amnesic period can be incorporated as memories. Often the "episodic time" of the memory involves previous amnesic intervals.

One anecdotal example of this process involved a woman who felt she had been abducted by an extraterrestrial alien after her car had been struck by a large luminous display (that was very similar to the type of phenomena that precede some earthquakes). Because: 1) the alternator and other electrical components of the automobile no longer functioned subsequent to the "encounter," 2) there was strong evidence of current induction (when the luminous phenomena was apposed to the car) that could have evoked electrical seizures within the temporal lobes, and 3) an eyewitness (who only later reported seeing a "ball of light hit and glance from the car"), this case can be considered a candidate for an example of the neurocognitive consequences of direct current stimulation of the brain.

When the woman was first interviewed, she was clearly anxious, confused, disoriented, and exhibited partial amnesia; there were deficits in the recall of the temporal order of events that occurred before the episode. All of these symptoms were strongly indicative of transient dysfunction of both the temporal (memory) and frontal (serial order, anxiety, erratic organization of thought) lobes. During the interview, the woman could not recall any details following the collision except that she had experienced impulses of pain to her leg (and later whole body "stiffness") and floating sensations. She compared these experiential fragments to "a dream." Then one of the interviewers thrust a picture of a small, hydroencephalic humanoid into her view and stated: "isn't this how they looked." The women reported she could not recall. About one week later, during another interview, the woman stated that she had "suddenly" remembered the sequence of events: while driving home she had struck a spaceship, her body had been floated out of the car, and her leg had been examined by a "small large-headed humanoid."

Such modifications of memory would be expected in light of the enhanced anomalous activity within the temporal lobes; it would have disrupted normal memory consolidation on the one hand but would have enhanced the impact of imagery on the other. The concomitant interference with prefrontal activity would have promoted the misattribution of the picture as an actual event within auto-biographical memory. Once consolidated (within about 20 minutes) the recollection would have been as real as those acquired through mundane processes.

The fantasy-prone personality [25] can be considered a highly hypnotizable individual whose deep temporal lobe structures are more labile and active than those individuals who are less suggestible. A major consequence of this electrical lability would be the ability to generate (parahippocampal; fusiform gyrus) images with profound personal meaning (amygdala) in response to verbal instructions or to infer images from perceptual patterns. Because of the reciprocal inhibition between the orbitofrontal and temporal cortices, the experiential continuum of these individuals would also be more influenced by the *external* structure such as context or explanation. Several studies [26] have shown that 50 percent of highly hypnotizable subjects, given an appropriate context, will accept a suggested pseudomemory as actually having occurred. If the numbers of pseudomemories become significant and are integrated strategically within the person's constellation of memories, one would expect alterations in the self concept. Because memory is the reference by which the person experiences the existence of the self, these changes would not be discernible. However external observers, such as parents and friends, would perceive this "different" person.

Clinical Cases of "Sudden Remembering"

During the last few years of clinical practice I have encountered numerous reports of people [27] who suddenly recall early memories (never before experienced) of sexual abuse or alien abduction/visitation. Their performances on standardized tests indicated elevations (T score > 69) on scales that infer numbers of complex partial epileptic-like signs (CPES), anxiety specific to "lower ego-strength" and a capacity to engage in imagery. All of these individuals had felt that before the "sudden recall" there had been something "missing in their lives." Now they felt integrated and experienced an urge to proselytize (tell the world about sex abuse or the presence of aliens). In previous decades or centuries, comparable "memories" following a revelation (at a prayer meeting) and subsequent changes in behavior would have been called a religious conversion.

Careful evaluation of the clients' histories indicated that they had been involved in strong social contexts, such as self-help groups, that would have promoted submissiveness. There had been some point where the therapist, group leader or "New Age" minister had stated "perhaps you were abused" or "perhaps you too have been abducted." The sudden memories, first associated with anxiety, followed. However with each "new memory" the anxiety of daily living decreased because each person began to understand "the purpose" of his or her existence. The behavioral operations that evoked these sequences are the ecological equivalent of the procedures that are used to induce pseudomemories during hypnotic induction within laboratory settings; the primary difference is the time frame.

One illustrative case involved a forty-year-old Roman Catholic woman who had been receiving psychiatric support for depression and anxiety. While engaged in this alliance, the women suffered an aneurysm within the right temporal lobe and required surgery. Subsequent to her recovery, she attended an incest survivors' self-help group, which was suggested as a technique for social interaction. A few months later, even though she had stopped attending the group meetings, she revealed to the psychiatrist (for the first time) that she had been sexually abused, repeatedly, between the ages of four and nine years of age by her father. These contentions were baffling to all members of the woman's family who did not remember any of the settings or contingencies during which the abuse allegedly occurred. Such modifications (rather than eliminations) of memory would be expected following subcortical disruptions within the right temporal lobe.

Enhanced electrical activity of the mesiobasal structures would have increased the intensity of imagery induced by the verbal behavior of others. Once consolidated, these "pseudomemories" would appear as real as any other. If there were amnesic intervals, which are normally present in human memory for the transition period between infantile and adult memory (that begins between the ages of 4 to 5 years), the "pseudomemories" could be attributed to those periods. Concurrence of right frontal dysfunction, which would interfere with the ordering of memory, could facilitate the misattribution and could contribute to well-integrated beliefs [28] without significant alteration in logical sequencing (i.e., faulty premises but normal inferencing).

Consequently, 1) significantly elevated memory processing capacity relative to intellectual level (an inference of recently enhanced hippocampal activity), 2) enhanced CPES and/or the capacity for imaging, and 3) indicators of right hemispheric anomalies (severe left hemispheric dysfunction would interfere with the self-concept and encourage anxious self-preoccupation) should facilitate the occurrence of "sudden memories." Because of the greater relative representation of linguistic processes within the right hemisphere, normal women should be more prone to these experiences than normal men.

Analysis of the neuropsychological assessments of six people, who had been referred because of difficulties adapting, supported this hypothesis. All of these individuals had been attending either an incest survivor group or a New Age (reincarnation, alien communication themes) group when the instructors had suggested that the clients had been either abused or abducted, respectively. The sudden imagery began at this point and continued over several weeks to months.

According to the Minnesota Multiphasic Personality Inventory (MMPI), Wechsler Adult Intellectual Scale (Revised) and Halstead Impairment Index, all of these people were normal. Every one of them displayed a specific psychometric profile: 1) elevated ($T > 70$) CPES signs, 2) an elevated ($T > 70$) Wilson-Barber (Inventory of Childhood Memories and Imaginings [29]) score, and 3) a Memory Quotient (MQ) that was at least one standard deviation higher than the full scale IQ. There was mild impairment in left handed tactual performance time and either the tactile memory or localization scores. These clients displayed a mild impairment for the Category test as well as marginal performance on either the Design Fluency (relative to verbal fluency) or Conditioned Spatial Association Task.

Perhaps the most conspicuous difference between these individuals involved a history of low self-esteem that was followed, at the time of the "sudden memories," by the experience of a sensed presence (ego-alien intrusions into awareness). The presence (or entity) occurred along the (left) peripheral visual field. EEG activity revealed bursts of anomalous theta activity over the right temporal lobe or nonpathological spikes and sharp waves within frontotemporal comparisons.

These results were interpreted as support for the explanation that the "sudden memories" were induced by the context of the social group setting. The enhanced hippocampal activity would have encouraged strong imagery (which was evident by their psychometric test results) in response to instructions such as "perhaps you were. . . ." Because of the anomalous right frontal activity (which could have affected the temporal order of memory), these images, once consolidated, would have been revivified as memories and would not have been distinguished from memories that were acquired by more routine processes.

THE CONTINUUM OF TEMPORAL LOBE LABILITY

If hypnotizability is a continuum along which all people are distributed and is associated with enhanced activity within the deep temporal lobe, then 1) there should be a continuum of temporal lobe lability that is characterized by the phenomenological equivalents of complex partial epileptic-like signs (CPES), and 2) there should be a positive correlation between temporal lobe signs and hypnotizability in the normal population.

Complex Partial Epileptic-Like Signs and Subclinical Electrical Anomalies of the Temporal Lobes

Roberts et al. have argued that the phenomenology of partial seizure-like symptoms is remarkably frequent in people who have sustained mild to moderate brain injury, especially when the temporal and frontal lobes have been focally disrupted or diffusely recruited because of some insidious process [30]. These experiential reports occur without the stereotypical motor activity; often the only electroencephalographic correlate is spontaneous bursts of theta rhythm activity. Patients with suspected brain injuries who display enhanced complex partial epileptic-like signs show marked and extreme disruptions in proficiency during dichotic listening tasks [31]. That the dichotic listening difficulties and the frequency of occurrence of complex partial epileptic-like signs are markedly attenuated by the anticonvulsant carbamazepine (Tegretol) suggests that both domains are associated with an "electrical anomaly" within the brain.

The experiential phenomena that Roberts et al. attributed to the presence of subclinical partial complex epilepsy are remarkably similar to those associated with hypnosis. In addition to the propensity to display staring spells when looking at a shiny or bright object, memory gaps, unrecalled behaviors, automatic driving, confusional spells, hearing a telephone ring (when it doesn't), urinary urgency, illusions of movement, visual anomalies (e.g., perceiving stars, bugs, threads moving in the peripheral field), haptic illusions (as if something brushed against the skin, such as a cobweb), metallic tastes, and olfactory sensations are common experiences.

Although the normal person may experience any or all of these phenomeno-logical domains at least once in a lifetime, the person who displays complex partial epileptic-like signs reports these experiences more frequently (quantitative vs. qualitative measurement). Stated alternatively, these individuals exhibit a *lower threshold* for the display of subjective experiences and symptoms that are similar to those that are also exhibited by highly hypnotizable subjects. The phenomenology that has been attributed to both complex partial epilepsy and hypnosis does not demonstrate causality; however it does suggest that a third factor, which is hypothesized to be enhanced hippocampal-amygdaloid lability, is responsible for both.

The Temporal Lobe Continuum in the Normal Population

For the last ten years Kate Makarec and I [32, 33] have been pursuing the concept of the continuum of temporal lobe lability within the normal population. We have assumed that the experiences of a normal person actually reflect the metabolic matrix of the brain. Only at the extreme ends of the continuum, where verified epilepsy emerges and massive paroxysmal activity disrupts memory consolidation, would phenomenological (paper and pencil) profiles fail to reflect this continuum.

The Personal Philosophy Inventories (PPI) of approximately 1,200 adults have been collected. The PPI contains 140 true-false items that reflect information relevant to complex partial epilepsy, beliefs, preferences, control responses, and demographic information. The three a priori major clusters of items (examples in Table 1), based upon theoretical concepts of temporal lobe function, are ictal-like experiences, interictal-like experiences and temporal lobe relevant experiences. The score for each cluster is simply the number of items that were endorsed (percentage of total); endorsement profiles on clusters of control statements and items from "lie" scales are used to control for "yes" responding and exaggerated presentations.

Experiments designed to test both convergent and divergent construct validity have supported the use of these designations. For example a correlation of +0.50

Table 1. Sample Items from Various Clusters of Temporal Lobe Indicators from the Personal Philosophy Inventory

I. Complex Partial Epileptic-like Signs (CPELS) Cluster
   Item 23. There have been times when I have stared at an object and it appeared to become larger and larger.
   Item 29. While sitting quietly, I have had uplifting sensations as if I were driving quickly over a rolling road.

II. Interictal-like Behavior (ILB) Cluster
   Item 33. People tell me that I "blank out" sometimes when we are talking.
   Item 137. Two or three times in my life, there have been a few brief moments when I felt very close to a Universal Consciousness.

III. Temporal Lobe Relevant (TLR) Cluster
   Item 122. When I am alone or feel really low, reciting poetry or prose is a pleasant experience.
   Item 32. Sometimes I can read another person's thoughts.

IV. Left Hemispheric Cluster
   Item 63. Sometimes, in the early morning hours between midnight and 4:00 A.M., my experiences are very meaningful.
   Item 53. I keep a diary or notebook about my feelings and thoughts.

V. Right Hemispheric Cluster
   Item 102. Once, in a crowded area I suddenly could not recognize where I was.
   Item 123. At least once in my life, just before falling down, I had the intense sensations of a smell from childhood.

was observed between the numbers (variability) of alpha seconds over (T3/T4 bipolar) the temporal lobes (but not occipital-O1/O2 lobes) per unit time and the percentage of signs and symptoms that are similar to temporal lobe epileptic patients who report these experiences spontaneously or during surgical stimulation of this brain region [34, 35].

Personality Correlates and the Capacity for Imagination

We have found moderate strength (+0.55) correlations between CPES and experiences of a sensed presence [32], such as an "entity" or "another consciousness" (which is often attributed to mystical or god sources). These experiences which occurred in about 20 percent of our population usually occur late at night or in the early morning hours (0100 to 0400 hr). The numbers of CPES are also associated with the numbers of different types of paranormal experiences (mean r = +0.60) and the numbers of these experiences are significantly associated (mean r about +0.50) with sensations of a sensed presence. Consistent associations (rs between +0.40 and +0.50) between CPES scores and the Wilson-Barber Inventory of Childhood Memories and Imaginations have been observed [36].

The traditional personality characteristics that have been most strongly correlated with CPES are also those found in highly hypnotizable subjects. People who display elevated CPES (after controlling for yes responding, which in general is a minor factor) are more prone to spontaneous imagery and mild to moderate impulsivity [7, 37]; the latter variable, as reflected in the hypomania scale from the MMPI, is more important for women than it is for men [38]. Individuals who display phenomenology that is similar to the themes of individuals with verified electrical lability within the temporal lobes also display a propensity to write or to like poetry and prose and to maintain personal notes about their experiences.

Elevations in CPES are reported by people who are more intuitive than sensing and who are more perceiving than judging [39], as defined by the Myers-Briggs Type Indicator. These individuals are emotionally sensitive, are talkative, act on sensitive intuition, are attention-seeking, and expect affection. Because of a generally lower ego strength, they are more likely to experience free-floating anxiety. Compliance, especially with authority, occurs in stark contrast to the normal cautiousness about social interaction. Perhaps one of the most interesting features of individuals who display elevated CPES is their capacity to engage in forced thinking and repeated, perseverative behaviors.

Hypnosis and TLS

If the same source of (questionnaire) response variance is responsible for the +0.40 to +0.50 association between CPES and other hypnosis-relevant phenomenology, then a comparable strength of association might be expected with some objective criterion reference. In three separate studies over the last ten years, correlations of between +0.35 and +0.55 have been found between Spiegel's HIP (Hypnosis Induction Profile) and either the Inventory of Childhood Memories and Imaginings or our inferences of temporal lobe lability [36, 40]. Factor analyses have repeatedly shown a weak (eigen values between 1.5 and 2.5) but persistent factor that was strongly loaded ($r > 0.60$) by both induction scores and CPES. The most powerful subcomponent of the HIP that has been strongly correlated with CPES has been vestibular phenomenology, for example, the "float" score. Vestibular experiences (including vertigo, giddiness and clouding of the visual field) are often considered unique indicators of temporal lobe (medial to the transverse gyri) activity.

Dichotic Listening Errors and Exotic Beliefs

The most consistent findings in this area of research have been the correlations of between +0.50 and +0.65 between complex partial epileptic-like signs and endorsement of exotic beliefs that include statements such as "Although I am not sure, I think I lived a previous life," "Alien intelligence is the cause of UFO's" and "ESP is real." However CPES have never been significantly correlated (after covariance for general belief endorsement) with traditional religious beliefs. One of the most interesting characteristics of the highly suggestible person, regardless of intelligence, is the capacity to accept beliefs totally and without challenge.

Recent experimental evidence indicates (as suggested by Spinoza centuries ago) that in order for statements to be understood, they first must be accepted as true. During the subsequent seconds the brain then determines if the statement was false. If this process is disrupted or distracted, then the default option "true" is attributed to the statement or experience [41]. For example, when a loud noise followed the presentation of bogus statements (e.g., a dwirp is a four-legged animal), subjects were more likely to endorse it as true (than bogus statements after which there had been no disruption) when the statement was presented again.

Skirda had suspected that people who display more dichotic errors (but within the non-clinical range) should have had a long history of auditory disruptions [42]. Consequently they would be more likely to accept statements as true, even those that appeared to be odd or strange (an extension of David M. Bear's sensory-limbic hyperconnectionism). If this hypothesis was correct then there should be a positive correlation between numbers of suppressions (errors) during a dichotic word listening task and the intensity of endorsement of beliefs in paranormal phenomena such as witches and alien life forms. Both high school and university students displayed this association ($r = 0.47$); the correlation between dichotic listening errors and traditional religious beliefs was not statistically significant ($r = 0.18$).

This result is relevant when applied to hypnotic settings. If enhanced complex partial epileptic signs (as inferred directly or by dichotic listening errors) interfere with the falsification process then the propensity for subjects who are highly suggestible (and prone to CPES) to accept instructions that are offered as pseudo-memories becomes rational. These individuals would be less able, even though they might be aware of the process, to reject the experience as false (i.e., a non-memory). In the Skirda study, a cumulative history of these experiences would contribute to the person's beliefs.

From the perspective of dynamic neuroanatomy, the utility of dichotic listening tasks to infer activity in the deep structures would appear limited. Dichotic listening capacity involves primarily the superior temporal gyrus whose inter-hemispheric neurons are projected primarily through the corpus callosum to the homologous contralateral region [43]. On the other hand, the hippocampal and amygdaloid regions are connected interhemispherically by the anterior commissure, the hippocampal commissure or its variants (except in epileptic patients, where the commissure of the dentate gyrus may be missing or reorganized by reactive synaptogenesis). Our working hypothesis is that enhanced mesiobasal activity enhances the *affective* component of information processing with the consequence of reducing the cognitive (number of bites) component; this is reflected as alterations in dichotic word list proficiency.

HEMISPHERICITY AND HYPNOSIS

Susceptibility to hypnosis has been associated with neuropsychological processes that are traditionally attributed to right hemispheric functions [44]. They have included the capacity to engage in spatial processing, the frequency of left (lateralized) eye movements and the predominance of affective experiences. Clinically, the special role of right hemispheric processes in dissociative phenomena has been inferred by the prevalence of left-sided somatic and motor dysfunctions in putative hysterical and conversion patients. Even the preferred tactile contact with the left hand during hypnotic induction implicates a right hemispheric mediation.

Right Hemispheric Indicators and the
Hypnosis Induction Profile

Canonical correlations between sets of items from the PPI with items from the Dissociative Experience Scale or DES [45] and the Hemispheric Questionnaire (HQ) by Vingiano [46] have suggested two major clusters of items. We have labeled them provisionally as "left hemispheric" and "right hemispheric." Example items for each of these clusters are shown in Table 1. The right hemispheric cluster is significantly correlated with scores on the DES and the HQ.

Young women who reported episodes of intense subjective pseudocyesis (the Roman Catholic: Protestant ratio was about 10:1) displayed significant elevations in right but not left hemispheric indicators. This pattern was considered support for the model that any organized belief system that encourages compartmentalization, such as statements like "men and women are equal but only men can be priests," would amplify the vectorial development of "right hemispheric" processes [11]; their details would be manifested by nonverbal expressions.

To test the hypothesis that right (temporal) phenomenology was more strongly associated with hypnosis, a total of forty-one women (18 to 28 years of age) and thirty-five men (similar age range) were given the PPI, the hemispheric quotient and the Dissociative Experience Scale. Within (plus/minus) one to ten days they were administered Spiegel's HIP by one of several senior undergraduate or graduate students (men and women) who were familiar with this procedure. Means and standard deviations for the various test scores demonstrated that sex differences were trivial and reflected the general consensus of minimal sex differences within the general domain of suggestibility.

However the association between the scores for the different inventories and the HIP revealed a stronger relationship for the women compared to the men. As shown in Table 2, the women displayed a consistent positive association between hypnotic susceptibility, right (but not left) hemisphericity as defined by the PPI cluster, a higher HQ (more right hemisphericity) score and more dissociation. (The differences between the weakest and strongest equivalent Pearson r values for men and women were not sufficient to be statistically different.)

Table 2. Spearman Rho Coefficients between the Major TLS Clusters, Factored Clusters, Hemispheric Quotient (HQ) and Dissociative Experience Scale (DES) and the "Float," "Dissociation" and HIP Scores of the Spiegel Procedure for Men (n = 35) and Women (n = 41)

Variable	Males			Females		
	Float	Dissoc	HIP	Float	Dissoc	HIP
Control	−0.03	0.10	0.03	−0.02	0.16	0.03
CPELS	0.20	−0.11	0.23	0.60**	0.35*	0.41**
Interictal-like	0.19	−0.10	0.32*	0.45**	0.26*	0.26*
Temporal Relevance	0.05	0.10	0.29*	0.56**	0.20	0.34*
Total	0.24	−0.02	0.30*	0.54**	0.32*	0.35**
Left Hemisphere	0.19	−0.03	0.15	0.29*	0.03	0.25
Right Hemisphere	0.13	0.10	0.33*	0.55**	0.46**	0.40**
HQ	0.06	0.16	0.18	0.13	0.36*	0.44**
DES	0.21	0.09	0.33*	0.54**	0.28*	0.47**

*$p < 0.05$
**$p < 0.01$

If the shared variance between scores for Vingiano's hemispheric question-naire, the DES and the PPI inferences of right hemisphericity is from the same source that is associated with hypnotizability, then they should load on the same factor. Factor analyses (varimax) showed that, for men, induction (0.70) right hemispheric PPI items (0.40) and the HQ (0.82; the higher the score the more right hemisphericity) were loaded on the same factor. For women, however, the capacity to dissociate as defined by the DES (0.88) was also loaded on the same factor that contained the induction score (0.70), right hemispheric PPI items (0.91) and the HQ (0.48).

Dichotic Listening Indicators of Suggestibility

If hemisphericity is a factor in hypnotizability, then dichotic word listen-ing performance immediately after the administration of the HIP (within the optimal context) should reflect this relationship. In a recent study twenty univer-sity men and twenty university women were tested individually in an acoustic chamber. After relaxing for about five minutes, each subject (in the presence of the experimenter) listened to an imaginative story. The HIP and Robert's dichotic word listening task were then administered.

Factor analyses of the numbers of left ear suppressions, right ear suppressions and HIP scores indicated an inverse loading ($rs > 0.60$) for right ear errors (left hemispheric proficiency) and hypnotic induction. For both sexes higher HIP scores were associated with fewer right ear suppressions. This result suggested that men and women who are most proficient in left hemispheric processing of simultaneous biaural linguistic information are also more suggestible within this specific context. Conversely (as predicted by the Spiegel model [5]), deterioration in left hemispheric processing, which would characterize cognitive disorders (e.g., obsessive compulsive, paranoid character disorders or the schizophrenias) would be associated with lower hypnotic capacity.

The major sex difference occurred with left ear errors (e.g., right hemispheric or corpus callosal processing). A positive relationship occurred between numbers of left ear errors and the right hemispheric factor for women. This was not observed for the men. This result is similar to that reported by Lavallee and Persinger, in which the numbers of right hemispheric indicators according to personal history were strongly associated with the numbers of left ear (but not right ear) suppres-sions during dichotic word listening tasks [47].

The Ego-Alien Intrusion Factor

We have been pursuing the concept that the sense of a presence, out-of-body experiences and related forms of mental diplopia are the right hemispheric homologues of the left hemispheric and highly linguistic sense of self [48]. We have assumed that in order to become "aware" of an experience, the neuroelec-trical substrate must be translated into linguistic images through left hemispheric processes. Because of the microstructural differences between the right and left hemisphere, especially within the temporal lobes, there would be substantial information that cannot be translated directly into left hemispheric sequences and hence cannot access "awareness" of the normal waking states.

When information from the right hemispheric homologue of left hemispheric processes (that generate the sense of self) surfaces into conscious awareness, the experience is that of a "presence" [49]. Effectively this "presence" is the limited syntactic and semantic information of the person's own right hemisphere. Because it subserves anxiety and vigilance, these experiences are more likely to occur when the person is apprehensive (e.g., alone) or when the right hemisphere is dominant (at night) and will contain a primarily negative affective theme.

If the sense of "presence" is primarily a right hemispheric process then its operation should generate these experiences as well as the negative affective theme. During normal dreaming when right laterality (as defined by Gordon et al. [50]) predominates, experiences of ego-alien intrusions such as the "stranger" or "the other" should be, and are, not only frequent but *normal*. The most dominant dream theme is apprehension or anxiety.

We have suspected that the normal (right-handed) woman is more prone to the sensed presence because: 1) the normal female brain is less lateralized, which increases the probability of intercalation between the two hemispheres, and 2) there is more representation of linguistic (language) processing within the right hemisphere. Thus any condition that enhances the coherence between the hemispheres (such as meditation, bilingualism, and particularly choir singing because of simultaneous activation of both temporal lobes) should facilitate the sensed presence and encourage dissociative states in the normally feminized brain.

IMPLICATIONS OF AN ASSOCIATION BETWEEN TEMPORAL LOBE HEMISPHERICITY AND HYPNOSIS

The empirical association between complex partial epileptic signs, specific hemisphericity, and hypnotic suggestibility implies the existence of a hypothetical construct that is strongly associated with a microneurostructural factor from which all three domains emerge. The effect size (r-squared) involves about 30 percent (20% to 40%) of the variance, which is large enough to meet the minimal criterion for clinical utility. Although there are clearly significant proportions of unexplained variability that suggests other factors must still be isolated (assuming it is not simply the "noise" of paper and pencil tests and individual variability), there are several implications if this factor exists.

The Hidden Observer Phenomenon

The concept of the hidden observer was introduced by Hilgard as a metaphor to describe the memory structure that appeared to have been registered without the person being "aware" of the consolidation [51]. Hilgard's hidden observer could be the initial process from which the ego-alien intrusion or sensed presence emerges. If this association is valid, then the information content for both the hidden observer and the sensed presence would be determined by the linguistic capacity of the person's right hemispheric processes.

Although one would expect most of the information that is stored by the hidden observer (right hemispheric process) to involve strong contextual patterns, such as visuospatial relationships, perceptual arrays and *especially* innuendo of speech presentations and facial expressions, the accessibility to "awareness" would reflect the accuracy of translation of this information into linguistic images. Thus the relative access to this translation should be directly related to the accuracy of the hidden observer.

Individuals who display more linguistic representation within right hemispheric processes should display stronger hidden observer effects and more frequent sensed presences. The normal woman, who displays more linguistic representation than the normal man within the right hemisphere, should display stronger hidden observer effects. Bilingual individuals, especially those who acquired the second language after the more or less complete syntactic acquisition of the first, should also display more intense "other" phenomenon.

Sex Differences

The sexual dimorphism of the human brain is expected on the bases of the powerful influences of hormonal stimuli on membrane function and the direct effects of steroids (androgens) upon the membrane of the cell nucleus. In most of our studies, the ego-alien intrusion cluster loaded positively on the same factor as the numbers of left ear suppressions and hypnotizability for women only. The ego-alien factor loaded negatively on this factor for normal men. This constellation of characteristics is commensurate with the observation that greater electrical homogeneity (less lateralization or asymmetry [52]) in the normal female brain would promote the intrusion experience. The results indicate that although men and women may display comparable hypnotizability, the processes that mediate this capacity may differ. This conclusion is similar to Ken and Patricia Bowers' observation that creativity, hypnotic susceptibility and spontaneous trance-like experiences are interrelated in women but not in men [53]. Men and women may be the same but this absence of difference is for different reasons.

The second gender difference involves sexual ideation. If hypnotizability is derived from the same source as is complex partial epileptic-like signs, then sexual ideation and its physiological correlates should be easier to evoke in women than in men. This hypothesis is based upon the conspicuous incidence of orgasmic and intense sexual ictal experiences that have been observed almost exclusively in female temporal lobe epileptics [54]. An extension of this capacity into the normal population may explain the 5:1 female (14%):male (3%) ratio of yes responses for item 28 "I have had an orgasm (or orgasms) just by imagining only" for the Inventory of Childhood Memories and Imaginings.

Although we would predict that right hemispheric electrical loci would predominate in cases of intrusive sexual ideation, the involvement of the amygdala-hippocampal complex as well as the hormonal modulation (including pseudocyesis) should be mediated by the anterior and hippocampal commissures. Because of the minimal cognitive correlates (via the corpus callosum) that would be associated with these experiences, they would appear to be more intrusive and consequently would be attributed to either real or imagined extrapersonal sources.

Ontogenetic Features

Classic studies have suggested that within the age range of six years to twenty-two years, normal eight- to ten-year-old children display the greatest hypnotizability [55]. This period would be expected in light of the dichotic listening results that were collected in the Neuroscience Laboratory by Drew Moulden. Although the numbers of right ear suppressions (left hemispheric function) during dichotic word listening displayed minimally (clinically) significant changes after seven years of age, there was a strong, statistically significant lag for left ear suppressions. These scores approached adult levels in children between nine and ten years of age.

We interpreted these results to suggest that during the initial stages of maturation (9 to 10 years of age) of the corpus callosum (which is associated with adult performance levels), there is greater intercalation between the right and left temporal lobes [56]. This would allow more intense intrusiveness from right hemispheric processes and enhanced hypnotizability. The expected increase in correlative apprehensiveness could explain the sudden increase in emotional responses to death stimuli and the general enhancement of death fear. The latter would be an indicator of the negative impact of right hemispheric intrusion upon the fragile left hemispheric process: the self concept.

As the corpus callosum matures and the reciprocal inhibitory interhemispheric fibers innervate the upper cortical layers, the baseline frequency of intrusive events should gradually decrease. The time span for this change would be reflected in the maturation range of interhemispheric processing (7 to 15 years) but could continue into the early portion of the third decade. These young adults, even those who display above average intelligence and proficiency, should be very prone to acquiring odd or exotic beliefs [42].

Finally, there is one unique event in neuroanatomical development that may be associated with perhaps the greatest of all amnesias: infantile amnesia. Douglas studied the sudden shift in the capacity to alternate rather than perseverate tasks; it occurs between the ages of four and five years (range 2.5 to 6 years) [57]. He argued that this shift is associated with maturation of the dentate gyrus component of the hippocampal formation.

This ontogenetic interval is important for several reasons. First, it is associated with the asymptote in electrical maturity of the left (linguistic) hemisphere [58]. Second, it is frequently the "age range" within which anomalous "memories," often obtained through regression hypnosis, appear to have occurred. Third, this is also the same period when children, in dozens of different human cultures, experience "ego-alien memories." Often they have been explained as evidence of "reincarnation" or "possession" by other personalities [59].

During this relatively brief developmental interval, children can suddenly report complex details of what appears to be information that has been acquired through adult perceptions. For example the child may relate specific characteristics concerning a dead relative or describe adult sexual acts and experiences, even though the level of understanding is limited and reflects the cognitive stage of the child. This interesting phenomenon, which has been largely ignored in western psychology, suggests an important species-specific transient that emerges during ontogenesis. The ultimate explanation for its emergence may be a structural artifact of brain function rather than a proof of spirituality.

This same region of the hippocampal formation is also prone to significant restructuring in temporal lobe epileptic patients [60, 61]. Neurochemical analyses of synaptic organization in the brains of patients who display idiopathic complex partial seizures reveal that the commissure of the dentate gyrus may be absent. The recent evidence that complex partial epilepsy may *promote* reactive synaptogenesis implies that the portions of the brain that mediate memory and experience can be, metaphorically speaking, rewired. Most neuroscientists assume that the structural subtlety of microbrain arrangement determines how each person experiences reality. The persistent intercorrelations between CPES and hypnotizability suggest that any process that encourages temporal lobe lability could modify memory, change the sense of self and alter perceptions of reality.

REFERENCES

1. G. Pawlik and W.-D. Weiss, Positron Emission Tomography and Neuropsychological Function, in *Neuropsychological Function and Brain Imaging,* E. D. Bigler, R. A. Yeo, and E. Turkheimer (eds.), Plenum, New York, pp. 65-138, 1989.
2. N. C. Andreasen, Brain Imaging: Application in Psychiatry, *Science, 239,* pp. 1381-1388, 1988.
3. J.-R. Laurence and C. Perry, Hypnotically Created Memory among Highly Hypnotizable Subjects, *Science, 222,* pp. 523-524, 1983.
4. N. P. Spanos, M. I. Gwynn, S. L. Comer, W. J. Baltruweit, and M. de Groh, Are Hypnotically Induced Pseudomemories Resistant to Cross-examination?, *Law and Human Behavior, 13,* pp. 271-289, 1989.
5. H. Spiegel and D. Spiegel, *Trance and Treatment,* Basic Books, New York, 1978.
6. M. A. Persinger and C. F. DeSano, Temporal Lobe Signs: Positive Correlations with Imaginings and Hypnosis Induction Profiles, *Perceptual and Motor Skills, 58,* pp. 347-350, 1986.

7. M. A. Persinger and K. Makarec, Temporal Lobe Epileptic Signs and Correlative Behaviors Displayed by Normal Populations, *The Journal of General Psychology, 114,* pp. 179-195, 1987.

8. J. R. Gates and R. J. Gunnit, Partial Seizures of Temporal Lobe Origin, in *Comprehensive Epileptology,* M. Gram and L. Dam (eds.), Raven, New York, pp. 187-195, 1990.

9. T. L. Babb, C. L. Wilson, and M. Isokawa-Akesson, Firing Patterns of Human Limbic Neurons during Stereoencephalography (SSEG) and Clinical Temporal Lobe Seizures, *Electroencephalography and Clinical Neurophysiology, 66,* pp. 467-482, 1987.

10. B. B. Galagher, H. F. Flanigin, D. W. King, J. R. Smith, A. M. Murro, and W. Littleton, ACTH Secretion in Human Temporal Lobe Epilepsy, in *Fundamental Mechanisms of Brain Function,* J. Engles and G. A. Ojemann, H. O. Luders, and P. D. Williamson (eds.), Raven, New York, pp. 201-208, 1987.

11. M. A. Persinger, Subjective Pseudocyesis (False Pregnancy) and Elevated Temporal Lobe Signs: An Implication, *Perceptual and Motor Skills, 72,* pp. 499-503, 1991.

12. B. Ramamruthi, M. Mascreen, and K. Valmikinathan, Role of the Amygdala and Hypothalamus in the Control of Gastric Secretion in Human Beings, *Acta Neurochirurgica,* Suppl. *24,* pp. 187-190, 1977.

13. B. E. Elftheriou (ed.), *The Neurobiology of the Amygdala,* Plenum, New York, 1972.

14. H. O. Besedovsky and E. Sorkin, Immunologic-neuroendocrine Circuits: Physiological Approaches, in *Psychoneuroimmunology,* R. Ader (ed.), Academic, New York, pp. 545-573, 1981.

15. P. Gloor, A. Olivier, L. F. Quensey, F. Andermann, and S. Horowitz, The Role of the Limbic System in Experiential Phenomena of Temporal Lobe Epilepsy, *Annals of Neurology, 12,* pp. 129-144, 1982.

16. W. Penfield and H. Jasper, *Epilepsy and the Functional Anatomy of the Human Brain,* Little, Brown, Boston, 1954.

17. M. J. Horowitz and J. E. Adams, Hallucinations on Brain Stimulation: Evidence for Revision of the Penfield Hypothesis, in *Origin and Mechanisms of Hallucinations,* W. Keup (ed.), Plenum, New York, pp. 13-20, 1970.

18. J. R. Stevens, V. H. Mark, F. Erwin, and K. Suematsu, Deep Temporal Stimulation in Man, *Archives of Neurology, 21,* pp. 157-169, 1969.

19. P. D. MacLean, *The Triune Brain in Evolution,* Plenum, New York, 1990.

20. N. Geschwind, Interictal Behavioral Changes in Epilepsy, *Epilepsia, 24,* pp. 23-40, 1983.

21. D. M. Bear and P. Fedio, Quantitative Analyses of Interictal Behavioral Temporal Lobe Epilepsy, *Archives of Neurology, 24,* pp. 454-467, 1977.

22. M. A. Persinger and K. Makarec, Interactions between Temporal Lobe Signs, Imaginings, Beliefs and Gender: Their Effect Upon Logical Inference, *Imagination, Cognition and Personality, 11,* pp. 149-166, 1991-92.

23. R. M. Post, Does Limbic System Dysfunction Play a Role in Affective Illness?, in *The Limbic System: Functional Organization and Clinical Disorders,* B. K. Doane and K. E. Livingston (eds.), Raven, New York, pp. 229-249, 1986.

24. G. F. Mahl, A. Rothenberg, J. M. R. Delgado, and H. Hamlin, Psychological Responses in the Human to Intercerebral Electrical Stimulation, *Psychosomatic Medicine, 26,* pp. 337-368, 1964.

25. R. E. Bartholomew, K. Basterfield, and G. S. Howard, UFO Abductees and Contactees: Psychopathology or Fantasy Proneness?, *Professional Psychology: Research and Practice, 22,* pp. 215-222, 1991.

26. L. Labelle, J-R. Laurence, R. Nadon, and C. Perry, Hypnotizability, Preference for an Imagic Cognitive Style and Memory Creation in Hypnosis, *Journal of Abnormal Psychology, 99,* pp. 222-228, 1990.

27. M. A. Persinger, "Sudden Remembering" of Early Childhood Memories and Specific Neuropsychological Indicators: Implications for Claims of Sexual Abuse and Alien Visitation/Abduction Experiences, *Perceptual and Motor Skills, 75,* pp. 259-266, 1992.
28. J. L. Cummings, *Clinical Neuropsychiatry,* Grune and Stratton, New York, 1985.
29. S. C. Wilson and T. X. Barber, The Creative Imagination Scale as a Measure of Hypnotic Responsiveness: Applications to Experimental and Clinical Hypnosis, *American Journal of Clinical Hypnosis, 20,* pp. 235-249, 1978.
30. R. J. Roberts, N. R. Varney, J. R. Hulbert, J. S. Paulsen, E. D. Richardson, J. A. Springer, J. M. Sheperd, C. M. Swan, J. A. Legrand, J. H. Harvey, and M. A. Struchen, The Neuropathology of Everyday Life: The Frequency of Partial Seizure Symptoms among Normals, *Neuropsychology,* pp. 65-85, 1990.
31. J. S. Springer, M. J. Garvey, N. R. Varney, and R. Roberts, Dichotic Listening Failure in Dysphoric Neuropsychiatric Patients Who Endorse Multiple Seizure-like Symptoms, *The Journal of Nervous and Mental Disease, 179,* pp. 459-467, 1991.
32. M. A. Persinger and K. Makarec, Complex Partial Epileptic-like Signs as a Continuum from Normal to Epileptics: Normative Data and Clinical Populations, *Journal of Clinical Psychology, 49,* pp. 33-45, 1993.
33. M. A. Persinger and K. Makarec, The Sensed Presence and Verbal Meaningfulness as Temporal Lobe Signs: Factor Analytic Verification of the Muses?, *Brain and Cognition,* in press.
34. K. Makarec and M. A. Persinger, Electroencephalographic Validation of a Temporal Lobe Signs Inventory in a Normal Population, *Journal of Research in Personality, 34,* pp. 323-327, 1990.
35. K. Makarec and M. A. Persinger, Temporal Lobe Signs: Electroencephalographic Validity and Enhanced Scores in Special Populations, *Perceptual and Motor Skills, 57,* pp. 1255-1262, 1985.
36. K. Makarec and M. A. Persinger, Electrocephalographic Correlates of Temporal Lobe Signs and Imaginings, *Perceptual and Motor Skills, 64,* pp. 1124-1126, 1987.
37. M. A. Persinger, Temporal Lobe Signs and Personality Characteristics, *Perceptual and Motor Skills, 66,* pp. 49-50, 1988.
38. M. A. Persinger, Canonical Correlation of Temporal Lobe Signs with Schizoid and Hypomania Scales in a Normal Population: Men and Women are Similar but for Different Reasons, *Perceptual and Motor Skills, 73,* pp. 615-618, 1991.
39. B. Huot, K. Makarec and M. A. Persinger, Temporal Lobe Signs and Jungian Dimensions of Personality, *Perceptual and Motor Skills, 69,* pp. 841-842, 1989.
40. J. Ross and M. A. Persinger, Positive Correlations between Temporal Lobe Signs and Hypnosis Induction Profiles: A Replication, *Perceptual and Motor Skills, 64,* pp. 828-830, 1987.
41. D. T. Gilbert, P. S. Malone, and D. S. Krull, Unbelieving the Unbelievable: Some Problems in the Rejection of False Information, *Journal of Personality and Social Psychology, 59,* pp. 601-613, 1990.
42. R. Skirda and M. A. Persinger, Positive Associations between Dichotic Word Listening Errors, Complex Partial Epileptic-like Signs and Paranormal Beliefs, *Journal of Nervous and Mental Disease, 181,* pp. 663-667, 1993.
43. F. E. Musiek, Neuroanatomy, Neurophysiology, and Central Auditory Assessment. Part III: Corpus Callosum and Efferent Pathways, *Ear and Hearing, 7,* pp. 349-358, 1986.
44. T. H. Budzynski, Clinical Applications of Non-drug-induced States, in *Handbook of States of Consciousness,* B. B. Wolman and M. Ullman (eds.), Van Nostrand, New York, pp. 428-460, 1986.

45. O. Devinsky, F. Putnam, J. Grafman, E. Bromfield, and W. H. Theodore, Dissociative States and Epilepsy, *Neurology, 39,* pp. 835-840, 1989.
46. W. Vingiano, Hemisphericity and Personality, *International Journal of Neuroscience, 44,* pp. 263-274, 1989.
47. M. Lavallee and M. A. Persinger, Left Ear Suppressions during Dichotic Listening, Ego Alien Intrusion Experiences and Spiritualistic Beliefs in Normal Women, *Perceptual and Motor Skills, 75,* pp. 547-551, 1992.
48. M. A. Persinger, Vectorial Cerebral Hemisphericity as Differential Sources for the Sensed Presence, Mystical Experiences and Religious Conversions, *Psychological Reports, 76,* pp. 915-930, 1993.
49. C. Munro and M. A. Persinger, Relative Right Temporal-lobe Theta Activity Correlates with Vingiano's Hemispheric Quotient and the Sensed Presence, *Perceptual and Motor Skills, 75,* pp. 899-903, 1992.
50. H. W. Gordon, B. Frooman, and P. Lavie, Shifts in Cognitive Asymmetries between Waking from REM and NREM Sleep, *Neuropsychologia, 20,* pp. 99-103, 1982.
51. E. R. Hilgard, The Hidden Observer and Multiple Personality, *The International Journal of Clinical and Experimental Hypnosis, 32,* pp. 248-253, 1984.
52. M. Corsi-Carrera, P. Herrera, and M. Malvido, Correlation between EEG and Cognitive Abilities: Sex Differences, *International Journal of Neuroscience, 45,* pp. 133-141, 1989.
53. K. S. Bowers and P. G. Bowers, Hypnosis and Creativity: A Theoretical Approach and Empirical Rapprochement, in *Hypnosis, Research Developments and Perspectives,* E. Fromm and R. E. Shor (eds.), Aldine, Chicago, pp. 255-291, 1972.
54. G. M. Remmillard, F. Andermann, G. F. Testa, P. Gloor, M. Aube, J. B. Martin, W. Feindel, A. Guberman, and C. Simpson, Sexual Ictal Manifestations Predominate in Women with Temporal Lobe Epilepsy: A Finding Suggesting Sexual Dimorphism in the Human Brain, *Neurology, 33,* pp. 323-330, 1983.
55. E. R. Hilgard, Individual Differences in Hypnotizability, in *Handbook of Clinical and Experimental Hypnosis,* J. E. Gordon (ed.), Macmillan, New York, pp. 391-443, 1967.
56. J. A. Drew Moulden and M. A. Persinger, Differential Ontogenetic Development of Left and Right Ear Suppressions a Dichotic Word Listening Task, in preparation.
57. R. J. Douglas, The Development of Hippocampal Function: Implications for Theory and for Therapy, in *The Hippocampus. Vol. 2: Neurophysiology and Behavior,* R. L. Issacson and K. H. Pribram (eds.), Plenum, New York, pp. 327-361, 1975.
58. R. W. Thatcher, R. A. Walker, and S. Giudice, Human Cerebral Hemispheres Develop at Different Rates and Ages, *Science, 236,* pp. 1110-1113, 1987.
59. I. Stevenson and G. Samararatne, Three New Cases of the Reincarnation Type in Sri Lanka with Written Records Made before Verification, *Journal of Scientific Exploration, 2,* pp. 217-238, 1988.
60. T. Sutula, G. Cascino, J. Cavazos, I. Parada, and L. Ramirez, Mossy Fiber Synaptic Reorganization in the Epileptic Human Temporal Lobe, *Annals of Neurology, 26,* pp. 321-330, 1989.
61. N. C. de Lanerolle, J. H. Kim, R. J. Robbins, and D. D. Spencer, Hippocampal Interneuron Loss and Plasticity in Human Temporal Lobe Epilepsy, *Brain Research, 495,* p. 387-395, 1989.

[Thanks to Pauline Richards and Yves Bureau for their comments. Portions of this research were supported by the Friends of Laurentian, Inc.]

Contributors

DEIRDRE BARRETT is Assistant Professor at Harvard Medical School and is President-Elect of the Association for the Study of Dreams. She has edited the book *Trauma and Dreams,* to be published by Harvard University Press, and has authored numerous chapters and articles on hypnosis, dreams, and dissociation.

PATRICIA BOISVERT recently graduated from the undergraduate psychology program at the University of Massachusetts Lowell. Presently, she works in marketing research and analysis.

CARLENE CARRABINO is a graduate student in public health at Loma Linda University and a recent graduate of the undergraduate psychology program at the University of Massachusetts Lowell. She has co-authored two published articles on reality testing.

WILLIAM C. COE is Professor of Psychology at California State University, Fresno where he was named "Outstanding Professor of the Year" in 1988. He was awarded the "Best Theoretical Paper" by the Society for Clinical and Experimental Hypnosis (SCEH) in 1979. Dr. Coe's research has focused on various aspects of hypnosis and also on applications of behavior theory. He has reviewed and edited for many journals and publishers, contributed many chapters, written several books, and published over sixty journal articles.

JAMES R. COUNCIL is Associate Professor of Psychology at North Dakota State University. He is a Fellow of the American Psychological Association, and received the 1993 Distinguished Early Career Contribution Award from APA Division 30, Psychological Hypnosis. He has authored over thirty publications and numerous conference presentations in the areas of hypnosis, imagination, personality, and behavioral medicine. His current research focuses on context effects in personality research, a methodological issue which emerged from his work on personality correlates of hypnotizability.

HELEN J. CRAWFORD is presently a psychologist in the Applied Experimental Program, Department of Psychology, Virginia Polytechnic Institute and State University, Blacksburg, Virginia. After receiving her Ph.D. at the University of California, Davis, she worked with Ernest R. Hilgard at Stanford University and then taught at the University of Wyoming. She has been president of the Society for Clinical and Experimental Hypnosis, as well as president and secretary of Division 30 (Psychological Hypnosis), American Psychological Association. She is a Fellow in the American Psychological Association, the American Psychological Society, the Society for Clinical and Experimental Hypnosis, and the International Organization of Psychophysiology. Her work in the fields of hypnosis and psychophysiology has been honored by the Society for Clinical and Experimental Hypnosis with two major awards: The Henry Guze Award for the Best Hypnosis Research Article in 1990, and the Bernard B. Raginsky Award for Leadership and Achievement.

DONALD R. GORASSINI is Associate Professor and Chair of Psychology at King's College, London, Canada. His research interests include the psychology of social influence and the psychology of conviction management.

DEBORA L. GRANT is a recent graduate of the undergraduate psychology program at North Dakota State University. She is currently coordinating a research grant awarded by the National Science Foundation to J. R. Council. She has co-authored five scientific papers on context effects in personality research.

JOSEPH P. GREEN, Ph.D., is an Assistant Professor of Psychology at the Ohio State University Campus at Lima, Ohio. Dr. Green has been the recipient of an American Psychological Association award for excellence in research and has written many articles and chapters on hypnotizability, fantasy, dissociation, and hypnotic phenomena.

MAXWELL I. GWYNN received his Ph.D. from Carleton University, Ottawa, followed by a S.S.H.R.C. (Canada) postdoctoral fellowship held at California State University, Fresno. His research interests include experimental hypnosis, eyewitness testimony, and social influence. He is currently an Assistant Professor in the Department of Psychology at Wilfrid Laurier University in Waterloo, Canada.

BILL JONES, Ph.D., is Professor and Chairman of the Department of Psychology at Carleton University, Ottawa. His areas of research interest include organizational psychology, stress management, psychophysics, cerebral laterality, pain and hypnosis. He also has scholarly interests in the philosophy of science and the history of psychoanalysis.

IRVING KIRSCH is Professor of Psychology at the University of Connecticut. He is North American Editor of *Contemporary Hypnosis* and an advisory editor of the *International Journal of Clinical and Experimental Hypnosis*. A diplomate of the American Board of Psychological Hypnosis and a Fellow of the American Psychological Association, American Psychological Society, and Society for Clinical and Experimental Hypnosis, Dr. Kirsch has served as President of the American Psychological Association Division of Psychological Hypnosis. He is the author of *Changing Expectations: A Key to Effective Psychotherapy* and an editor of the *Handbook of Clinical Hypnosis*. Dr. Kirsch has published more than eighty journal articles and book chapters on hypnosis, behavior therapy, anxiety disorders, depression, and expectancy effects.

ROBERT G. KUNZENDORF is Professor of Psychology at the University of Massachusetts Lowell. He has served as President of the American Association for the Study of Mental Imagery, and as Research Advanced Fellow in behavioral medicine at Harvard Medical School and Cambridge Hospital. Dr. Kunzendorf's research has focused on materialistic interpretations of conscious phenomena, particularly mental images and hypnotic phenomena, and has generated over fifty scientific publications, including two edited books entitled *The Psychophysiology of Mental Imagery* and *Mental Imagery.*

STEVEN JAY LYNN is a Professor of Psychology at Ohio University and has a private practice. He is a former president of the American Psychological Association's (APA) Division of Psychological Hypnosis; a Fellow in the APA, the American Psychological Society, and the Society for Clinical and Experimental Hypnosis; and a diplomate of the American Board of Psychological Hypnosis. He has received an award from the Society for Clinical and Experimental Hypnosis for the best hypnosis book published during 1991 (*Theories of Hypnosis: Current Models and Perspectives*); he has written or edited textbooks on abnormal psychology, psychotherapy, dissociation; and he has published more than 120 articles and book chapters. Dr. Lynn is on a number of editorial boards including the *Journal of Abnormal Psychology* and the *International Journal of Clinical and Experimental Hypnosis,* and is the North American Editor of *Contemporary Hypnosis.*

VICTOR NEUFELD, Ph.D., is a Psychologist at Penrose Hospital, Colorado Springs. He works with neurologically impaired, elderly, and chronic pain patients. Dr. Neufeld has published many articles and chapters on fantasy, imagination, direct versus indirect suggestions, and smoking cessation.

ARTHUR H. PERLINI is an Assistant Professor of Psychology at Algoma University in Ontario, Canada. His experience with hypnosis began when he assisted Donald Gorassini with his research on involuntariness and hypnosis at King's College, U.W.O. He underwent advanced training in experimental psychology and hypnosis under the tutelage of Dr. Nicholas P. Spanos at the Laboratory for Experimental Hypnosis at Carleton University. He received his M.A. (1987) and Ph.D. from Carleton University in 1991. He has co-authored a number of papers with Spanos and his research group, most notably research on compliance and hypnosis. His research interests have focused on the generic problems of experimental methods in psychology and the objectification of subjective experience. His tenure at a small liberal arts university has compelled him to broaden his teaching and research areas considerably. In addition to his commitment to research and teaching, he is currently undertaking an externship in clinical psychology.

MICHAEL A. PERSINGER is Professor of Psychology and Coordinator of the Behavioral Neuroscience Program at Laurentian University in Sudbury, Ontario (Canada). He has published over 200 technical articles and six books within the areas of neuroscience, parapsychology, biometeorology, geophysics, and psychology. Recent research has focused upon the materialistic interpretations of the relationship between the continuum of limbic lobe electrical (seizure) lability, memory modification and altered (mystical/religious) states and their elicitation by geophysical/meteorological stimuli.

CHARLES M. RADER is a Senior Clinical Psychologist, Director of the Student Training Program, and Coordinator of Psychological Evaluations at Ramsey County Mental Health Clinic in St. Paul, Minnesota. He obtained his Ph.D. in 1979 from the University of Minnesota (Clinical Psychology Training Program) under the direction of Dr. Auke Tellegen. Dr. Rader has published in the area of hypnosis, synesthesia, and personality evaluation.

JUDITH RHUE, Ph.D., is a Professor of Family Medicine at the Ohio University College of Osteopathic Medicine and has a private practice. She is a Fellow of the American Psychological Association's (APA) Division of Psychological Hypnosis. She has received awards for excellence in research from APA, as well as an award for the best hypnosis book published during 1991 (*Theories of Hypnosis: Current Models and Perspectives*), bestowed by the Society for Clinical and Experimental Hypnosis. Dr. Rhue serves on the editorial boards of the *International Journal of Clinical and Experimental Hypnosis* and *Contemporary Hypnosis*. She is coeditor of two hypnosis books and a forthcoming book on dissociation (with Steven Jay Lynn), and she has written numerous articles and book chapters on hypnosis, fantasy, and child abuse.

ROSEMARY ROBERTSON is a graduate of the University of Queensland, Brisbane, Australia. She has co-authored a number of research papers in the field of hypnosis, and most recently has worked and published in the area of rapport and hypnosis. She has also been actively involved in hypnosis research for some four years.

DAVID SANDBERG, Ph.D., is a Doctoral Candidate in Clinical Psychology at Ohio University. He is the author of a number of articles on sexual abuse, maltreatment, and dissociation.

PETER W. SHEEHAN is Professor of Psychology and Pro-Vice-Chancellor (Research and Postgraduate Studies) at the University of Queensland, Australia. He is past president of the Australian Psychological Society, and was president of the International Congress of Psychology in 1988. He is currently President of the Academy of the Social Sciences in Australia, and is a Fellow of the Australian Psychological Society, the American Psychological Association, and the New York Academy of Sciences. His special fields of research interest are hypnosis, imagery, and the effects of media violence on children. He is author or editor of many books and research monographs and has authored some 140 separate research publications.

NICHOLAS P. SPANOS, Ph.D., was Professor of Psychology and Director of the Laboratory for Experimental Hypnosis at Carleton University, Ottawa. His areas of research interest included hypnosis, pain control, anomalous experience, psychopathology, law and psychology, and the history of psychology and psychopathology.

DEANNA D. TUROSKY completed her M.A. degree in experimental psychology at Cleveland State University. She has co-authored two published articles on imagery.

GRAHAM F. WAGSTAFF is Senior Lecturer in Psychology at the University of Liverpool, England. He is a past member of Council of the British Society of Experimental and Clinical Hypnosis, and serves on the editorial boards of *Contemporary Hypnosis* and *Experimentelle und Klinische Hypnose*. His research has focused mainly on social psychological influences on hypnotic responding, and forensic hypnosis. He is author of the book *Hypnosis, Compliance and Belief,* and has published widely in the areas of hypnosis and the psychology of justice and law.

BENJAMIN WALLACE is Professor of Psychology at Cleveland State University. Dr. Wallace's research has focused on visual perception, and individual differences in hypnosis and imaging ability. He is the author of over 100 scientific publications, including two books, *Applied Hypnosis* and *Consciousness and Behavior.*

Index

Absorption, 7, 10-12, 19, 36, 47-60, 75, 78-80, 84, 88, 99-106, 111-116, 123, 125-127, 132-133, 253, 255, 267 (*see also* Fantasy proneness, Imaginative involvement)

Abuse, physical or sexual, 23, 80, 82-89, 124, 289-290

Adaptive regression, 82, 116

Afterimagery, 2, 233, 248, 255-256, 272

Alcohol and drugs, 75, 78

Alpha wave of the EEG, 240, 243, 246, 248-249, 262, 294

Altered state of consciousness, 12, 19-22, 43, 224-225, 264, 284-285

Androgyny, 73, 104

Artistic involvement, 31-32, 224, 231

Attention, 9, 12, 19, 68, 71, 74-75, 79, 87, 89, 101, 149, 156, 185, 188-189, 207-208, 213-216, 253-257, 261, 263, 266, 269, 271-272

Autokinetic movement, 158-159, 255

Automatic writing/talking, 129-131, 179, 227, 232, 302

Belief in the image, 7-8, 30, 50, 79, 88, 194-195, 295 (*see also* Hallucination, Reality testing)

Bizarreness of the image, 72, 77-78, 82, 125, 129

Boundary thinness, 9, 99-100, 103-104, 106, 115-116

Cerebral blood flow, 259, 262-273

Childhood, 4, 30, 32, 41, 48, 73, 80, 86-89, 124-127, 131-133, 224, 231, 291, 294-295, 301-302 (*see also* Developmental differences)

Compliance, 19, 22-37, 45-46, 155-167, 199-207, 294 (*see also* Social desirability)

Computational model of the image, 236

Contextual effects, 5, 8, 10-12, 27, 50-60, 101, 162-163, 167-168, 201-207, 225, 232, 288, 290 (*see also* Demand characteristics, Expectancy in hypnosis)

Control of the image, 3-5, 8-9, 76

Corticofugal innervation, 224, 260

Creativity, 67-70, 79, 106, 189, 245, 300

Demand characteristics, 2-6, 12, 21, 34, 49, 199-207, 225, 254 (*see also* Contextual effects, Expectancy in hypnosis)

Depression, 74-79, 82, 85-86, 133, 267, 287

Developmental differences, 73, 165, 224, 231, 301-302 (*see also* Childhood)

Dissociation, 5, 9, 13, 20-23, 28, 53, 69, 75, 77, 84-90, 123-124, 126-130, 133-134, 140, 150-152, 193, 231-232, 254-255, 271, 284, 286-287, 296-298 (*see also* Hidden observer)

Dreaming, 68-70, 77-78, 100, 103, 124, 131, 286-287

Paranormal experience, 31, 53, 79-80, 125, 127, 131, 165, 286, 294-295, 298-302 (*see also* Magical thinking)

Perception, 1-3, 152-156, 158-159, 182-185, 199-203, 223-232, 236-238, 253, 256-260 (*see also* Afterimagery, Attention, Autokinetic movement, Gestalt closure, Reality testing, Signal detection, Subjective contours)

Personality disorders, 83-85, 104

Phobic imagery, 90

Placebos, 41-43, 49

Positron emission tomography, 259, 263, 266, 269, 273

Posthypnotic amnesia, 27, 29-30, 34-35, 41, 44, 123-124, 126, 128-131, 133, 137-144, 232

Primary process thinking, 46-47, 70, 82, 99-104, 106, 115-116

Pseudomemory, 7, 46, 161-168, 181, 289-291, 296

Psychiatric inpatients, 76, 83

Psychosis, 67-69, 76, 84, 99, 165

Psychopathology (*see* Depression, Dissociation, Neurosis, Personality disorders, Phobic imagery, Psychiatric inpatients, Psychosis, Primary process thinking, Reality testing, Repression)

Psychosomatics (*see* Hypnotic analgesia, False pregnancy, Placebos, Sexual fantasy, Tumor regression)

Racial differences, 73

Reality construction, 151, 302

Reality testing, 79, 88, 99-107, 109-113, 115-116, 181, 223-232, 253, 287-288, 301 (*see* Belief in the image, Hallucination)

Relaxation, 5, 19, 29-30, 43, 87, 271

Repression, 70, 75, 100 (*see* Hidden observer, Self-deception, the Subconscious)

Rotation of the image, 2, 81, 243, 245, 259

Scanning of the image, 9, 259

Schemas, 71, 182-186, 189, 196

Self-consciousness, 100, 224, 226, 232, 254, 271

Self-esteem, 28, 73, 83-84, 165, 291

Self-deception, 177, 179-197, 204 (*see also* Hidden observer, Repression, the Subconscious)

Sensation, 68-69, 88, 99-100, 104, 106, 182, 223-225, 231-232, 236, 287, 292

Sexual fantasy, 72, 79, 125, 127, 131, 300-301

Signal detection, 159

Single photon emission computer tomography, 259, 263-266, 271, 273

Sleep, lack of, 78, 107, 112-113, 116, 232

Social desirability, 11, 49, 147-149, 155-161, 165, 180, 254, 290 (*see also* Compliance)

Spatial/holistic reasoning, 239, 247, 256, 259-261, 265, 291

Subjective contours, 2

Subconscious, the, 70, 101, 223-232, 255-256 (*see also* Hidden observer, Repression, Self-deception)

Subcortical processing, 208-209, 223-224, 228-230, 254-255, 261, 264-266, 272-273, 284-285, 301

Synesthesia, 99-102, 104-109, 113-115

Temporal-lobe epilepsy, 53, 264, 284-302

Theta wave of the EEG, 269, 271, 292

Tumor regression, 231, 256

Ultradian rhythms, 9

Vividness of the image, 4-9, 13, 30-31, 48, 74, 76, 79, 82, 99, 102-116, 124-126, 134, 223-226, 228-232, 237-238, 248, 254-255, 257, 265-267, 284-286

Volition, 5, 10, 12, 20, 23-26, 34-36, 42-43, 47, 88, 90, 100, 128-129, 134, 139-140, 142-144, 149-153, 186-187, 190-193

Waking suggestibility, 152-165, 167-168